Second Edition

Essentia CATARACT SURGERY

Edited by

Bonnie An Henderson, MD
Ophthalmic Consultants of Boston
Tufts University School of Medicine
Boston, Massachusetts

Associate Editors
Roberto Pineda II, MD
Massachusetts Eye and Ear Infirmary
Harvard Medical School
Boston, Massachusetts

Sherleen H. Chen, MD, FACS
Massachusetts Eye and Ear Infirmary
Harvard Medical School
Boston, Massachusetts

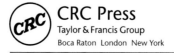

CRC Press
Taylor & Francis Group
Boca Raton London New York

CRC Press is an imprint of the
Taylor & Francis Group, an **informa** business

First Published in 2014 by SLACK Incorporated

Published 2024 by CRC Press
2385 NW Executive Center Drive, Suite 320, Boca Raton FL 33431

and by CRC Press
4 Park Square, Milton Park, Abingdon, Oxon, OX14 4RN

CRC Press is an imprint of Taylor & Francis Group, an informa business

© 2014 by Taylor & Francis Group

Library of Congress Cataloging-in-Publication Data
Essentials of cataract surgery / edited by Bonnie An Henderson ; associate editors, Roberto Pineda, II, Sherleen H. Chen. -- Second edition.
    p. ; cm.
  Includes bibliographical references and index.
  ISBN 978-1-61711-067-2 (paperback : alk. paper)
  I. Henderson, Bonnie An, editor of compilation. II. Pineda, Roberto, II, editor of compila-tion. III. Chen, Sherleen H., editor of compilation.
  [DNLM: 1. Cataract Extraction. WW 260]
  RE451
  617.7'42059--dc23

                    2013042970

ISBN: 9781617110672 (pbk)
ISBN: 9781003524038 (ebk)

DOI: 10.1201/9781003524038

Second Edition

Essentials of
CATARACT
SURGERY

DEDICATION

To our mentors for inspiring us;
To our students for challenging us;
To our families for supporting us.

CONTENTS

About the Editor

Bonnie An Henderson, MD is a partner at Ophthalmic Consultants of Boston and a Clinical Professor at Tufts University School of Medicine. Her career focus has been on education. She created and organized the annual Harvard Intensive Cataract Surgical Training Course, which focuses on teaching surgery to US residents. She was the lead investigator for the development of a computer software program that simulates surgery for training purposes. She has been the recipient of the "Teacher of the Year" award by the Harvard Medical School Department of Ophthalmology and nominated for Harvard's Excellence in Teaching Award.

The former Director of Comprehensive Ophthalmology and Cataract Consultation at the Massachusetts Eye and Ear Infirmary, Dr. Henderson has authored over 100 articles, papers, book chapters, and abstracts and has delivered over 250 invited lectures worldwide. Dr. Henderson is the Associate Editor for the *Journal of Refractive Surgery* and Associate Editor for *Eyeworld* for the American Society of Cataract and Refractive Surgery. She serves on the editorial advisory board of *Eyenet Magazine* of the American Academy of Ophthalmology, and serves on the editorial boards of 3 other journals. She serves on a number of committees for the American Academy of Ophthalmology and the American Society of Cataract and Refractive Society. She is a reviewer for eight ophthalmic journals.

Dr. Henderson has been awarded an Achievement Award and Secretariat Award by the American Academy of Ophthalmology, and "Best of" awards from the American Society of Cataract and Refractive Surgery for her research and films. Dr. Henderson completed her ophthalmology residency at Harvard Medical School, Massachusetts Eye and Ear Infirmary. She graduated from Dartmouth College and from Dartmouth Medical School with high honors. She serves on the Board of Overseers at the Geisel School of Medicine at Dartmouth, the Executive Committee of American Society of Cataract and Refractive Surgery, the Executive Board of the Massachusetts Society of Eye Physicians and Surgeons, the Executive Board of Women In Ophthalmology, and has served on the Physician Board of Directors at the Massachusetts Eye and Ear Infirmary. Married with three children, her interests include culinary arts and competing in triathlons.

ABOUT THE ASSOCIATE EDITORS

Roberto Pineda II, MD completed his ophthalmology residency, chief residency, and cornea fellowship at the Massachusetts Eye and Ear Infirmary. He is currently Director of Refractive Surgery and is on the cornea service at the Massachusetts Eye and Ear Infirmary. He has coauthored several books and has received the "Teacher of the Year" award from Massachusetts Eye and Ear Infirmary. He has been involved in resident education and teaching for over a decade and routinely participates in ORBIS International, a nonprofit organization with a flying eye hospital, helping to train and educate ophthalmologists as well as establish eye banks in developing countries.

Sherleen H. Chen, MD is Assistant Professor of Ophthalmology at Harvard Medical School and Director of the Comprehensive Ophthalmology and Cataract Consultation Service at the Massachusetts Eye and Ear Infirmary. Dr. Chen graduated from Stanford University with distinction and was elected to Phi Beta Kappa. She was a Howard Hughes Scholar while at Harvard Medical School. Dr. Chen then completed her ophthalmology residency at the Massachusetts Eye and Ear Infirmary and was selected from her residency class to serve as Chief Resident and Director of the Trauma Service. She is actively involved in resident education and surgical teaching. She has mentored many cataract surgeons graduating from the Massachusetts Eye and Ear Infirmary.

CONTRIBUTING AUTHORS

Maria Aaron, MD (Chapter 21)
Professor of Ophthalmology
Emory University School of Medicine
Atlanta, Georgia

John D. Au, MD (Chapter 11)
Cole Eye Institute
Cleveland Clinic Foundation
Cleveland, Ohio

Joseph Bayes, MD (Chapter 4)
Assistant Professor of Anesthesia
Harvard Medical School
Boston, Massachusetts

Hilary Beaver, MD (Chapter 17)
Associate Professor of Clinical
 Ophthalmology
Weill Cornell Medical College
Houston Methodist Hospital
Adjunct Associate Professor
The University of Texas Medical
 Branch at Galveston
Houston, Texas

John P. Berdahl, MD (Chapter 2)
Vance Thompson Vision
Assistant Clinical Professor of
 Ophthalmology
Sanford School of Medicine
University of South Dakota
Sioux Falls, South Dakota

Kathryn Bollinger, MD, PhD
 (Chapter 8)
Medical College of Georgia
Georgia Regents University
August, Georgia

Geoffrey Broocker, MD (Chapter 21)
Walthour-DeLaPerriere Professor of
 Ophthalmology
Program Consultant
Emory University School of Medicine
Atlanta, Georgia

David F. Chang, MD (Chapter 14)
Clinical Professor
University of California, San
 Francisco
Altos Eye Physicians
Los Altos, California

Dongmei Chen, MD, PhD
 (Chapter 18)

Jessica Chow, MD (Chapter 30)
Assistant Professor
Yale Eye Center
New Haven, Connecticut

Jessica B. Ciralsky, MD (Chapter 29)
Assistant Professor, Ophthalmology
Weill Cornell Medical College
New York, New York

Kenneth L. Cohen, MD (Chapter 23)
Sterling A. Barrett Distinguished
 Professor of Ophthalmology
University of North Carolina School
 of Medicine
The Kittner Eye Center
Chapel Hill, North Carolina

John J. DeStafeno, MD (Chapter 20)
Clinical Instructor
Wills Eye Hospital
Chester County Eye Care Associates
Philadelphia, Pennsylvania

James P. Dunn, MD (Chapter 3)
Associate Professor of
  Ophthalmology
The Wilmer Eye Institute
The Johns Hopkins School of
  Medicine
Baltimore, Maryland

*Bryan D. Edgington, MD
  (Chapter 19)*
Portland VA Medical Center
Casey Eye Institute
Portland, Oregon

Ryan Fante, MD (Chapter 26)
Ophthalmology Resident
University of Michigan Kellogg Eye
  Center
Ann Arbor, Michigan

*Tamiesha A. Frempong, MD, MPH
  (Chapter 5)*
Icahn School of Medicine
Mount Sinai
New York, New York

*Michael H. Goldstein, MD, MBA
  (Chapter 19)*
Co-Director, Cornea and External
  Disease Service
New England Eye Center
Assistant Professor
Tufts University School of Medicine
Boston, Massachusetts

B. David Gorman, MD (Chapter 7)
Fifth Ave EyeCare & Surgery
Assistant Clinical Professor of
  Ophthalmology
Columbia Presbyterian Medical
  School
New York, New York

*Artem Grush, MD, MBA
  (Chapter 4)*
Director of the Surgicenter
Massachusetts Eye and Ear
  Infirmary
Instructor in Anesthesia
Harvard Medical School
Boston, Massachusetts

*John C. Hart, Jr, MD, FACS
  (Chapter 24)*
Co-Chief of Anterior Segment Surgery
William Beaumont Hospital
Royal Oak, Michigan
Professor of Ophthalmology
William Beaumont/Oakland
  University School of Medicine
Rochester, Michigan

*A. Tim Johnson, PhD, MD
  (Chapter 17)*
Clinical Professor of Ophthalmology
University of Iowa
Iowa City, Iowa

Sandra M. Johnson, MD (Chapter 28)
Associate Professor of Ophthalmology
University of Virginia Department of
  Ophthalmology
Charlottesville, Virginia

Carol L. Karp, MD (Chapter 15)
Professor of Ophthalmology
Bascom Palmer Eye Institute
University of Miami School of Medicine
Miami, Florida

Terry Kim, MD (Chapter 20)
Professor of Ophthalmology
Duke University School of Medicine
Director of Fellowship Programs
Associate Director, Cornea and
  Refractive Surgery
Duke University Eye Center
Durham, North Carolina

Lynda Z. Kleiman, MD (Chapter 7)
Eye Physicians of Central Florida
Maitland, Florida

Talia Kolin, MD (Chapter 13)
Associate Clinical Professor of
  Ophthalmology
University of Southern California
Chief of Ophthalmology
Department of Veterans Affairs,
  Los Angeles Ambulatory Care
  Center
Los Angeles, California

*Roger H. S. Langston, MD
  (Chapter 11)*
Cole Eye Institute
Cleveland Clinic
Cleveland, Ohio

Francis S. Mah, MD (Chapter 27)
Director, Cornea and External Diseases
Co-Director, Refractive Surgery
Scripps Clinic
La Jolla, California

*Sankaranarayana Mahesh, MD
  (Chapter 19)*
Faculty
The George Washington University
Washington, DC

Jack Manns, MD (Chapter 28)

Scott M. McClintic, MD (Chapter 6)
University of California, San Francisco
San Francisco, California

Mario A. Meallet, MD (Chapter 13)
Clinical Professor of Ophthalmology
Doheny Eye Institute/LAC+USC
A Center for Vision Care
Los Angeles, California

Shahzad I. Mian, MD (Chapter 26)
Terry J. Bergstrom Professor
Associate Chair, Education
Associate Professor
Residency Program Director
Department of Ophthalmology and
  Visual Sciences
University of Michigan
Ann Arbor, Michigan

Kevin M. Miller, MD (Chapter 9)
Kolokotrones Professor of Clinical
  Ophthalmology
Jules Stein Eye Institute
David Geffen School of Medicine
  at UCLA
Los Angeles, California

Eydie Miller-Ellis, MD (Chapter 10)
Clinical Associate Professor of
  Ophthalmology
University of Pennsylvania School of
  Medicine
Director, Glaucoma Service
Director, Glaucoma Fellowship
Scheie Eye Institute
Philadelphia, Pennsylvania

Wuqaas M. Munir, MD (Chapter 15)
Assistant Professor
Boston University School of
    Medicine
Boston, Massachusetts

Ayman Naseri, MD (Chapter 6)
University of California, San
    Francisco
San Francisco VA Medical Center
San Francisco, California

*Peter A. Netland, MD, PhD
    (Chapter 28)*
Vernah Scott Moyston Professor and
    Chair
Department of Ophthalmology
University of Virginia School of Medicine
Charlottesville, Virginia

*Thomas A. Oetting, MS, MD
    (Chapter 17)*
Clinical Professor of Ophthalmology
University of Iowa
Iowa City, Iowa

*Yuri S. Oleynikov, MD, PhD
    (Chapter 7)*
Columbia University
    Ophthalmology
New York, New York
Jules Stein Eye Institute
University of California, Los Angeles
Los Angeles, California

Lisa Park, MD (Chapter 16)
Clinical Associate Professor
Residency Program Associate Director
Department of Ophthalmology
NYU School of Medicine
Chief of Ophthalmology
Bellevue Hospital Center
New York, New York

Jeff Pettey, MD (Chapter 21)
Residency Program Director
Moran Eye Center
University of Utah
Salt Lake City, Utah

*Saraswathy Ramanathan, MD
    (Chapter 12)*
Associate Professor
Department of Ophthalmology
University of California, San Francisco
San Francisco, California

*Susannah Rowe, MD, MPH
    (Chapter 1)*
Assistant Professor of Ophthalmology
Boston University School of Medicine
Vice Chair for Patient Safety and
    Quality
Department of Ophthalmology
Boston Medical Center
Boston, Massachusetts

Nisha V. Shah, MD (Chapter 30)

Brett Shapiro, MD (Chapter 6)
School of Medicine
University of California, San
    Francisco
San Francisco, California

*Stephen G. Slade, MD, FACS
    (Chapter 31)*
Surgeon
Slade & Baker Vision
Houston, Texas

*Scott D. Smith, MD, MPH
    (Chapter 8)*
Cole Eye Institute
Cleveland Clinic
Cleveland, Ohio

Priyanka Sood, MD (Chapter 29)
Assistant Professor
Weill Cornell Medical College
New York, New York

Clark Springs, MD (Chapter 18)
Assistant Professor of
  Ophthalmology
Indiana University School of
  Medicine
Indianapolis, Indiana

Michael E. Sulewski, MD (Chapter 5)
Clinical Associate Professor of
  Ophthalmology
Chief of Ophthalmology at the
  Veterans Affairs Medical Center of
  Philadelphia
Co-Director of the Cornea Service
  and Director of Refractive Surgery
University of Pennsylvania
Philadelphia, Pennsylvania

Geoffrey Tabin, MD (Chapter 21)
Professor of Ophthalmology and
  Visual Sciences
Director of the Division of
  International Ophthalmology
John A. Moran Eye Center, University
  of Utah
Salt Lake City, Utah

Diamond Y. Tam, MD (Chapter 6)
Clinical Assistant Professor
University of Toronto
Toronto, Canada

Robin R. Vann, MD (Chapter 2)
Assistant Clinical Professor of
  Ophthalmology
Chief, Comprehensive
  Ophthalmology Service
Duke University Eye Center
Durham, North Carolina

*Evan Waxman, MD, PhD
  (Chapter 25)*
Associate Professor of
  Ophthalmology
University of Pittsburgh School of
  Medicine
UPMC Eye Center
Pittsburgh, Philadelphia

Sonia H. Yoo, MD (Chapter 30)
Professor of Ophthalmology
Bascom Palmer Eye Institute
University of Miami Miller School of
  Medicine
Miami, Florida

*Chi-Wah (Rudy) Yung, MD, FACS
  (Chapter 18)*
Professor of Ophthalmology
Chief, Ophthalmology Service
Eskenazi Health Services
Medical Director of Student Education
Eugene and Marilyn Glick Eye Institute
Indiana University School of Medicine
Indianapolis, Indiana

INTRODUCTION

The idea for the first edition of this book originated with the creation of the first Harvard Medical School Intensive Cataract Surgical Training Course at the Massachusetts Eye and Ear Infirmary in 2005. The authors of this textbook are the faculty members from this course. The authors are distinguished ophthalmologists who were nominated as the best cataract surgery teachers by the Chairperson at their respective academic institutions. As such, this compilation of work represents the viewpoints of the most well-respected cataract surgery educators in the United States.

Mastering phacoemulsification surgery is arduous and arguably the most difficult surgery to learn during residency. We have attempted to dissect each step and dedicate an entire chapter to each individual building block of the surgery. Each chapter outlines the important aspects of the surgical step with personal tips from an experienced mentor. This second edition has been updated with the newest developments in laser technology, intraocular lenses, and surgical techniques. We hope that you will find this book useful while developing competence in cataract surgery and also as a reference once you have mastered it.

The completion of this project required great effort from many people. We do not have enough space in this book to properly express our gratitude. We hope we have properly named all those who have contributed to every aspect of this work.

First and foremost, we are grateful to all the contributing authors. We understand that writing yet another book chapter is not high on the priority list. We share the same passion for teaching and therefore appreciate the authors' acquiescence to participate in this undertaking.

We are grateful to our industry partners from Alcon, Abbott Medical Optics, and Bausch & Lomb for supporting the Harvard Cataract Course and development of this book.

This project would still be just an idea without the help and hard work of Erika Gonzalez, April Billick, Veronica Moul, and John Bond from SLACK Incorporated publishers. Their hours of dedication have made the book a reality.

We are indebted to our family and friends for generously allowing us to burn the midnight oil for the past 2 years.

Bonnie An Henderson, MD

1

APPROPRIATENESS OF CATARACT SURGERY

Susannah Rowe, MD, MPH

Cataracts are prevalent among older adults, and the incidence of cataract-related vision loss increases with age.[1] When performed appropriately, cataract extraction usually improves quality of life, reduces injury, and attenuates functional declines. Cataract extraction has proven to be generally safe and highly successful; however, it is important to ensure that surgery is performed for the appropriate indications because vision-threatening complications can occur.

I. GUIDELINES

The American Academy of Ophthalmology Preferred Practice Pattern for Cataract in the Adult Eye offers general parameters for ethical decision-making in cataract surgery:

The primary indication for surgery is visual function that no longer meets the patient's needs and for which cataract surgery provides a reasonable likelihood of improvement, or when the lens opacity inhibits optimal management of posterior segment disease or the lens causes (inflammation, angle closure, etc) medically unmanageable open-angle glaucoma.[2]

II. ACADEMIC STUDIES OF APPROPRIATENESS

In 1996, an expert panel of both ophthalmologists and nonophthalmologists first applied well-established standardized criteria for evaluating the appropriateness of medical interventions to assess 1139 cataract surgeries performed in 10 US academic centers during 1990.[3] Based on expert review of available medical records, researchers deemed the overwhelming majority

Henderson BA. *Essentials of Cataract Surgery, Second Edition (pp 1-7).*
© 2014 Taylor & Francis Group.

of surgeries to be "appropriate" (52%) or "appropriate and crucial" (39%). A small minority of surgeries was considered to be either "uncertain" (7%) or "inappropriate" (2%). Subsequent to this study, a White Paper jointly published by the American Academy of Ophthalmology, the American Society of Cataract and Refractive Surgery, and the European Society of Cataract and Refractive Surgeons highlighted evidence that cataract surgery as performed in the United States is generally appropriate and beneficial to the patient.[4] These findings are in general agreement with subsequent studies showing cataract surgery is generally appropriate.[5]

III. Visual Disability From Cataracts Reduces Overall Function and Quality of Life

Visual disability from any cause can profoundly affect quality of life and can reduce a person's ability to function safely and independently. Studies show that visual disability reduces global quality of life (based on the SF-36) more than chronic headache, type 2 diabetes, or a history of myocardial infarction.[6]

The visual acuity threshold for functional difficulties varies from patient to patient, but some population-based studies suggest that even mild reductions in vision can be symptomatic. Klein et al demonstrated in a large population-based study that early lens opacities associated with mildly reduced visual acuity are often associated with difficulty reading, driving, and recognizing faces.[7] Cataract surgeons can advise patients regarding the impact of decreased distance vision as summarized in Table 1-1.[7-10]

IV. Appropriate Cataract Surgery Improves Safety and Quality of Life

Removing visually significant cataracts usually reduces the risk of injury and improves a patient's quality of life.[11-20] Even when surgery is successful in the first eye, second-eye cataract surgery offers additional benefits.[15] In one study, patients aged 65 and older who had significant functional limitations due to cataracts had an 85% likelihood of substantial subjective functional improvement after cataract surgery.[13]

In addition to subjective benefits, research shows that appropriate cataract surgery impacts numerous objective measures of quality of life. Specific improvements include better night vision, enhanced ability to drive, fewer falls and fractures, fewer motor vehicle accidents, better cognitive functioning on standardized tests, greater ability to live independently, and attenuated declines in overall functioning and well-being.[13-20]

TABLE 1-1. IMPACT OF DECREASED DISTANCE VISION	
Visual Acuity	*Impact*
Worse than 20/25	More falls and fractures
Worse than 20/40	Decreased overall quality of life Functional declines in global health status (mobility, activities of daily living, and physical performance)
Worse than 20/50	Greater risk of death Impaired visual field, contrast sensitivity, and distance vision Greater risk of motor vehicle accidents

V. ASSESSING THE IMPACT OF CATARACTS ON PATIENTS' QUALITY OF LIFE

Deciding to proceed with cataract surgery represents a collaborative process between the patient and the surgeon as well as other family members and caregivers as indicated. This process should include a careful assessment of the patient's subjective visual function. Preoperative vision-specific quality of life and glare disability remain the most reliable predictors of patient satisfaction with cataract surgery, whereas preoperative visual acuity is only weakly predictive of patient satisfaction.[14,21] Patients with the poorest preoperative subjective visual function are generally the most satisfied after cataract surgery.

To appropriately advise patients regarding the risks and benefits of cataract surgery, ophthalmologists must clearly understand their patients' needs, desires, and priorities. During this process, surgeons should take into account possibly inaccurate expectations regarding functional decline with age (too high/too low) and some patients' inability to recognize and acknowledge gradual decreases in vision and visual function. Finally, surgeons have a responsibility to educate patients regarding the ways in which decreased vision can limit abilities, safety, and quality of life and to help them balance these risks with the potential risks of surgery.

VI. OTHER PREDICTORS OF GOOD OUTCOME FROM CATARACT SURGERY

In addition to worse vision-associated quality of life, other predictors of good outcome after cataract surgery include age <75 years, posterior subcapsular cataract and glare disability, and the absence of age-related macular degeneration or diabetes.[21]

VII. DOMAINS OF SUBJECTIVE VISUAL FUNCTION

In order to understand a patient's subjective visual function, surgeons should ask specific questions about vision as it relates to activities of daily living. Quality-of-life studies have identified several important domains of vision-targeted quality of life and include the following[22,23]:

Difficulty with near vision activities, such as:
- Reading small print such as newspaper, telephone book
- Reading letters from friends and family
- Identifying medicines
- Reading legal forms
- Managing bills
- Sewing, cooking, using tools such as scissors
- Finding things on a shelf
- Performing make-up, hairstyling, shaving

Difficulty with distance vision tasks, such as:
- Going up and down stairs or curbs
- Playing games, exercising, bowling, etc
- Recognizing signs across a hall
- Recognizing people across a room
- Going to see movies, plays
- Watching TV

Vision needs for social functioning, such as:
- Entertaining friends or family in home/room
- Visiting people in their rooms, homes, or restaurants
- Seeing faces and how people react to things

Role limitations from visual impairment, such as:
- Limitations in how long activities can be done
- Accomplishing less than desired
- Needing more help than desired
- Limitations in kinds of activities possible

Dependency from visual impairment, such as:
- Needing lots of help
- Needing to rely on what others say
- Not being able to go out alone
- Staying in a room because of eyesight

Feelings of reduced well-being/distress, such as:
- Worrying about vision
- Feeling frustrated with vision
- Experiencing loss of control
- Fearing embarrassing self or others
- Feeling irritable because of poor vision

Peripheral and color vision tasks, such as:
- Seeing objects off to the side
- Picking out and matching clothes

VIII. SPECIAL CASES

A. Monocular Patients

Cataract surgery outcomes for monocular patients have not been formally assessed in large studies. For patients without good visual potential in the fellow eye, careful assessment of subjective visual function is especially critical to help patients and surgeons balance the risks of proceeding with surgery versus the risks of deferring intervention. Recommendations for the surgeon include taking extra time with the decision-making and consent processes and being realistic about the surgical skills and resources necessary for a good outcome. Many surgeons consider referring monocular patients for a subspecialty consult to assess any additional ocular pathology that could influence the outcome of surgery.

B. Patients With Low Visual Potential

Many low-vision patients are very satisfied with the results of cataract surgery if they understand in advance the goals of the surgery and have realistic expectations. Therefore, even when the visual potential is limited by factors other than cataracts, it is reasonable to consider surgery if the cataract is advanced and if the patient is well informed and motivated to undergo surgery. In these cases it can be useful to focus on functions related to peripheral vision, improved colors, and brightness, rather than on central visual acuity. It is important to consider the increased threat of surgical complications posed by other pathology, as well as the potential need to remove the cataract in order to diagnose and treat other ocular disorders. Finally, it is critical to evaluate carefully and optimize treatment of disorders such as glaucoma and diabetic retinopathy prior to surgery.

IX. CONCLUSION

Cataract surgery is an appropriate option to consider whenever a patient has decreased ability to perform needed or desired activities due to cataract. In addition, patients who are not aware of subjective visual deficits may benefit from surgery if they have reduced vision from cataract and have elevated risks for falls, motor vehicle accidents, or other injuries. Patients with cataract obscuring the view of the posterior segment may also benefit from cataract surgery. Appropriate decision making for cataract surgery is a collaborative effort between the patient and the surgeon and requires an understanding of the patient's vision-related quality of life and visual function.

KEY POINTS

1. Cataract surgery is indicated when visual function no longer meets the patient's needs or when the lens opacity inhibits optimal management of other ocular disease.
2. Overall, studies report that cataract surgery is performed appropriately in the United States and is beneficial to patients.
3. Visual disability from cataracts reduces overall function and quality of life while appropriate cataract surgery improves safety and quality of life.
4. To appropriately advise patients regarding the risks and benefits of cataract surgery, ophthalmologists must clearly understand their patients' needs, desires, and priorities.
5. Special attention and care must be taken in special circumstances such as monocular patients or those with limited visual potential.

REFERENCES

1. Congdon N, Vingerling JR, Klein BE, et al. Eye Diseases Prevalence Research Group. Prevalence of cataract and pseudophakia/aphakia among adults in the United States. *Arch Ophthalmol.* 2004;122(4):487-494.
2. American Academy of Ophthalmology: The Eye M.D. Association. Cataract in the Adult Eye. American Academy of Ophthalmology, 2011. (Preferred Practice Pattern).
3. Tobacman JK, Lee P, Zimmerman B, Kolder H, Hilborne L, Brook R. Assessment of appropriateness of cataract surgery at ten academic medical centers in 1990. *Ophthalmology.* 1996;103(2):207-215.
4. Obstbaum SA. American Academy of Ophthalmology, American Society of Cataract and Refractive Surgery, and European Society of Refractive Surgeons. White paper: utilization, appropriate care, and quality of life for patients with cataracts. *Ophthalmology.* 2006;113(10):1878-1881.

5. Escobar A, Bilbao A, Blasco JA, Lacalle J, Bare M, Begiristain JM, Quintana JM. IRYSS-Cataract Group Validity of Newly Developed Appropriateness Criteria for Cataract Surgery. *Ophthalmology* 2009;116(3):409-417.
6. Lee PP, Spritzer K, Hays RD. The impact of blurred vision on functioning and well-being. *Ophthalmology*. 1997;104(3):390-396.
7. Klein BE, Klein R, Knudtson MD. Lens opacities associated with performance-based and self-assessed visual functions [see comment]. *Ophthalmology*. 2006;113(8):1257-1263.
8. Scott IU, Schein OD, West S, Bandeen-Roche K, Enger C, Folstein MF. Functional status and quality of life measurement among ophthalmic patients. *Arch Ophthalmol.* 1994;112(3):329-335.
9. Chia EM, Mitchell P, Rochtchina E, Foran S, Wang JJ. Unilateral visual impairment and health related quality of life: the Blue Mountains Eye Study. *Br J Ophthalmol.* 2003;87(4):392-395.
10. McGwin G Jr, Owsley C, Gauthreaux S. The association between cataract and mortality among older adults. *Ophthalmic Epidemiol.* 2003;10(2):107-119.
11. Tielsch JM, Steinberg EP, Cassard SD, et al. Preoperative functional expectations and postoperative outcomes among patients undergoing first eye cataract surgery. *Arch Ophthalmol.* 1995;113(10):1312-1318.
12. Groessl EJ, Liu L, Sklar M, Tally SR, Kaplan RM, Ganiats TG Measuring the impact of cataract surgery on generic and vision-specific quality of life. *J Cataract Refract Surg.* 2013;39(5):673-9.
13. Mangione CM, Phillips RS, Lawrence MG, Seddon JM, Orav EJ, Goldman L. Improved visual function and attenuation of declines in health-related quality of life after cataract extraction. *Arch Ophthalmol.* 1994;112(11):1419-1425.
14. Rubin GS, Adamsons IA, Stark WJ. Comparison of acuity, contrast sensitivity, and disability glare before and after cataract surgery. Arch *Ophthalmol.* 1993;111(1):56-61.
15. Lee BS, Munoz BE, West SK, Gower EW. Functional improvement after one- and two-eye cataract surgery in the Salisbury Eye Evaluation. *Ophthalmology*. 2013;120(5):949-55.
16. Gillespie LD, Robertson MC, Gillespie WJ, Sherrington C, Gates S, Clemson LM, Lamb SE. Interventions for preventing falls in older people living in the community. *Cochrane Database Syst Rev.* 2012 Sep 12;9:CD007146
17. Meuleners LB, Hendrie D, LeeAH, Ng JQ, Morlet N. The Effectiveness of Cataract Surgery in Reducing Motor Vehicle Crashes: A Whole Population Study Using Linked Data. *Ophthalmic Epidemiol.* 2012;19(1):23-28
18. Owsley C, McGwin G Jr, Sloane M, Wells J, Stalvey BT, Gauthreaux S. Impact of cataract surgery on motor vehicle crash involvement by older adults. *JAMA*. 2002;288(7):841-849.
19. Sloan FA, Ostermann J, Brown DS, Lee PP. Effects of changes in self-reported vision on cognitive, affective, and functional status and living arrangements among the elderly. *Am J Ophthalmol.* 2005;140(4):618-627.
20. Mangione CM, Orav EJ, Lawrence MG, Phillips RS, Seddon JM, Goldman L. Prediction of visual function after cataract surgery: a prospectively validated model. *Arch Ophthalmol.* 1995;113(10):1305-1311.
21. Mangione CM, Lee PP, Gutierrez PR, Spritzer K, Berry S, Hays RD. National Eye Institute Visual Function Questionnaire Field Test Investigators. Development of the 25-item National Eye Institute Visual Function Questionnaire. *Arch Ophthalmol.* 2001;119(7):1050-1058.
22. Cassard SD, Patrick DL, Damiano AM, et al. Reproducibility and responsiveness of the VF-14: an index of functional impairment in patients with cataracts. *Arch Ophthalmol.* 1995;113(12):1508-1513.

2

CATARACT SURGERY
PREOPERATIVE EVALUATION

John P. Berdahl, MD and Robin R. Vann, MD

I. INTRODUCTION

There are 4 main goals in the preoperative evaluation of cataract surgery:
1. Ensure symptoms are consistent with cataracts.
2. Preoperatively identify and avoid potential sources of intraoperative complications.
3. Clarify surgeon and patient goals regarding the course and outcome of surgery.
4. Match the proper technology to the patient.

The best way to achieve these goals is by a complete ophthalmologic history and physical.

As cataract surgery has become safer with faster visual recovery and improved uncorrected visual outcomes, the risk/benefit ratio of this surgery has dramatically improved. As a result, we are relying on loss of visual function instead of visual acuity as the primary method of assessing the benefit of cataract surgery. Cataract surgeons, now more than ever before, must be diligent to ensure that the cataract is the cause (or at least partial cause) of the visual dysfunction. As discussed in Chapter 1, the appropriateness of cataract surgery for an individual patient may be the most important part of the preoperative assessment. Each patient has individual visual needs, and surgery should be determined on an individual basis after an individual risk/benefit analysis.[1,2] Documentation of the specific visual disturbance and impact on the patient is crucial. Because technology is improving, our ability to create spectacle independence is improving as well. Multifocal, accommodating, and toric intraocular lenses (IOLs) all require special testing and consideration but can leave patients much more functional without spectacles after

Henderson BA. *Essentials of Cataract Surgery, Second Edition (pp 9-24).* © 2014 Taylor & Francis Group.

surgery. Other technologies such as laser-assisted cataract surgery are just being developed that may also improve outcomes and increase safety.

II. HISTORY

A. History of Present Illness

Pertinent features of the history of present illness include the patient's age, symptoms, duration of symptoms, and impact on quality of life. Common symptoms of cataracts follow:

- Visual decline (blurred, clouded, a film, a skim) over weeks to years
- Glasses no longer improve eyesight
- Decreased distance vision, near vision, or both
- Decreased color perception (harder to distinguish blues and blacks, yellow is dim)
- Disabling glare
- Starbursts or halos around lights
- Worse during different periods of the day (day, dusk, and night)
- Monocular diplopia or polyopia

B. Ocular History

The ocular history includes both preexisting and concurrent conditions. Preoperative identification of these conditions allows the surgeon to give the patient realistic expectations, identify and avoid potential complications, suggest combined procedures, or suggest surgery be delayed or even avoided altogether.

1. Preexisting conditions that should be identified

- Amblyopia/strabismus
- Anterior basement membrane dystrophy, keratoconus, and corneal guttata
- Macular degeneration, epiretinal membrane, macular hole, and diabetic retinopathy
- Retinitis pigmentosa associated with posterior subcapsular cataracts and cystoid macular edema

2. Conditions with implications for cataract surgery

a. Glaucoma

The severity of the patient's glaucoma should be understood. Would the patient's optic nerve be able to withstand a perioperative

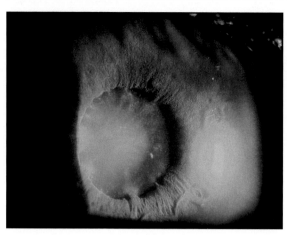

Figure 2-1. Posterior synechiae after uveitis limiting dilation. (Reprinted with permission of Joseph Halabis, OD.)

intraocular pressure (IOP) spike? Would this patient be a better candidate for a combined cataract and glaucoma procedure?[3] Is the patient using pilocarpine and will the pupils dilate intraoperatively? Recent studies have indicated that cataract surgery alone can create a significant and sustained reduction of IOP especially in patients with high preoperative IOP.[4,5]

b. Uveitis

Patients with uveitis are more prone to postoperative inflammation, cystoid macular edema (CME), epiretinal membrane, and posterior capsular opacification. A topical nonsteroidal anti-inflammatory drug (NSAID) or steroid is necessary to control inflammation prior to surgery. Often these patients have posterior synechiae leading to poor dilation (Figure 2-1).[6-8]

c. High myopia

Patients with high myopia have a higher risk of retinal detachment after cataract surgery, and their periphery should be closely examined for breaks prior to surgery. They also may have posterior staphyloma, making IOL calculations difficult. In addition, there is a higher risk of globe perforation with retrobulbar anesthesia due to an elongated globe.[9,10]

d. Prior retinal surgery

IOL calculation errors are more common in patients who have a scleral buckle. Patients who have had vitrectomy can have rapid progression of cataracts, and surgery is often more difficult due to loose zonules and posterior capsular instability.[11]

Figure 2-2. Lens dislocation following trauma. (Reprinted with permission of Joseph Halabis, OD.)

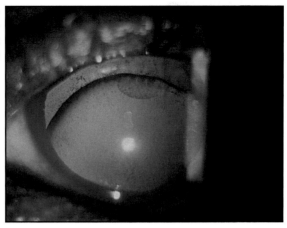

e. Prior ocular trauma

Trauma can impact any intraocular structures and complicate the approach to surgery. It is very important to realize and anticipate that zonular instability may complicate these cases (Figure 2-2).

f. Pseudoexfoliation

Pseudoexfoliation syndrome is well known to cause zonular instability, poor pupillary dilation, and increased risk of postoperative IOP spikes (Figure 2-3).[12]

g. Prior refractive surgery

Achieving accurate postoperative outcomes is difficult in patients who have had prior refractive surgery because keratometric data are inaccurate. All cataract patients should be specifically asked about prior refractive procedures. Specific strategies to deal with these cases will be discussed in a later chapter.

h. Contact lens wear

Soft contact lens wearers must stop lens use at least 1 week prior to keratometry and rigid lens wearers 3 weeks prior to keratometry.

C. Medical History

A complete past medical history can explain the cause of early onset cataracts and can help with planning the case.

1. Steroids

Patients with any condition requiring steroids, such as asthma, arthritis, or organ transplant, are at increased risk for early cataracts.

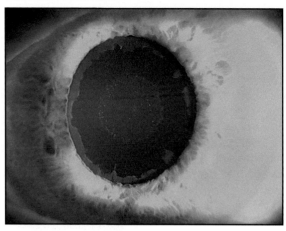

Figure 2-3. Pseudoexfoliation creates lenticular instability and poor dilation. (Reprinted with permission of Joseph Halabis, OD.)

2. Systemic diseases

Patients who have received radiation near the eye or have atopic dermatitis, diabetes, galactosemia, hypocalcemia, Wilson disease, or myotonic dystrophy have an increased risk of cataract formation. Marfan syndrome and homocystinuria are notorious causes of lenticular subluxation and zonular weakness.

3. Conditions that compromise a patient's ability to cooperate or position during surgery

Patients with chronic obstructive pulmonary disease, congestive heart failure, obesity, arthritis, kyphosis, dementia, Parkinson's disease, head tremors, or language barriers may be unable to lie still for surgery without a general anesthetic.

4. Ocular conditions that may worsen after surgery

Patients with diabetic retinopathy are at risk for progression of disease following cataract surgery.[13,14]

D. Medications

1. Medications that are known to cause cataracts

The medications that are known to cause cataracts are corticosteroids, phenothiazines, anticholinesterases, amiodarone, and statins.

2. Medications that compromise the cataract surgery itself

Tamsulosin HCl (Flomax) is known to cause intraoperative floppy iris syndrome (IFIS), causing poor pupillary dilation and an unstable iris with tendencies to prolapse into the wound. Progressive intraoperative miosis is also common. Studies are continuing to further elucidate the role of tamsulosin and other medications with IFIS.[15]

3. Anticoagulants

Anticoagulants do not increase the incidence of bleeding; however, if bleeding occurs it tends to be larger and can complicate retrobulbar anesthesia and visualization. Over-the-counter products (aspirin, ibuprofen, and naproxen) should also be included in this group. Although anticoagulants are generally not stopped for cataract surgery even when retrobulbar anesthesia is used, the surgeon should be aware that these medications are being used.[16-18]

As an aside, it is important to remind patients to continue chronic eye medications, such as glaucoma drops, during the perioperative period.

E. Allergies/Adverse Reactions

Allergies and adverse reactions should be documented. The patient should be specifically questioned about latex and iodine allergies as well as anesthesia difficulties. Often patients have reactions to systemic medications such as NSAIDs or fluoroquinolones. In these cases, it is important to understand the exact reaction and determine if the topical medications pose a significant risk.

F. Family History

Some patients have a strong family history of cataracts that can explain early onset cataract formation.

G. Social History

1. Alcohol and sedative use or abuse may require further intraoperative sedative medications.
2. Smoking may cause early onset cataract.
3. It is important to know if the patient will be able to perform postoperative instructions such as restrictions on lifting and instillation of eye medications.

III. EXAM

A. Introduction

A general overall view of the patient to determine surgically limiting factors such as body habitus, kyphosis, or tremor should be observed. A complete dilated eye exam is necessary in all patients to determine surgical necessity and surgical planning. Special attention should be paid to lenticular stability.

B. Vision

1. Visual acuity

Snellen visual acuity has traditionally been one of the main indicators of the necessity of cataract surgery. However, Snellen acuity measures only high contrast discrimination in controlled lighting situations. This is not an accurate metric for patients who experience real world symptomatology such as glare or decreased color vision. Although poor Snellen acuity alone may be an indication for surgery, good Snellen acuity is not a contraindication for surgery. A complete assessment of visual function could include any or all of the following based on an individual's symptoms: distance acuity, near acuity, binocular function to test anisometropia, glare testing, light testing, and contrast sensitivity. A potential acuity meter or interferometry may be used to determine visual potential.

C. Keratometry

Keratometry is used for IOL calculations and must be performed in both eyes as an internal control. Keratometric measurements also help determine corneal astigmatism and provide the basis for discussion of astigmatic treatments. As discussed previously, it is imperative to inquire about contact lens wear and previous refractive surgery before keratometric measurements.

D. Corneal Topography

Topography might be indicated in some circumstances:
1. If keratometry values differ from the past, between eyes, or from the refraction.
2. If corneal astigmatic procedures are planned (limbal relaxing incisions and astigmatic keratotomy).
3. If considering a presbyopia-correcting or astigmatic-correcting lens.

E. Pupils

1. Afferent pupillary defect

Check all patients for an afferent pupillary defect (APD). Should a new APD be found, further work-up is warranted prior to surgery. Cataracts generally do not cause an APD; however, it has been reported that dense cataracts can cause a contralateral APD.[19]

2. Dilation

Poor dilation in the clinic suggests poor dilation during surgery and the surgeon should be prepared for this eventuality. Extremely large pupils predispose patients to glare and dysphotopsia. Appropriate IOLs should be chosen in these cases.

F. Intraocular Pressure

Significantly elevated intraocular pressures or narrow angles may require treatment before surgery.

G. Motility

1. Tropias

Patients with severe longstanding cataracts can develop tropias from sensory deprivation. If the deprivation is cured (ie, cataract removal), the patient may develop diplopia with his or her new binocularity and need prism glasses or additional strabismus surgery to treat the diplopia.

2. Trauma

Traumatic cataracts may also create a tropia; however, it may be traumatic and not sensory in origin.

3. Diplopia and ptosis

Diplopia and ptosis are known complications of cataract surgery, including topical surgery. It is important to document preexisting motility disorders.

H. External

A prominent forehead and/or deeply recessed globe may pose a technical challenge to the cataract surgery procedure especially when performed superiorly.

I. Slit Lamp

A complete slit lamp examination with specific attention paid to the following conditions will aid in the preoperative planning.

1. Lids/lashes

Blepharitis or meibomitis may increase risk of endophthalmitis and should be treated before surgery. Blepharophimosis can limit surgical exposure. Ptosis can be exacerbated by speculum use.

2. Conjunctiva/sclera

The presence of prior surgery such as filtering blebs may alter the approach to surgery. Symblepharon, conjunctival scarring, or scleral thinning may alter the surgical approach as well. Conjunctivochalasis may make suction difficult to obtain if performing laser-assisted cataract surgery.

3. Cornea

Guttata may represent early Fuchs' dystrophy, which can be made worse with cataract surgery, especially with extended phacoemulsification times. Corneal pathology such as scars or peripheral degenerations may alter the surgical approach. Pigment on the endothelial surface may be a clue to pseudoexfoliation.

4. Anterior chamber

Narrow angles with elevated IOP may require laser peripheral iridotomy before cataract surgery. If anterior chamber IOL placement is likely, gonioscopy is necessary to look for peripheral anterior synechiae or angle neovascularization.

5. Iris

Determine maximal dilation and check for posterior synechiae. Debris present at the pupillary margin may represent pseudoexfoliation.

6. Lens

Determine cataract density to plan the surgical approach. Check for lenticular stability by either having the patient look back and forth quickly or hitting the slit lamp table while observing the lens. Identify lenticular dislocation or subluxation. Pseudoexfoliation is most obvious on the anterior lens capsule. In addition, check for posterior polar cataracts as they are associated with increased risk of posterior capsular rupture with vitreous loss.

7. Anterior vitreous

Asteroid hyalosis and vitreous hemorrhage can make visualization very difficult in the operating room.

As an adjunct to complete slit lamp examination, retinoscopy can provide valuable information regarding the visual impact of cataracts that are unimpressive at the slit lamp.

J. Fundus

Patients need to be dilated for a cataract evaluation.

1. Retina

Any retinal pathology such as age-related macular degeneration (AMD), epiretinal membrane (ERM), vitreomacular traction, macular hole, scars, or diabetic retinopathy that could be responsible for decreased vision should be identified and discussed with the patient to give him or her appropriate expectations for postoperative vision.

2. Optic nerve

The optic nerve should also be thoroughly evaluated for pallor or cupping and treated or referred appropriately.

3. Ultrasonography

Should cataract density prevent adequate visualization of the posterior pole, B-scan ultrasonography should be used to rule out gross abnormalities such as tumors or retinal detachments.

K. Orbit

The orbit should be examined and the surgeon should visualize the ideal approach for surgery when making the preoperative plan. Deep orbits may preclude a superior or superonasal incision, limiting the ability to operate on the steep keratometric axis. In addition, excessively deep or narrow orbits may prevent suction in conjunction with laser-assisted cataract surgery.

L. Neuropsychiatric

Comprehension and ability to follow commands during the examination are clues to how the patient will behave in the operating room. Patients who are not able to follow commands should be offered general anesthesia. Patients who are extremely visually demanding or prone to bitter complaints of glare and halo inconsistent with the exam should probably avoid multifocal lenses.

IV. PATIENT EXPECTATIONS

As discussed throughout this chapter, individualized surgical planning must occur for each patient. Patients have varying visual requirements and expectations regarding cataract surgery. The most important conversation between the patient and the surgeon is to adequately address patient expectations. Key issues to address include postoperative visual expectations, visual potential, uncorrected visual goal and the need for visual aids outside that range, the surgical experience, surgical and postoperative risks, and postoperative care.

In order to meet or exceed patient expectations of surgical outcomes, the surgeon needs to know what symptoms have brought the patient to seek surgery. It is best to summarize and focus on addressing specific objective symptoms such as eliminating glare while driving at night or improving the ability to read road signs. If the patient has concurrent ocular pathology, it is important to remind him or her of how this condition may limit the postoperative visual outcome of cataract surgery. It is up to the surgeon to ensure that the patient has a realistic expectation of the visual outcome prior to consenting for surgery.

In addition, cataract surgery has the unique opportunity to change the patient's uncorrected refraction postoperatively. It is therefore important to include in the preoperative discussion the uncorrected visual goal for each surgery. Each patient has individual interests resulting in individual visual needs. For example, some myopic patients may prefer to remain myopic for near work, such as avid readers; while distance vision may be more important to golfers. Other patients prefer spectacle independence with monovision correction or the use of accommodative or multifocal lenses. If these issues are not addressed preoperatively, an otherwise successful surgery can lead to an unsatisfied patient. Identifying the patient's visual needs and then choosing the correct lens and postoperative refractive goal is crucial to meet the expectations of the patient.

Although cataract surgery is a very successful operation, there are risks associated with the operation that may complicate the outcome of surgery. We believe that patients should be informed of the potential complications associated with the surgery before they commit to consenting for the operation. During the surgery discussion, we review the potential for ptosis, endophthalmitis, corneal decompensation, retinal detachment, CME, and suprachoroidal hemorrhage in layman's terms for them. If they have concurrent ocular conditions that increase the risks of surgery, we try to emphasize and review that risk to the individual as well.

The surgical experience is typically well tolerated for most patients. However, the uninformed patient is likely to have much more anxiety about surgery. Specific information that should be provided include where and when to report for surgery, expected duration of the surgery, expected total time at the surgical center, method of anesthesia and sedation and how patients tolerate it, expected amount and duration of pain, patient responsibilities the evening after surgery, when and where to report the day after surgery, and future appointments. Often a typed sheet with the above information is helpful to the patient.

Most patients have a friend or relative who had a wonderful experience with cataract surgery. While this is a credit to the profession of ophthalmology, it may create difficulties for the surgeon to match the patient's experience to that of his or her peers. Patients should realize that cataract surgery is indeed surgery and although it usually proceeds without difficulty, complications can occur even if the surgery goes perfectly. This conversation is delicate because the surgeon must not induce unnecessary fears while providing an accurate representation of the risks. As always an honest approach is best.

V. SPECIAL CONSIDERATION FOR SPECTACLE INDEPENDENCE

Recent advances in multifocal and accommodative IOL design have led to a tremendous increase in patient satisfaction with spectacle independence. However, the most critical part of ensuring success with these lenses is the preoperative evaluation. Appropriately identifying patient's visual goals is always the first step to choosing the best IOL. However, the patient's goals must be consistent with the capabilities of the patient's optical system. In the following section, we will discuss objective measurements that can help surgeons determine if accommodative, multifocal, or toric lenses are indicated.

A. The Ocular Surface

The microenvironment of the tear film changes as we age. Ocular surface disease is very common in an older population and the air/tear interface is responsible for 70% of the eyes' refractive power. Maximizing the quality of the tear film and the ocular surface is critical to IOL performance. When considering these lenses, the surgeon needs to evaluate and treat for dry eye syndrome. Objective testing includes tear breakup time, Schirmer testing, osmolality testing, and physical exam. Treatment regimens including cyclosporine, omega-3 fatty acids, punctal occlusion, topical azithromycin, and others can help maximize quality of the ocular surface.

B. Corneal and Lenticular Astigmatism

Multifocal IOLs or accommodative IOLs are very sensitive to even mild amounts of astigmatism and the surgeon needs to try to limit the postoperative astigmatism to less than 0.5 diopters. For mild astigmatism, the surgeon may simply choose to operate on the steep axis to reduce astigmatism to acceptable levels. If mild-to-moderate amounts of astigmatism are present, a concurrent limbal relaxing incision or astigmatic keratotomy can be performed to reduce the astigmatism. In patients with high amounts of astigmatism, the toric IOLs are the best option for achieving good distance vision. Although these lenses do not correct for presbyopia, patients can still achieve spectacle independence through targeting a monovision with these toric lenses. If residual astigmatism is present postoperatively, excimer laser treatment is the most accurate way to remove residual astigmatism. However, if the spherical equivalent is near plano, astigmatic keratotomies or limbal relaxing incisions can be used to decrease the astigmatism.

C. Topography and Tomography

Irregular astigmatism has a tremendous effect on the ability of presbyopia-correcting lenses to function well. Topography is important in all patients

undergoing presbyopia-correcting lenses to make sure that irregular astigmatism is not present and to quantify and confirm the amount of regular
astigmatism that is present.

D. Higher-Order Aberrations

Irregular astigmatism, anterior basement membrane dystrophy, and
other factors can cause higher-order aberrations. Because both presbyopia-
correcting IOLs and higher-order aberrations decrease contrast sensitivity,
it is important to avoid multifocals in the setting of excessive higher-order
aberrations. Wavefront aberrometers are able to predict how much of the
higher-order aberrations come from the corneal surface and avoid multifocals in such scenarios. For example, the Nidek OPD III scan can perform
this function and if the root means square is greater than 0.3, multifocals are
generally avoided.

E. Angle Kappa

Angle kappa is the distance between the center of the pupil and the visual
axis. If angle kappa is greater than half the diameter of the central optical
zone of a multifocal IOL, the primary path of light may traverse one of the
multifocal rings instead of the central optic, leading to unwanted glare. The
ReSTOR 3.0 lens has a central optical zone of 0.8 mm and a Tecnis multifocal
has a central optical zone of 1.0 mm. Therefore, an angle kappa of less than
0.4 for the ReSTOR (Alcon Laboratories) 3.0 or 0.5 for the Tecnis (Abbott
Medical Optics) multifocal is probably acceptable (Figure 2-4).[20,21]

F. 3-mm and 5-mm Refractive Zones

Patients can experience a phenomenon known as night myopia that is due
to the increased curvature of the peripheral cornea. This is particularly true
in patients who have had prior refractive surgery with smaller ablation zones.
Instruments such as the Nidek OPD III scan and the iTrace (Tracey Technologies) systems can measure refractions at differing optical zones. If the 3-mm
and 5-mm optical zone is different, then presbyopia-correcting lenses are often avoided (Figure 2-5).

G. Optical Coherence Tomography of the Macula

Trying to achieve spectacle independence after cataract surgery is dependent on a healthy macula. Although a good funduscopic exam can pick up
most subtle pathology of the macula, sometimes a small change in the foveal
contour or an epiretinal membrane or posterior vitreous detachment or a
subtle subfoveal drusen is picked up on optical coherence tomography (OCT)
while missed on the exam. In these settings, we often avoid presbyopia-
correcting lenses.

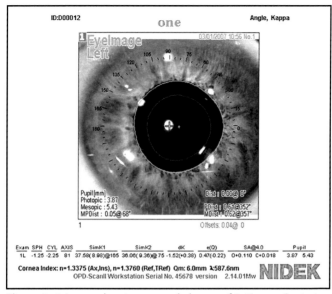

Figure 2-4. Image showing an angle kappa of 0.61 mm. Centering the IOL on the pupil may result in glare because the visual axis and the pupil center are significantly different.

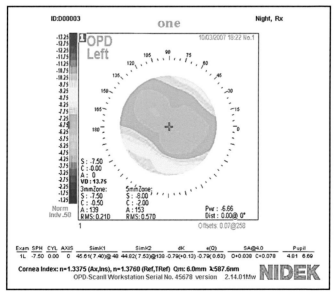

Figure 2-5. Image demonstrating a different refraction at the 3-mm and 5-mm refractive zones. The change in refraction could lead to nighttime defocus and glare in a multifocal patient. Further, notice the elevated higher order aberrations, at the 5-mm zone, which could degrade image quality.

H. Ability to Use Laser Vision Correction in the Future

Despite the best preoperative evaluation and IOL calculations, a small percentage of patient will not achieve the refractive goal. The surgeon should consider any possible contraindications to laser vision correction prior to implanting a lens to minimize spectacle independence.

VI. SPECIAL CONSIDERATION FOR LASER CATARACT SURGERY

As of this writing refractive laser-assisted cataract surgery (ReLACS) is just entering the marketplace. Although much is yet to be learned, the authors have significant early experience with ReLACS and can share some preoperative evaluative thoughts.

The biggest difference using ReLACS is docking the patient interface to the eye with suction. Although, not difficult, it is a new approach for nonrefractive surgeons. Factors that limit the ability to achieve an adequate dock include deep orbits, flat corneas, irregular corneas, pterygia, narrow interpalpebral fissures, excessive conjunctiva, or a patient who squeezes his or her eyes.

ReLACS can be used in cases with loose zonules to minimize lens manipulation and in the setting of Fuchs' dystrophy to minimize phacoemulsification energy to help preserve endothelial cells.

KEY POINTS

1. Documentation of the specific visual disturbance and impact on the patient is crucial.
2. There is no substitute for a complete ophthalmologic history and physical.
3. Specifically ask if a patient has worn contact lenses or had prior refractive surgery.
4. Physician-patient communication of goals, realistic outcomes, and limitations due to preexisting conditions are necessary to ensure patient and surgeon satisfaction.
5. Special testing such as topography and OCT is usually necessary when choosing multifocal and accommodating lenses.
6. Laser-assisted cataract surgery may not be suitable in all situations, but may be advantageous in others.

REFERENCES

1. Cinotti AA. Evaluation of indications for cataract surgery. *Ophthalmic Surg.* 1979;10(12):25-31.

2. Hess R, Woo G. Vision through cataracts. *Invest Ophthalmol Vis Sci.* 1978;17(5):428-435.

3. Gianoli F, Schnyder CC, Bovey E, Mermoud A. Combined surgery for cataract and glaucoma: phacoemulsification and deep sclerectomy compared with phacoemulsification and trabeculectomy. *J Cataract Refract Surg.* 1999;25(3):340-346.

4. Berdahl JP. Cataract surgery to lower intraocular pressure. *Middle East Afr J Ophthalmol.* 2009;16(3):119-122.

5. Poley BJ, Lindstrom RL, Samuelson TW. Long-term effects of phacoemulsification with intraocular lens implantation in normotensive and ocular hypertensive eyes. *J Cataract Refract Surg.* 2008;34(5):735-742.

6. Estafanous MF, Lowder CY, Meisler DM, Chauhan R. Phacoemulsification cataract extraction and posterior chamber lens implantation in patients with uveitis. *Am J Ophthalmol.* 2001;131(5):620-625.

7. Foster CS, Fong LP, Singh G. Cataract surgery and intraocular lens implantation in patients with uveitis. *Ophthalmology.* 1989;96(3):281-288.

8. Krishna R, Meisler DM, Lowder CY, et al. Long-term follow-up of extracapsular cataract extraction and posterior chamber intraocular lens implantation in patients with uveitis. *Ophthalmology.* 1998;105(9):1765-1769.

9. Alldredge CD, Elkins B, Alldredge Jr OC. Retinal detachment following phacoemulsification in highly myopic cataract patients. *J Cataract Refract Surg.* 1998;24(6):777-780.

10. Lyle WA, Jin GJ. Phacoemulsification with intraocular lens implantation in high myopia. *J Cataract Refract Surg.* 1996;22(2):238-242.

11. Pinter SM, Sugar A. Phacoemulsification in eyes with past pars plana vitrectomy: case-control study. *J Cataract Refract Surg.* 1999;25(4):556-561.

12. Naumann GO, Schlotzer-Schrehardt U, Kuchle M. Pseudoexfoliation syndrome for the comprehensive ophthalmologist. Intraocular and systemic manifestations. *Ophthalmology.* 1998;105(6):951-968.

13. Mittra RA, Borrillo JL, Dev S, et al. Retinopathy progression and visual outcomes after phacoemulsification in patients with diabetes mellitus. *Arch Ophthalmol.* 2000;118(7):912-917.

14. Jaffe GJ, Burton TC, Kuhn E, et al. Progression of nonproliferative diabetic retinopathy and visual outcome after extracapsular cataract extraction and intraocular lens implantation. *Am J Ophthalmol.* 1992;114(4):448-456.

15. Chang DF, Campbell JR. Intraoperative floppy iris syndrome associated with tamsulosin. *J Cataract Refract Surg.* 2005;31(4):664-673.

16. Carter K, Miller KM. Phacoemulsification and lens implantation in patients treated with aspirin or warfarin. *J Cataract Refract Surg.* 1998;24(10):1361-1364.

17. Kallio H, Paloheimo M, Maunuksela EL. Haemorrhage and risk factors associated with retrobulbar/peribulbar block: a prospective study in 1383 patients. *Br J Anaesth.* 2000;85(5):708-711.

18. Katz J, Feldman MA, Bass EB, et al. Risks and benefits of anticoagulant and antiplatelet medication use before cataract surgery. *Ophthalmology.* 2003;110(9):1784-1788.

19. Lam BL, Thompson HS. A unilateral cataract produces a relative afferent pupillary defect in the contralateral eye. *Ophthalmology.* 1990;97(3):334-338.

20. Hayashi K, Hayashi H, Nakao F, Hayashi F. Correlation between pupillary size and intraocular lens decentration and visual acuity of a zonal-progressive multifocal lens and a monofocal lens. *Ophthalmology.* 2001;108(11):2011-2017.

21. McKelvie J, McArdle B, McGhee C. The influence of tilt, decentration, and pupil size on the higher-order aberration profile of aspheric intraocular lenses. *Ophthalmology.* 118(9):1724-1731.

3

PREOPERATIVE EYEDROPS AND OTHER MEDICATIONS

James P. Dunn, MD

I. INTRODUCTION

Appropriate use of preoperative eyedrops is essential in providing a well-dilated pupil prior to cataract surgery and in minimizing the risk of endophthalmitis. Residents should develop a consistent approach to their preoperative regimen based on fundamental principles and the specific characteristics of a given procedure.

- Most cases of endophthalmitis following cataract surgery result from inoculation of bacteria into the eye from endogenous lid flora.[1] Maximal reduction of bacteria on the ocular surface and control of blepharitis are therefore essential.
- Blepharitis should be addressed well before the day of surgery with warm compresses, lid hygiene, and systemic treatment with doxycycline, azithromycin, or similar medication as necessary.
- The goal is not to sterilize the eye but to reduce bacterial counts to a sufficiently low level so that the anterior chamber is exposed to no more than a small inoculum during insertion of instruments into the eye without development of infection.

II. GENERAL PRINCIPLES

- It is important that eyedrops are instilled in a way that does not dilute their concentration. A common mistake is to rapidly instill a whole series of eyedrops, including antibiotics, cycloplegics, adrenergic agents, and possibly nonsteroidal anti-inflammatory drugs (NSAIDs) immediately after one another. Such a technique may induce reflex

Henderson BA. *Essentials of Cataract Surgery, Second Edition (pp 25-30).* © 2014 Taylor & Francis Group.

tearing from irritation, or simply overfill the fornix so that the drops spill onto the eyelids. In either case, the efficacy is likely to be reduced.

- Patients should be instructed to gently close their eyelids (or apply punctual occlusion) for a minute or more or so after a single drop of each drug is instilled.

- Use of a pledget (eg, 1 cm × 2 mm cellulose sponge), soaked in the combination of drops and placed in the inferior fornix, may be more economical and efficient and provide better dilation than standard eyedrop instillation.[2]

III. ANTIBIOTICS

Endophthalmitis is a fortunately rare complication of cataract surgery and for that reason it is unlikely that a randomized controlled clinical trial will ever be done that definitively demonstrates efficacy of a particular prophylactic antibiotic regimen. However, several large studies have shown that povidone-iodine 5% is safe and effective in reducing the risk of endophthalmitis,[1,3] regardless of other antibiotics used.

- Most cases of postoperative endophthalmitis are due to gram-positive organisms, with increasing resistance among coagulase-negative staphylococci to ciprofloxacin.[4] The fourth-generation fluoroquinolones provide better gram-positive coverage than ciprofloxacin or ofloxacin. Surgeons may need to modify their prophylactic regimen depending on the patterns of resistance in their own population base.

- While povidone-iodine is a broad-spectrum antibiotic, it does have some holes in coverage, such as *Serratia*. Both moxifloxacin 0.5% and gatifloxacin 0.3% provide broad-spectrum coverage against gram-positive and gram-negative organisms. Both gatifloxacin and moxifloxacin are well tolerated by the eye.[5]

- A combination of povidone-iodine and a fourth-generation fluoroquinolone is therefore most commonly used for endophthalmitis prophylaxis. Povidone-iodine should be diluted from the stock 10% solution to 5% with balanced salt solution for the ocular surface because the higher concentration can cause significant corneal epitheliopathy due to its low pH. The periocular skin can be treated with either concentration.

- Paradoxically, lower concentrations of povidone-iodine (0.05% to 0.5%) are actually more bactericidal than the standard 5% solution because the dilution increases the release of the active free iodine; a much longer contact time is required for the 5% solution to achieve the same kill rate. However, the stock 5% solution is stable for a much longer period of time. The use of intraoperative irrigation with freshly diluted povidone-iodine 0.25% during cataract surgery has been shown to be highly effective at reducing anterior chamber bacterial contamination at the conclusion of surgery without ocular toxicity.[6]

- Never use povidone-iodine scrub around the eyes, as the surfactant is toxic to the corneal epithelium.

- Some investigators believe that a preoperative antibiotic regimen is best started 24 to 72 hours before surgery in order to achieve adequate drug levels in the eye.[7] Others feel that such an approach may be logistically difficult and feel it is sufficient to initiate antibiotic drops 1 to 2 hours before surgery (eg, 1 drop every 10 to 15 minutes for 4 doses),[8] especially if followed by povidone-iodine.

- Studies indicate that moxifloxacin 0.5% achieves higher intraocular levels than gatifloxacin 0.3%, whether started the day before surgery[9] or 1 hour before surgery[8]; however, there are no controlled clinical trials that indicate superior clinical efficacy of moxifloxacin. Both drugs are relatively expensive.

IV. DILATING DROPS

- Adequate dilation of the pupil prior to cataract surgery is critical in providing the surgeon a good red reflex, the opportunity to create an adequately sized capsulorrhexis, and safer phacoemulsification.

- While a number of different dilating drops can be used, a typical regimen consists of a moderately long-acting anticholinergic agent (eg, cyclopentolate 1% to 2%) and an adrenergic agonist (phenylephrine 2.5%).

- Preoperative atropine 1% combined with intraoperative epinephrine may reduce the risk of intraoperative floppy iris syndrome in patients taking tamsulosin.[10]

- It is best to avoid dilating the patient on the day before surgery if possible, as this can result in suboptimal dilation on the day of surgery ("pupil fatigue").[11]

- Phenylephrine 10% does not provide additional pupillary dilation compared with phenylephrine 2.5%[6] and should not be used because of the greater risk of cardiovascular side effects.

V. NONSTEROIDAL ANTI-INFLAMMATORY DRUGS

There are a number of different FDA-approved topical NSAIDs available for ophthalmic use. Most of these drugs are approved for the treatment of inflammation associated with cataract surgery (Table 3-1) but are also used off-label to help prevent intraoperative miosis,[12,13] and may also reduce postoperative cystoid macular edema (CME).

TABLE 3-1. TOPICAL NONSTEROIDAL ANTI-INFLAMMATORY DRUGS USED IN CATARACT SURGERY	
Drug	*FDA-Approved Indication*
Flurbiprofen 0.03%	Inhibition of intraoperative miosis
Ketorolac 0.5%	Treatment of inflammation associated with cataract surgery
Diclofenac 0.1%	Treatment of inflammation associated with cataract surgery
Nepafenac 0.1%	Treatment of inflammation associated with cataract surgery
Bromfenac 0.09%	Treatment of inflammation associated with cataract surgery

- If used for prevention of miosis, it is reasonable to begin instilling the NSAID drops several hours prior to surgery along with antibiotics and dilating agents.
- The routine use of NSAIDs to reduce intraoperative miosis may not be necessary in those cases in which epinephrine is added to the irrigating fluid,[14] but it may be more helpful in patients in whom mechanical dilation of the pupil intraoperatively (posterior synechiae, prior pilocarpine therapy) may be necessary.
- If the goal is to reduce CME, it is better to start using the NSAIDs several days preoperatively, especially in patients with uveitic cataracts.

VI. CORTICOSTEROIDS

Preoperative topical and oral corticosteroids are not indicated for routine cataract surgery. However, in patients with a history of uveitis or scleritis, some combination of these medications may be necessary.[15]

- Patients with uveitic cataracts should defer surgery for at least several months after the uveitis is quiet in order to minimize the chances of a postoperative flare. Some patients will require ongoing corticosteroid therapy or the addition of steroid-sparing immunomodulatory drugs to maintain control of the uveitis.
- One regimen for patients with a history of severe uveitis is as follows:
  - ¤ Begin prednisolone acetate 1% every 2 hours while awake beginning the week before surgery.
  - ¤ Begin oral prednisone 1 mg/kg (up to 60 mg) per day for the 2 days before surgery.
  - ¤ Intravenous Solu-Medrol (methylprednisolone) 62.5 to 500 mg is given at the time of surgery; be sure to clear this with the anesthesiologist prior to starting the operation, as there are potential risks of intravenous corticosteroids.

    ¤ The oral prednisone is then tapered off or down to the baseline suppressive dose over the first 2 to 6 weeks postoperatively, depending on the degree of inflammation.

VII. MISCELLANEOUS COMMENTS

- A common mistake for the beginning surgeon is to scrub the eyelashes and fornices of patients with blepharitis vigorously during the prep and drape phase of surgery in the hopes of eliminating the problem. Such an approach is actually more likely to increase the bacterial load. Instead, the lashes should be "painted" gently with povidone-iodine solution. One study found that thorough irrigation of the fornix with povidone-iodine was more effective in reducing bacterial counts than simply dripping the solution onto the eye.[16]

- After the prep is completed, the drapes are applied. The sterile drape should be applied so as to completely isolate the lashes of the upper and lower lids from the surgical field. The speculum should then be rotated slightly as necessary to provide unobstructed access of the phacoemulsification probe to the wound.

- In vascularized eyes undergoing scleral tunnel phacoemulsification or combined phacoemulsification/trabeculectomy, the use of preoperative apraclonidine 1% 30 minutes before surgery can help blanch conjunctiva and Tenon capsule.[17]

KEY POINTS

1. Proper selection and use of preoperative eyedrops reduces the chance of postoperative infection and provides a well-dilated pupil to enhance the surgeon's view during surgery.

2. Instill preoperative eyedrops at appropriate intervals to ensure maximal effectiveness.

3. The use of povidone-iodine solution is the only preoperative regimen proven to reduce the risk of endophthalmitis.

4. Fourth-generation fluoroquinolones provide better gram-positive coverage than third-generation fluoroquinolones and are therefore usually used in combination with povidone-iodine solution preoperatively, although their cost-effectiveness has yet to be proven.

5. Topical corticosteroids are not indicated preoperatively for routine cataract surgery, but may be necessary (along with oral corticosteroids) in patients with uveitic cataracts.

REFERENCES

1. Speaker MG, Menikoff JA. Prophylaxis of endophthalmitis with topical povidone-iodine. *Ophthalmology*. 1991;98:1769-1775.
2. Sengupta S, Subramoney K, Srinivasan R. Use of a mydriatic cocktail with a wick for preoperative mydriasis in cataract surgery: a prospective randomised controlled trial. *Eye (London)*. 2010;24:118-122.
3. Wu PC, Li M, Chang SJ, et al. Risk of endophthalmitis after cataract surgery using different protocols for povidone-iodine preoperative disinfection. *J Ocul Pharmacol Ther*. 2006;22:54-61.
4. Recchia FM, Busbee BG, Pearlman RB, et al. Changing trends in the microbiologic aspects of postcataract endophthalmitis. *Arch Ophthalmol*. 2005;123:341-346.
5. Herrygers LA, Noecker RJ, Lane LC, Levine JM. Comparison of corneal surface effects of gatifloxacin and moxifloxacin using intensive and prolonged dosing protocols. *Cornea*. 2005;24:66-71.
6. Shimada H, Arai S, Nakashizuka H, et al. Reduction of anterior chamber contamination rate after cataract surgery by intraoperative surface irrigation with 0.25% povidone-iodine. *Am J Ophthalmol*. 2011;151:11-17.
7. Ta CN, Egbert PR, Singh K, Shriver EM, Blumenkranz MS, Mino de Kaspar H. Prospective randomized comparison of 3-day versus 1-hour preoperative ofloxacin prophylaxis for cataract surgery. *Ophthalmology*. 2002;109:2036-2040; discussion 2040-2041.
8. Kim D, Stark WJ, O'Brien TP, Dick JD. Aqueous penetration and biologic activity of moxifloxacin 0.5% ophthalmic solution and gatifloxacin 0.3% solution in cataract surgery patients. *Ophthalmology*. 2005;112:1992-1996.
9. McCulley JP, Caudle D, Aronowicz JD, Shine WE. Fourth-generation fluoroquinolone penetration into the aqueous humor in humans. *Ophthalmology*. 2006;113:955-959.
10. Masket S, Belani S. Combined preoperative topical atropine sulfate 1% and intracameral nonpreserved epinephrine hydrochloride 1:4000 [corrected] for management of intraoperative floppy-iris syndrome. *J Cataract Refract Surg*. 2007;33:580-582.
11. Power WJ, Hope-Ross M, Mooney DJ. Preoperative pupil fatigue. *J Cataract Refract Surg*. 1992;18:306-309.
12. Ozturk F, Kurt E, Inan UU, Ilker SS. The efficacy of 2.5% phenylephrine and flurbiprofen combined in inducing and maintaining pupillary dilatation during cataract surgery. *Eur J Ophthalmol*. 2000;10:144-148.
13. Solomon KD, Turkalj JW, Whiteside SB, Stewart JA, Apple DJ. Topical 0.5% ketorolac vs 0.03% flurbiprofen for inhibition of miosis during cataract surgery. *Arch Ophthalmol*. 1997;115:1119-1122.
14. Shaikh MY, Mars JS, Heaven CJ. Prednisolone and flurbiprofen drops to maintain mydriasis during phacoemulsification cataract surgery. *J Cataract Refract Surg*. 2003;29:2372-2377.
15. Foster CS, Rashid S. Management of coincident cataract and uveitis. *Curr Opin Ophthalmol*. 2003;14:1-6.
16. Mino de Kaspar H, Chang RT, Singh K, et al. Prospective randomized comparison of 2 different methods of 5% povidone-iodine applications for anterior segment intraocular surgery. *Arch Ophthalmol*. 2005;123:161-165.
17. Sii F, Todd B, Shah P, Chiang M. Reduction of anterior-segment vascularity with preoperative topical apraclonidine 1%. *J Cataract Refract Surg*. 2006;32:692-693.

4

ANESTHESIA FOR CATARACT SURGERY

Artem Grush, MD, MBA and Joseph Bayes, MD

I. INTRODUCTION

There are several commonly used techniques for providing analgesia, sedation, and anesthesia for patients undergoing cataract surgery. Anesthetists and ophthalmologists caring for these patients should be familiar with the benefits, risks, and technical considerations of these techniques.

II. TOPICAL ANESTHESIA

Topical anesthesia involves placing a local anesthetic eyedrop(s) on the cornea and conjunctiva, thereby anesthetizing that area. Topical anesthesia is best suited for patients who are having brief procedures in or near the anterior chamber. Topical anesthesia may be used as the sole anesthetic for cataract surgery or to supplement another anesthetic technique (eg, an incomplete block or a block that has worn off).

A. Patient Requirements

Patients receiving topical anesthesia must be able to cooperate, communicate, and lie supine and motionless during surgery. Surgeons must be able to tolerate some eye movement, as topical anesthesia will not provide akinesia of the extraocular muscles (EOM).

B. Common Usage

Topical anesthesia is a widely used form of analgesia in the United States for cataract surgery.[1] Commonly used local anesthetics include lidocaine 2% jelly, proparacaine 0.5%, and tetracaine 0.75%.

Henderson BA. *Essentials of Cataract Surgery, Second Edition (pp 31-43)*.
© 2014 Taylor & Francis Group.

C. Sedation

To facilitate patient cooperation, it is wise to give sedatives only to patients who require them for anxiety and cannot be relaxed by verbal reassurance. For many anxious patients, holding their hand has a calming effect. It is important to remember that no amount of sedation, short of general anesthesia (GA), will compensate for inadequate analgesia. Therefore, it is necessary to ensure that the eye is anesthetized during the entire operation.

D. Sedative Requirements

If sedatives are required, they should be used in the smallest dose needed (eg, midazolam 0.5 to 1 mg intravenously). If sedatives (or regional blocks) are administered, pulse oximetry, blood pressure, and electrocardiogram monitors should be used by appropriately trained personnel. Supplementary oxygen and appropriately trained resuscitation personnel and equipment must be immediately available. If oxygen is administered, starting it at a concentration of 30% and increasing it to the lowest concentration clinically required will reduce the rare but serious risk of fire. If >30% oxygen is required, the surgeon should be warned not to use any heat source for at least 60 seconds after discontinuing oxygen to allow the high concentration of oxygen to dissipate.

E. Complications

Topical anesthesia has the lowest local complication rate of any anesthetic technique. Rarely serious systemic complications such as arrhythmias or pulmonary edema can occur. Eke and Thompson reported a 0.2% serious systemic complication rate of patients undergoing eye surgery with topical anesthesia.[2] Interestingly, this rate was similar to the serious systemic complication rate of most other anesthetic techniques in their review.

III. INTRACONAL BLOCK (RETROBULBAR BLOCK)

Intraconal block was first described over 125 years ago and has been the predominant technique of providing regional anesthesia to the globe during the 20th century.[3] The goal of the block is to deposit about 5 mL of local anesthetic in the anterior half of the muscle cone formed by the 4 recti muscles (the intraconal space). From this location, it spreads and anesthetizes the sensory and motor nerves to the eye. Patient requirements to undergo surgery with sedation and an intraconal block are similar to those of topical anesthesia.

A. Commonly Used Anesthetics

Commonly used local anesthetics include lidocaine 2%, bupivacaine 0.75%, and equal ratio mixtures of the two. Lidocaine can be myotoxic in concentrations greater than 2% and should not be used.[4] Epinephrine is not usually required to prolong the duration of lidocaine if bupivacaine and lidocaine are combined. For patients with vascular disease, epinephrine might increase the risk of inadequate blood flow to the eye.[5] Analgesia from intraconal block usually lasts 1 hour to several hours, depending on the local anesthetic(s) used.

B. Hyaluronidase

The bulk of evidence suggests hyaluronidase increases the speed of onset of ophthalmic blocks and reduces the chance of EOM injuries.[6-8] Several pharmaceutical companies now manufacture hyaluronidase that is approved for use by the US FDA. Although higher concentrations of hyaluronidase had been suggested in the past,[9] there is evidence that it is effective in concentrations as low as 0.75 unit/mL.[10]

C. Effects of Intraconal Block

Unlike topical anesthesia, an intraconal block is effective in anesthetizing the posterior chamber of the eye and causing akinesis of EOM. In experienced hands, intraconal block has a success rate of >90%.[11] Intraconal blocks may occasionally require supplementation with a Van Lint block (a peripheral facial nerve block) if blinking interferes with surgery.

D. Long Axial Lengths

Patients with long axial lengths (ALs) are at significantly higher risk of globe perforation if an intraconal block is performed.[12-14] Therefore, the AL (obtained from the preoperative ultrasound report) should be determined before attempting an intraconal block on cataract patients. If the AL is greater than 25 to 26 mm, other techniques (eg, topical, extraconal block, sub-Tenon block [STB], or GA) should be considered.

E. Staphylomas

Staphylomas are outpouches of a weakened sclera. They are usually located posteriorly and inferiorly on the globe. The presence of a staphyloma dramatically increases the risk of globe perforation from an intraconal block.[15,16] The incidence of staphylomas increases with AL. In one study, 15% of patients with AL of 27 mm had a staphyloma. The incidence increased to 60% of patients who had AL >31 mm.[16]

F. Preparation and Sedation

At our institution we administer a topical anesthetic, then swab a 10% povidone-iodine solution over the injection site. The solution is wiped off several minutes after application for optimal antibacterial effect. The patient is usually lightly sedated. Common adult dosages of medications administered are 0.5 to 1 mg of midazolam, followed by 30 mcg of remifentanil. Patients who are <60 years of age will usually receive larger doses (up to 2 mg of

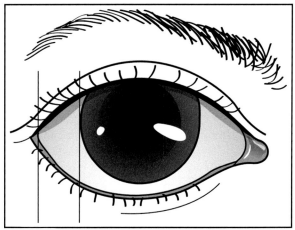

Figure 4-1. Needles inserted deep in the orbit may perforate the optic nerve and other structures tightly packed near the orbital apex. (Reprinted from ClipArt ETC, an online service of the Florida Center for Instructional Technology.)

midazolam and 60 mcg of remifentanil). Patients older than 80 years of age usually receive only remifentanil 0.5 to 1 mcg/mL. We think remifentanil has advantages over other narcotics because of its intense but brief effect, and the fact that patients given the drug can usually cooperate during the block. Our pharmacy will dilute a 1-mg vial of remifentanil to make about 33 syringes, each containing 30 mcg of the drug (10 mcg/mL).

G. Technique Continued and Complications

We request patients to look straight ahead during the block (primary gaze position). Looking up and in (Atkinson position) brings the optic nerve closer to the midline and increases the risk of injury from the needle tip.[17] We promote the use of needles 1 inch (25 mm) or less instead of traditionally used long needles. Using needles ≤1.25 inches seems to reduce the risk of several complications including central nervous system spread of local anesthesia,[18] injury to the optic nerve,[19] injury to the superior rectus muscle,[20] and retrobulbar hemorrhage[2] (Figure 4-1). The success rate of intraconal blocks seems to be similar whether inserting needles 1 inch, or 1.5 inches, from the inferiolateral orbit to the intraconal space.[11]

H. Insertion Point of Needle

A palpating finger identifies the lower part of the globe, the inferior orbital rim, and pushes the globe slightly up. The needle is inserted, bevel toward the globe, 0.25 to 0.5 inch below the lateral canthus, and just above the inferior orbital rim. There is evidence the insertion at this "modified" insertion point,

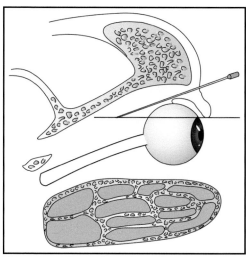

Figure 4-2. The traditional needle insertion point is at the junction of medial and lateral third of the inferior orbital rim of the right eye. By inserting the needle at the modified insertion point, 0.25- to 0.5-inch inferior to the lateral canthus and just above the inferior orbital rim, the risk of injuring the inferior rectus and inferior oblique muscles may be reduced. (Reprinted from ClipArt ETC, an online service of the Florida Center for Instructional Technology.)

instead of the "traditional" insertion point at the junction of the middle and lateral third of the orbital rim, reduces the risk of injury to the inferior rectus, and possibly the inferior oblique muscle[4] (Figure 4-2).

I. Direction of Needle Approach

The needle is initially directed perpendicular to all planes of the skin. In order to minimize the chance of entering the globe one of the authors (AG) attempts to visualize the lower rim of the eyeball by displacing the lower lid caudally. Simultaneous retraction of the upper eyelid by an experienced assistant helps to achieve better exposure of the field.

To reduce the chance of inadvertently perforating the globe, one of the authors (JB) wiggles the needle when the needle is through the skin, parallel to the globe at a frequency of about 3 times per second, to help identify if the sclera is inadvertently encountered. (If so, the globe would be expected to move at the same frequency as the wiggling motion.) If this occurs, the needle is withdrawn and redirected slightly more inferiorly.

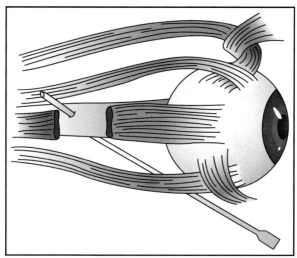

Figure 4-3. The 7/8- to 1-inch needle is advanced under the most inferior aspect of the globe (the inferior equator) with the tip of the needle directed to lie, when fully inserted, in the plane projecting posterior from the lateral limbus (the junction of the colored part of the lateral iris and the white of the sclera). (Reprinted with permission of Dr. Gary Fanning.)

The needle is advanced under the most inferior aspect of the globe (the inferior equator). One author (JB) directs the tip of the needle directed to lie, when fully inserted, in the plane projecting posterior from the lateral limbus (the junction of the colored part of the lateral iris and the white of the sclera; Figure 4-3). The other author (AG) directs the needle tip, when fully inserted, to be in a plane projected backward from the center of the iris. There may be slight resistance as the needle pierces the skin and a slight "pop" after penetration through the orbital septum several millimeters below the skin (Figure 4-4).

J. Reducing Risk of Complications

To reduce the chance of the needle injuring the optic nerve, the tip should not cross the midline. When the tip of the needle is thought to be in the intraconal space, aspirate for signs of blood. If blood is identified, withdraw the needle, apply intermittent digital pressure and reevaluate the orbit before attempting to proceed. Injection into the globe of <2 mL of local anesthesia will cause the globe to rupture, a devastating injury.[21]

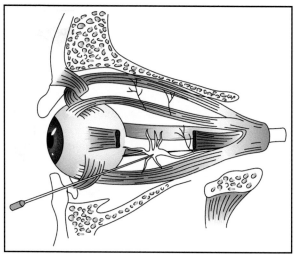

Figure 4-4. An injection of local anesthesia with a 7/8- to 1.25-inch (22 to 32 mm) needle from the inferior orbital rim is sufficient to carry the anesthetic solution to the ciliary ganglion and motor nerves. Figure showing a 1¼-inch needle injecting local anesthetic into the intraconal space. (Reprinted from Yale University Center for Advanced Instructional Media Medical Illustrations by Patrick Lynch, medical illustrator; C. Carl Jaffe, MD, cardiologist. Generated for multimedia teaching projects by the Yale University School of Medicine, Center for Advanced Instructional Media, 1987 to 2000. http://patricklynch.net, Creative Commons Attribution 2.5 License 2006; no usage restrictions.)

K. Intraconal Block With Shorter Needles

It is of note that many anesthetists perform orbital blocks using a 7/8-inch or 1-inch "peribulbar" needle, an inferior-lateral insertion point and aim for the intraconal space. Despite the "peribulbar" needle name, we should be aware that with this technique the tip of the needle is likely to be in the anterior intraconal space.

IV. EXTRACONAL BLOCK (SOMETIMES CALLED PERIBULBAR BLOCK)

Several decades ago, when anesthesiologists began performing eye blocks more commonly, a technique was reported for placing local anesthetic purposely outside the EOM cone.[22] Proponents of extraconal block suggest that it would be safer to routinely keep the tip of the needle further from the globe and intraconal components. These blocks were called "peribulbar" blocks, although extraconal is perhaps a more accurate term.

A. Additional Indications for Extraconal Block

Extraconal blocks may be safer in situations in which intraconal blocks are contraindicated (eg, AL > 25 to 26 mm). Extraconal blocks should also be considered for patients with a scleral buckle or severe enophthalmos. Initially, 2 needles were placed in the extraconal space, one in the inferior lateral orbit, and the other in the superior orbit. Over time evidence has shown that one injection may be as effective as two.[23-25] In addition, a second injection in the superior orbit may increase the risk of globe perforation[21] due to the proximity of the globe to the superior orbital wall.

B. Single Injection and Supplementary Technique

Most practitioners now routinely use only a single inferior lateral extraconal injection. If an additional medial or superior block is required, many practitioners now use a "median orbital block," a technique for administering local anesthetic in the avascular space medial to the globe. Readers are referred to the original article for those interested in learning this technique.[26]

C. Success Rate

Although the reported success rates of 83% to 84% with extraconal block[23,27] are not quite as high as with retrobulbar technique, it is adequate to warrant use of an extraconal block when a retrobulbar block is contraindicated. Some practitioners use extraconal blocks as their primary block.

D. Local Anesthetic Requirements

The inferior lateral extraconal block requires a larger volume of local anesthetic (5 to 8 mL are commonly used), and takes slightly longer to be effective. These blocks are usually effective because there are no discrete septal barriers defining the intraconal space.[28] Local anesthetic placed near the intraconal space can diffuse into the intraconal space and anesthetize the sensory and motors nerves within the intraconal space.

E. Technique

The technique of extraconal block is similar to an intraconal block (see Intraconal Blocks Sections III F and G mentioned previously). Again the authors recommend a needle ≤1 inch in length with the bevel of the needle facing the globe. The insertion site is 0.25 to 0.5 inch below the lateral canthus just above the inferior orbital rim. The needle is directed below the inferior-lateral aspect of the globe and parallel to the floor of the orbit. Once through the skin, the needle is directed posteriorly, parallel to the intraconal space, without entering it. There will be some resistance as the needle pierces the skin and sometime a small "pop" is felt as the needle penetrates the orbital fascia a few millimeters posterior to skin. Care is taken to avoid the lateral and inferior wall of the globe as the needle is advanced. Further, 6 to 8 mL of local anesthetic are injected outside but in close proximity to the EOM cone.

V. SUPPLEMENTARY TECHNIQUES

If patients experience eye pain in the operating room despite a preoperative attempt(s) to obtain adequate analgesia or receive supplemental topical anesthesia, the surgeon can place a small amount of local anesthetic in the subconjunctival or anterior sub-Tenon space (STB). A fine gauge needle (eg, 30-gauge needle) is used. Care must be taken not to perforate the globe if this technique is used.

VI. SUB-TENON BLOCK

Turnbull introduced the concept of STB block in 1884.[29] Classic articles about its preoperative use appeared in the early 1990s.[30-32] Its use has increased rapidly in the United Kingdom and several other countries. It has been promoted by its practitioners, largely because they believe that STB reduces the risk of serious injury to the eye.

A. Complications

Minor complications, such as chemosis and subconjuntival hemorrhage, occur more frequently than with needle blocks.[33] However, as the popularity of this technique has increased, occasional case reports have appeared describing many of the same serious injuries that occur with needle techniques.[34-37]

B. Technique

The technique involves administering local anesthetic eye drops, followed by 5% povidone-iodine eyedrops. The conjuntiva is picked up with toothless forceps, usually in the inferior-medial quadrant 3 to 5 mm from the limbus. At this point, the conjunctiva and sub-Tenon capsule are fused. Using blunt scissors, a 1- to 2-mm incision is made in the conjunctiva. A curved blunt cannula (eg, a 1-inch Steven cannula) is inserted through the incision, and advanced posteriorly between the sclera and sub-Tenon capsule. Then, 3 to 5 mL of local anesthesia is injected into sub-Tenon space. Analgesia and akinesia of the EOM occur within minutes after the injection.

C. Contraindications

Absolute contraindications include infection and prior scleral buckle. (Scleral buckle prevents the posterior spread of local anesthetic.) Relative contraindications include coagulopathy, prior retinal surgery (can cause scarring and ineffective block), and glaucoma surgery (STB can interfere with the lifting of a flap required for some glaucoma operations).

VII. SPECIAL CONSIDERATIONS REGARDING ANTITHROMBOTICS

The concern that patients taking antithrombotics before surgery *might* be at higher risk or perioperative bleeding must be balanced against the risk of stopping these drugs and increasing the risk of a life-threatening clotting complication (eg, stroke, myocardial infarction, pulmonary embolism or deep vein thrombosis). There have been several recent articles addressing this issue for patients having cataract surgery.

After reviewing multiple studies on this issue, the most widely quoted review on the perioperative use of antithrombotics by Douketis et al in 2008 recommends continuing aspirin and warfarin (Coumadin) in therapeutic doses before cataract surgery.[38] At that time, the authors recommended continuing clopidogrel (Plavix) for patients who were at high risk of stopping it but also commented that there were few studies looking at the risks of continuing clopidogrel before cataract surgery.

However, a large retrospective study published in 2009[39] of patients taking aspirin, warfarin (Coumadin), and clopidogrel (Plavix) up to the time of cataract surgery found that although patients taking warfarin and clopidogrel had a slightly higher incidence of minor bleeding issues (eg, lid hematomas, subconjunctival bleeding), patients taking any of these 3 drugs did not have a higher incidence of sight-threatening bleeding complications (eg, retrobulbar or intraocular hemorrhage) from eye blocks or cataract surgery.

Patients taking aspirin and clopidogrel for the most common type of cardiac stent insertion (drug eluting stents) are at significantly increased risk of life-threatening stent clotting complications if these drugs are stopped before 12 months of therapy.[40] For these patients, these drugs should routinely be continued up to the time of cataract surgery.

VIII. GENERAL ANESTHESIA

A small percentage of patients undergoing cataract surgery will not be able to have their operation performed with topical anesthesia or a block. For these patients, GA should be considered.

A. Indications

Not all patients are candidates for regional anesthesia. Children for example would be expected to require GA for cataract surgery to remain motionless. On occasion, GA is necessary for adult patients who are unable to remain motionless because of pre-existing medical conditions (eg, severe Parkinson's disease, dementia, or claustrophobia) or cannot lie supine because of musculoskeletal, pulmonary, or cardiac disease. For patients with significant medical problems, it would be wise for the ophthalmologist to consult with the anesthesia personnel who will be caring for the patient, in advance of surgery, to determine if the benefits of proceeding with surgery outweigh the potential side effects and risks of GA.

B. Benefits and Risks

The advantages of GA include assurance that patients do not experience any pain and will be immobile. However, there are many disadvantages that include a much higher rate of postoperative nausea, vomiting, drowsiness, confusion, cough, cardiac and respiratory complications, and sore throat. In addition, rare but more serious complications related to GA can occur.

KEY POINTS

1. Anesthetists and ophthalmologists must be knowledgeable about a variety of techniques, and tailor the anesthetic to the needs of the patient and surgeon. New techniques are best learned under supervision of individuals with extensive experience with regional ophthalmic anesthesia.

2. Always determine the AL of the globe before performing a needle block. If the AL is >25 to 26 mm, or a scleral buckle or enophthalmos is present, other techniques (eg, topical, extraconal block, STB, or GA) should be considered.

3. Use of needles of 1 inch or less reduces the risks of local and systemic complications.

4. Use the "modified" inferior, far lateral insertion point for intraconal and extraconal needle blocks to reduce the risk of EOM injury.

5. All anesthetic techniques have a risk of serious local and/or systemic complications. Anesthetists and ophthalmologists need to be prepared to manage these uncommon but serious complications.

ref-0-.

REFERENCES

1. Leaming DV. Practice styles and preferences of ARCRS members: 2003 survey. *J Cataract Refract Surg.* 2004;30:892-900.
2. Eke T, Thompson JR. The national survey of local anesthesia for ocular surgery II. Safety profiles of local anaesthesia techniques. *Eye.* 1999;13:196-204.
3. Knapp H. On cocaine and its use in ophthalmic and general surgery. *Arch Ophthalmol.* 1884;13:402-448.
4. Hamilton RC. A discourse on the complications of retrobulbar and peribulbar blockade. *Can J Ophthalmol.* 2000;35:363-372.
5. Troll GF. Regional ophthalmic anesthesia: safe technique and avoidance of complications. *J Clin Anesth.* 1995;7:163-172.
6. Strouthidis NG, Sobha S, Lanigan LP, et al. Vertical diplopia following peribulbar anesthesia: The role of hyaluronidase. *J Pediatr Ophthalmol Strabismus.* 2004;41(1):25-30.
7. Jehan FS, Hagan III JC, Whittaker TJ, et al. Diplopia and ptosis following injection of local anesthesia without hyaluronidase. *J Cataract Refract Surg.* 2001;27(11):1876-1879.
8. Brown SM, Brooks SE, Mazow ML, et al. Cluster of diplopia cases after periocular anesthesia without hyaluronidase. *J Cataract Refract Surg.* 1999;25:1245-1249.
9. Wong DHW. Regional anaesthesia for intraocular surgery. *Can J Anaesth.* 1993;40(7):635-657.
10. Debroff BM, Hamilton RC, Loken RG, et al. Retrobulbar anesthesia with 7.5 unit vs. 0.75 units/mL of hyaluronidase. *Can J Ophthalmol.* 1995;30(5):262-264.
11. Hamilton RC, Gimbel HV, Strunin L. Regional anesthesia for 12,000 cataract extraction and intraocular lens implantation procedures. *Can J Anaesth.* 1988;35(6):615-623.
12. Duker JS, Belmont JB, Benson WE, et al. Inadvertent globe perforation during retrobulbar and peribulbar anesthesia. *Ophthalmology.* 1991;98(4):519-526.
13. Berglin L, Stenkula S, Algvere PV. Ocular perforation during retrobulbar and peribulbar injections. *Ophthalmic Surg Lasers.* 1995;26:429-434.
14. McCombe M, Heriot W. Penetrating ocular injury following local anesthesia. *Aust N Z J Ophthalmol.* 1995;23(1):33-36.
15. Edge R, Navon S. Scleral perforation during retrobulbar and peribulbar anesthesia: Risk factors and outcomes in 50,000 consecutive injections. *J Cataract Refract Surg.* 1999;25:1237-1244.
16. Vohra SB, Good PA. Altered globe dimensions of axial myopia as risk factors for penetrating ocular injury during peribulbar anaesthesia. *Br J Anaesth.* 2000;85(2):242-245.
17. Pautler SE, Grizzard WS, Thompson LN, Wing GL. Blindness from retrobulbar injection into the optic nerve. *Ophthalmic Surg.* 1986;17(6):334-337.
18. Nicoll JM, Acharya PA, Ahlen K, et al. Central nervous system complications after 6,000 retrobulbar blocks. *Anesth Analg.* 1987;66:1298-1302.
19. Katsev DA, Drews RC, Rose BT. An anatomical study of retrobulbar needle path length. *Ophthalmology.* 1989;96(8):1221-1224.
20. Hamilton RC. Retrobulbar block revisited and revised. *J Cataract Refract Surg.* 1996;22:1147-1150.
21. Bullock JD, Warwar RE, Green WR. Ocular explosion from periocular anesthetic injections. *Ophthalmolgy.* 1999;106:2341-2353.
22. Davis II DB, Mandel MR. Posterior peribulbar anesthesia: an alternative to retrobulbar anesthesia. *J Cataract Refract Surg.* 1986;12:182-184.
23. Demirok A, Simsek S, Cinal A, et al. Peribulbar anesthesia: one versus two injections. *Ophthalmic Surg Lasers.* 1997;28:998-1001.
24. Saini IS, Roysarker K, Grawal SPS, et al. Efficacy and time sequence analysis of modified single injection peribulbar anesthesia. *J Cataract Refract Surg.* 1993;19:646-650.
25. Agrawal V, Athanikar AS. Single injection, low volume periocular anesthesia in 1000 cases. *J Cataract Refract Surg.* 1994;20:61-63.

26. Hustead RF, Hamilton RC, Loken RG. Periocular local anesthesia: median orbital as an alternative to superior nasal injection. *J Cataract Refract Surg.* 1994;20:197-201.
27. Budd J, Hardwick M, Barber K et al. A single-centre study *of 1000 consecutive* peribulbar blocks. *Eye.* 2001;15:464-468.
28. Koornneef I. Orbital septa: anatomy and function. *Ophthalmology.* 1979;86:876-880.
29. Turnbull CS. *Med Surg Rep.* 1884;29:628.
30. Hansen EA, Mein CE, Mazzoli R. Ocular anesthesia for cataract surgery: a direct sub-Tenon's approach. *Ophthalmic Surg.* 1990;21(10):696-699.
31. Friedberg MA, Spellman FA, Pilkerton R, et al. An alternative technique of local anesthesia for vitreoretinal surgery. *Arch Ophthalmol.* 1991;109:1615.
32. Stevens JD. A new local anaesthesia technique for cataract extraction by one quadrant sub-Tenon's infiltration. *Br J Ophthalmol.* 1992;76:670-674.
33. Kumar CM. How to do a sub-Tenon's block. CPD *Anaesthesia.* 2001;3(2):56-61.
34. Ruschen H, Bremner FD, Carr C. Complications after sub-Tenon's eye block. *Anesth Analg.* 2003;96:273-277.
35. Olitsky SE, Juneja RG. Orbital hemorrhage after the administration of sub-Tenon's infusion anesthesia. *Ophthalmic Surg Lasers.* 1997;28(2):145-146.
36. Jaycock PD, Mather CM, Ferris JD, Kirkpatrick JN. Rectus muscle trauma complicating sub-Tenon's local anaesthesia. *Eye.* 2001;15:583-586.
37. Spierer A, Schwalb E. Superior oblique muscle paresis after sub-Tenon's anesthesia for cataract surgery. *J Cataract Refract Surg.* 1999;25:144-145.
38. Douketis JD, Berger PB, Dunn AS, et al. The perioperative management of antithrombotic therapy, American College of Chest Physicians Evidence-Based Clinical Practice Guidelines (8th edition). *Chest.* 2008;133:299-339S.
39. Benzimra JD, Johnston RL, Jaycock P, et al. The cataract national dataset electronic multicenter audit of 55567 operations: antiplatelet and anticoagulant medications. *Eye.* 2009;23:10-16.
40. American Society of Anesthesiologists Committee on Standards and Practice Parameters. Practice alert for the perioperative management of patients with coronary artery stents. *Anesthesiology.* 2009;110:22-23.

5

INTRACAMERAL ANESTHESIA
CONSIDERATIONS ON EFFECTIVENESS, TOXICITIES, AND COMPLICATIONS

Michael E. Sulewski, MD and
Tamiesha A. Frempong, MD, MPH

I. INTRODUCTION

Intracameral anesthesia, an anesthetic modality involving the injection of a small volume of an amide anesthetic into the anterior chamber, is among the newest modalities in ocular surgery. It was introduced as an adjunct to topical anesthesia as a possible method for providing additional anesthetic effect by blocking the sensory nerves in the iris and ciliary body. In this way, intracameral anesthesia would reduce discomfort during iris and lens manipulation and intraocular lens (IOL) implantation in cataract surgery.[1-3]

II. EFFECTIVENESS OF INTRACAMERAL ANESTHESIA

Several studies have shown significantly decreased pain and improved comfort with the addition of intracameral anesthesia to topical anesthetics. However, many reports have also demonstrated minimal pain with or without intracameral anesthesia and therefore marginal pain control benefit with this modality as an adjunct to topical anesthesia.[2-6]

A. Preparing the Patient

To maximize patient comfort, careful and detailed preoperative counseling should be given to patients regarding what to expect during cataract surgery while under topical anesthesia with or without an intracameral agent. Being informed that they may be aware of tissue manipulation or the microscope

Henderson BA. *Essentials of Cataract Surgery, Second Edition (pp 45-49).*
© 2014 Taylor & Francis Group.

light may help mitigate intraoperative anxiety experienced by patients. Patients may mistakenly interpret these experiences or sensations as pain.

B. Anesthesia in Routine and Complex Cases

It has been the authors' experience that in over 90% of the cases, topical lidocaine 2% jelly given within 10 minutes prior to the surgery is all that is necessary in routine cases. Adjunctive sub-Tenon, intracameral, or even perior retrobulbar anesthesia may be necessary if there are more complexities in the case such as a small pupil requiring stretching maneuvers, combined glaucoma procedures, dense nuclei, Flomax (Boehringer Ingelheim Pharmaceuticals, Inc) cases, or other such issues.

III. INTRACAMERAL ANESTHETIC AGENTS

A. Volume and Method of Administration

There is no standard regarding the volume of intracameral anesthesia; however, the use of between 0.1 and 0.5 mL is reported in the literature without event.[5,6] The anesthetic agent should be directed near the iris or through the pupil and under the iris to allow for diffusion around the iris tissue and ciliary body. No study has evaluated the optimal point in the procedure to administer the intracameral anesthetic. Generally, most surgeons inject the anesthetic agent through the paracentesis prior to the start of the capsulorrhexis and before the viscoelastic agent is injected. Others may inject prior to the phaco portion of the procedure or in response to the patient having discomfort with topical anesthesia alone at any point in the procedure.

B. Concentration and Corneal Toxicity

Preservative-free (PF) lidocaine 2% or more concentrated dosages are associated with corneal endothelial changes.[2,7] Therefore, PF lidocaine 1% is likely the safest choice for an intracameral anesthetic agent. Bupivacaine 0.5% diluted with 1:1 glutathione bicarbonate has no associated corneal changes compared to the corneal swelling associated with bupivacaine 0.5% alone.[2] Tetracaine hydrochloride 0.5% has been demonstrated to be without corneal toxicity; however, bupivacaine 0.75% and proparacaine hydrochloride 0.5% cause corneal thickening and opacification.[2,8]

C. Retinal Toxicity

Regarding retinal toxicity, published research has demonstrated that there was no diffusion to the posterior segment by intracameral anesthetic agents.[9]

In addition, using electroretinogram (ERG) measurements, numerous reports found no significant reduction in ERG amplitudes after use of intracameral lidocaine 1%.[10] No systemic concentration of lidocaine has been detected with intracameral use of an amide anesthetic, and cardiac and respiratory functions remain stable throughout the surgical procedure.[11] However, long-term sequelae have not been studied and so remain unknown.

IV. OPTIMAL CONDITIONS AND INTRACAMERAL ANESTHESIA

A. Operative Time

Cases should be completed in 30 minutes or less and thus, early resident surgery may require retrobulbar, peribulbar, or sub-Tenon anesthesia until surgical skill and operative times are reduced. It may take 30 or more cases for residents to become skilled and efficient enough to finish cases from start to finish in less than 30 minutes. I believe topical and intracameral anesthesia cases should only be reserved for surgeons who have proven that they are far along the learning curve and are beyond the stage of stumbling over various stages of the case.

B. Relative Contraindications

Topical anesthesia is also not ideal when there is an anticipated need to enlarge the incision. Examples of these situations include potential conversion of a phaco case to an extracapsular cataract extraction with a dense brunescent cataract, in complex cases such as small pupil cases, traumatic cataracts, or those surgeries involving a combined cataract and glaucoma procedure. Thus, this underscores the gradual transition from more invasive anesthesia to topical with or without intracameral anesthesia in accordance with the resident surgeon's progression.

C. Transitioning to Intracameral Anesthesia

The posterior capsular tear incidence should be under 10% before a resident surgeon should consider converting to topical/intracameral anesthesia. There is no urgency to transition to topical anesthesia until the surgeon is entirely comfortable with his or her technique and able to operate efficiently and safely. It is much more difficult to manage a capsular tear issue under topical anesthesia. The goal of anesthesia is to enable the cataract surgery to be performed safely and successfully, while providing comfort to the patient in a relatively stress-free environment for the surgeon. Sometimes the authors find that the residents forget that there is a patient under the drape and that their experience, comfort, and ultimate result are the most important aspects of the surgery. The transition to topical/intracameral anesthetic cases will come with time and may arrive sooner for some than others.

V. CONCLUSION

Modern cataract surgery involving self-sealing sutureless incisions, femtosecond lasers, advanced phacoemulsification technology, and premium IOLs has pushed the degree of anesthesia needed for this now rapid, minimally invasive procedure to even further heights. In fact, it has made topical and/or intracameral anesthesia for cataract surgery the standard of care in most places once beyond the early stages of the learning curve.[1] Conclusions about the effectiveness of intracameral anesthesia as an adjunct to a topical agent are mixed. This combination is likely to be most beneficial to the 10% of the population undergoing phacoemulsification that have pain during the course of surgery.[12] Perhaps the "as needed" approach is the most prudent and resource-sensitive approach at this time. Overall, conservative use of these agents regarding their concentrations and the volume administered is advised.

It seems the short-term safety of intracameral anesthesia, particularly a small volume (0.1 to 0.5 mL) of PF lidocaine 1% with regard to the lack of corneal, retinal, and systemic toxicity, has been established.

Deciding whether or not intracameral anesthesia would be appropriate to use in cataract surgery depends on the surgeon's level of comfort and experience. Some objective benchmarks to consider are a surgeon's posterior capsular tear rate to be less than 10% for residents in training, and less than 5% for more experienced surgeons, and a surgical time of less than 20 to 30 minutes. In addition, the patient's ability to cooperate and communicate pain or problems to the surgeon, the anticipated possibility of increased complexities or complications, the axial length, the anticoagulation status, the use of alpha blockers, dense lenses, pseudoexfoliation, and traumatic cataracts are factors to consider in deciding the appropriateness of a certain anesthetic modality in cataract surgery.[13]

Anesthesia in cataract surgery can optimize the potential for success by minimizing patient discomfort and the surgeon's stress. Adjunctive intracameral anesthesia can be useful when used appropriately.

KEY POINTS

1. Conclusions about the effectiveness of intracameral anesthesia in cataract surgery have been mixed.
2. PF lidocaine 1% 0.1 to 0.5 mL is the anesthetic type and volume most frequently used intracamerally in cataract surgery.
3. There are no significant short-term or systemic toxicities from minimally concentrated, low-volume intracameral anesthesia.
4. The success of topical and intracameral anesthesia is related to the surgical duration, which is dependent on the surgeon's experience, skill, and comfort.
5. The posterior capsular tear incidence should be under 10% before a resident surgeon should consider converting to topical anesthesia.

REFERENCES

1. Crandall AS. Anesthesia modalities for cataract surgery. *Curr Opin Ophthalmol.* 2001;12(1):9-11.
2. Karp CL, Cox TA, Wagoner MD, Ariyasu RG, Jacobs DS. Intracameral anesthesia: a report by the American Academy of Ophthalmology. *Ophthalmology.* 2001;108(9):1704-1710.
3. Gills JP, Cherchio M, Raanan MG. Unpreserved lidocaine to control discomfort during cataract surgery using topical anesthesia. *J Cataract Refract Surg.* 1997;23:545-550.
4. Carino NS, Slomovic AR, Chung F, Marcovich AL. Topical tetracaine versus topical tetracaine plus intracameral lidocaine for cataract surgery. *J Cataract Refract Surg.* 1998;24:1602-1608.
5. Masket S, Gokmen F. Efficacy and safety of intracameral lidocaine as a supplement to topical anesthesia. *J Cataract Refract Surg.* 1998;24(7):956-960.
6. Boulton JE, Lopatazidis A, Luck J, Baer RM. A randomized control trial of intracameral lidocaine during phacoemulsification under topical anesthesia. *Ophthalmology.* 2000;107(1):68-71.
7. Eggeling P, Pleyer U, Hartmann C, Rieck PW. Corneal endothelial toxicity of different lidocaine concentrations. *J Cataract Refract Surg.* 2000;26:1403-1408.
8. Judge AJ, Najafi K, Lee DA, Miller KM. Corneal endothelial toxicity of topical anesthesia. *Ophthalmology.* 1997;104:1373-1379.
9. Rigal-Sastourne JC, Huart B, Pariselle G, et al. Diffusion of lidocaine after intracameral injection. *J Fr Ophtalmol.* 1999;22(1):21-24.
10. Pang MP, Fujimoto DK, Wilkens LR. Pain, photophobia, and retinal and optic nerve function after phacoemulsification with intracameral lidocaine. *Ophthalmology.* 2001;108(11):2018-2025.
11. Wibrelauer C, Iven H, Bastian C, Laqua H. Systemic levels of lidocaine after intracameral injection during cataract surgery. *J Cataract Refract Surg.* 1999;25(5):648-651.
12. Malecaze FA, Deneuville SF, Julia BJ, et al. Pain relief with intracameral mepivacaine during phacoemulsification. *Br J Ophthalmol.* 2000;84(2):171-174.
13. Pandey SK, Werner L, Apple DJ, Agarwal A, Agarwal A, Agarwal S. No-anesthesia clear corneal phacoemulsification versus topical and topical plus intracameral anesthesia. *J Cataract Refract Surg.* 2001;27:1643-1650.

6

INCISION CONSTRUCTION

Scott M. McClintic, MD; Brett Shapiro, MD;
Diamond Y. Tam, MD; and Ayman Naseri, MD

I. INTRODUCTION

Beginning surgeons should learn the essential aspects of wound construction in cataract surgery, including wound type, location, and architecture. This chapter focuses on the 2 types of wounds commonly used in cataract surgery today: the scleral tunnel and clear corneal incisions. We will also discuss the significance of wound location and wound architecture for modern phacoemulsification.

II. WOUND TYPE

The 2 principal types of wounds in cataract surgery are the scleral tunnel and the clear corneal incisions. In the last decade, the clear cornea incision has eclipsed the scleral tunnel as the preferred wound type for most surgeons, with reported use of clear cornea incisions rising from 1.5% in 1992 to 87.1% in 2010.[1,2] Nonetheless, the scleral tunnel incision is a versatile wound that may be particularly useful during the early stages of learning phacoemulsification.

A. Scleral Tunnel Incision

1. Technique

Although a scleral tunnel wound can be fashioned under topical anesthesia alone,[3] a retrobulbar block provides akinesia and improved analgesia[3-7] for facilitation of conjunctival and scleral dissection (Figure 6-1). There are several steps in scleral tunnel wound construction, including conjunctival

Henderson BA. *Essentials of Cataract Surgery, Second Edition (pp 51-67).*
© 2014 Taylor & Francis Group.

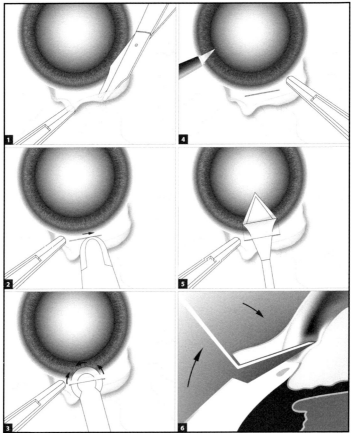

Figure 6-1. The scleral tunnel wound. (1) A conjunctival peritomy is performed using toothed grasping forceps and Westcott scissors. (2) A blade angled perpendicular to the scleral surface is used to create an approximately half-thickness groove. (3) A pocket or crescent blade is placed into the base of the scleral groove and advanced into the clear cornea with circular motions. (4) A paracentesis port is created with a superblade approximately 2 clock hours away from the scleral tunnel. (5) A keratome is used to "dimple down" into the cornea and enter the anterior chamber. (6) A cross-sectional view of the "dimple down" maneuver performed by the keratome.

peritomy, scleral groove, tunnel creation, formation of a paracentesis port, injection of viscoelastic, and keratome entry into the anterior chamber.

a. Step 1

Once the eye is anesthetized, the first step is the conjunctival peritomy. Although the wound can theoretically be placed anywhere, many surgeons choose the superotemporal sclera. The conjunctival incision should be slightly longer than the planned scleral tunnel length, with or without a radial conjunctival cut to facilitate adequate exposure. The incision is followed by blunt dissection through Tenon fascia, using electrocautery for hemostasis as necessary.

b. Step 2

The scleral groove incision site is marked 1 to 2 mm posterior to the limbus. After fixating the globe with toothed grasping forceps, a blade (commonly a #69 beaver blade) angled perpendicular to the scleral surface is used to create an approximately half-thickness scleral groove.

c. Step 3

The scleral tunnel is then extended anteriorly with a pocket or crescent blade. First, the blade is placed into the groove with the heel of the blade off of the sclera to ensure the plane of the tunnel is at the full depth of the groove. Once adequately within the groove, the heel of the blade is lowered to be flush with the scleral surface, and the blade is advanced with circular motions tunneling toward the cornea, stopping once the tip has reached the limbus. As the curvature of the globe changes at the cornea, the tip of the blade is then angled upward slightly in order to avoid an overly thin posterior corneal lip or premature entry into the anterior chamber.

d. Step 4

A limbal paracentesis port is then created approximately 2 to 3 clock hours from the planned location of the scleral tunnel. Viscoelastic is subsequently injected through the paracentesis to fill the anterior chamber.

e. Step 5

While globe fixation is maintained with grasping forceps, the keratome is gently placed into the scleral tunnel. Small side-to-side movements of the keratome are used to ensure that the blade remains within the plane of the tunnel, avoiding creation of a secondary scleral plane. When the keratome tip is visible in clear cornea at the most anterior aspect of the tunnel, the heel of the blade is then elevated off the sclera, directing the keratome toward the iris opposite the wound. This downward pressure at the tip of the keratome creates small, visible folds in the cornea, described by the term *dimple-down*. The keratome is then advanced into the anterior chamber such that the shoulders of the blade pass through the internal aspect of the wound, thus ensuring adequate internal wound width.

2. Advantages

There are advantages to scleral tunnel wounds over clear corneal incisions.

- A scleral tunnel incision can be safely enlarged for purposes such as insertion of nonfoldable intraocular lenses (IOLs) or conversion to extracapsular cataract extraction.

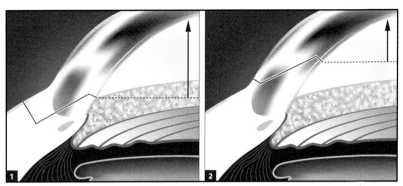

Figure 6-2. Cross-sectional view of scleral tunnel and clear corneal wounds. (1) An incision is made in the sclera with the tunnel extending forward into the cornea (solid line). (2) A grooved biplanar clear corneal incision is depicted (solid line). Note the more posterior corneal entry in the scleral tunnel wound. The anticipated position of the phacoemulsification probe (dotted line) also is further from the endothelium in the scleral tunnel wound as compared to the clear corneal wound (vertical arrow).

- Once the scleral tunnel incision is closed, conjunctiva covers these wounds, which may play a role in the lower reported incidence of endophthalmitis.[8,9]

- Scleral tunnels begin further posteriorly than clear corneal tunnels, and thus anterior chamber entry is also relatively more posterior. The resultant vertical distance between the phacoemulsification probe tip and the corneal endothelium is greater in the scleral tunnel than that of clear corneal wounds, leading to less endothelial damage by ultrasound phacoemulsification power[10,11] (Figure 6-2).

- As scleral tunnel wounds are created further from the optical center, a phaco-induced wound burn at this location would have less astigmatic consequence than a burn in the clear cornea.

- The magnitude of induced postoperative astigmatism increases with both incision length and proximity to the optical center.[12] Generally, larger incisions in the sclera induce less postoperative astigmatism than similar-sized clear corneal incisions, as they are further from the optical center.[13] However, while multiple studies[14-16] have suggested that smaller incisions may be astigmatically equivalent between wound types, there is some discrepancy regarding the wound size at which this occurs. While 2 prospective, randomized trials found no difference in keratometric astigmatism between 3- and 3.2-mm scleral tunnel and clear cornea incisions at 3 months,[14,15] another trial found that induced astigmatism as measured by vector analysis and videokeratography was higher in 3-mm clear corneal incisions compared to 3-mm scleral tunnels at 8 weeks.[16]

3. Disadvantages

There are disadvantages to using a scleral tunnel incision.

- The topography of the patient's face can restrict surgical exposure, making a scleral tunnel incision difficult. For example, a prominent brow, a narrow palpebral fissure, or a sunken globe in a deep orbit may obstruct access to the superior and superotemporal sclera, if chosen as the incision location.

- When tunneling forward with the pocket blade, failure to tilt the blade downward when creating the lateral aspect of the tunnel may result in severing the edge, creating a loose scleral flap at the posterolateral aspect of the wound.

- If the scleral groove incision is too deep, damage or disinsertion of the ciliary body may result. If the roof of the scleral tunnel is too thin, a blade entering the wound may cause an anterior buttonhole or perforation, creating an undesirable scleral defect.

- Globe perforation, premature posterior entry to the anterior chamber, iris prolapse, and poor wound apposition are other potential complications of a deep scleral groove.[17]

- The presence of a filtering bleb or conjunctival scarring preoperatively may complicate the creation of a conjunctival peritomy. Functionality of preexisting blebs may be affected; conjunctival manipulation may result in scar tissue that can decrease functionality of potential future filtering blebs.[18]

- Dissection and manipulation of vascular tissues such as the conjunctiva and sclera can cause blood to track forward through the tunneled wound into the anterior chamber, resulting in a hyphema. In addition, subconjunctival hemorrhages are more common with scleral tunnel wounds and may result in an inferior cosmetic outcome to that of the clear cornea phacoemulsification.

- Finally, while the surgically induced astigmatism of clear corneal incisions has been employed advantageously for astigmatic correction, the use of scleral tunnel wounds for this purpose has not been described.

B. Clear Corneal Incision

1. Technique

The steps in the construction of clear corneal incisions include anesthesia, paracentesis creation, corneal groove incision, and keratome entry into the

Figure 6-3. The clear corneal wound. (1) A Thornton ring fixates the eye, and a superblade is used to create a paracentesis port. (2) A guarded blade is angled perpendicular to the corneal surface and used to create a groove. (3) A diamond keratome is then advanced into the corneal stroma for approximately 2 mm. The heel of the blade is then elevated and advanced into the anterior chamber.

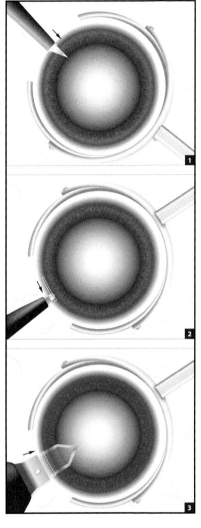

anterior chamber (Figure 6-3). Although various modes and combinations of anesthesia may be employed,[5,19-21] many surgeons use topical anesthesia for clear corneal incisions.[1,4,22,23]

a. Step 1

The paracentesis is created in the same manner as previously described for a scleral tunnel.

b. Step 2

The next step for some surgeons is the corneal groove incision, which is usually placed temporally at the limbus. A Thornton fixation ring is used to stabilize the globe, and a guarded knife is angled perpendicular to the cornea in order to achieve a consistent fixed groove depth. A groove can be chosen to be at the same depth as the tunnel, or deeper, with the latter resulting in a hinge at the base of the tunnel, which has been found to improve self-sealability of the wound upon application of external pressure.[24] Some surgeons skip this step completely, creating a single plane incision.

c. Step 3

The keratome is then placed in the corneal groove with the heel down flush with the ocular surface and advanced approximately 2 mm anteriorly, dissecting a plane through the corneal stroma. The heel of the blade is subsequently elevated off of the globe so that the tip of the keratome is directed toward the iris opposite the wound. Depending on the sharpness of the blade being used, this can create visual folds in the cornea as described above for scleral tunnel incisions. When using diamond blades or ultra-sharp metallic keratomes, some surgeons simply create a single plane incision without a limbal groove or a "dimple-down" maneuver. The keratome is advanced into the anterior chamber such that the shoulders of the blade penetrate the internal aspect of the wound, ensuring adequate internal wound width.

While some surgeons prefer the tactile tissue resistance during creation of the corneal tunnel afforded by metallic keratomes, diamond keratomes have been shown to cause less tissue disruption in corneal stroma.[25] Furthermore, diamond keratomes remain sharp and resist wear longer than their metal counterparts.

2. Advantages

Clear corneal incisions have some advantages over scleral tunnel wounds.

- As clear corneal incisions may be performed with topical anesthesia alone, a retrobulbar block is avoided.[21,26] This is an important consideration in patients who have a bleeding diathesis or who are highly myopic, as there is a higher risk of retrobulbar hemorrhage[27] or globe perforation,[28] respectively, from a retrobulbar block. A retrobulbar block can also cause complications inducing retinal vascular occlusion,[29,30] optic nerve injury,[31] strabismus,[32] and brainstem anesthesia.[33,34] Topical anesthesia allows for rapid visual rehabilitation following the surgical procedure while avoiding the risks of retrobulbar anesthesia.[35]

- A clear corneal incision is more time efficient and often has a better immediate cosmetic result.

- Since the conjunctiva is relatively untouched, it is left naïve for future filtering surgery if necessary. Similarly, a clear corneal approach leaves preexisting filtering blebs undisturbed.[36,37]
- With regard to refractive outcomes, preoperative astigmatism can be corrected at the time of cataract surgery through modifications in incision length, clock hour position, and proximity to the optical center.[38,39] For example, placement of the incision on the steep axis of astigmatism can be used to correct astigmatic errors of <1 D.[40] Furthermore, relatively simple modifications to the clear cornea incision such as limbal relaxing incisions can be employed.[40]

3. Disadvantages

There are disadvantages to clear corneal incisions.

- Preexisting corneal problems such as Fuchs' endothelial dystrophy, peripheral corneal degeneration, previous penetrating keratoplasty, or radial keratotomy scars are relative contraindications to corneal wounds.[41] In addition, in patients with impaired blinking, as seen in Parkinson's disease, exposed incisions in the cornea should be avoided due to the risk of corneal melt. The incision in these patients should generally be protected by conjunctiva.
- While conjunctiva covers the wound in scleral tunnel incisions, a clear corneal wound is exposed, and a postoperative wound leak allows for potential ingress of contaminated ocular surface fluid into the anterior chamber.[42,43] Several reviews in the literature have reported a 3- to 4-fold higher rate of endophthalmitis in sutureless clear corneal incisions compared to scleral tunnel incisions,[8,9] and yet other series have found no significant difference.[44-46] Stromal hydration and postoperative hypotony are thought to contribute to poor wound closure.[47,48]
- A corneal groove that is placed too posterior can cause an inadvertent incision in the conjunctiva and lead to ballooning as irrigation fluid collects in the subconjunctival space.[49,50]
- Instrument manipulation can cause corneal striae, which may result in death of corneal endothelial cells.[51,52]
- Incisions longer than 4 mm are preferentially made in the sclera, as unsutured corneal incisions of this size can gape and fail to self-seal.[53] Subsequent suture closure of such an incision may result in greater induced postoperative astigmatism. In addition, the recent use of optical coherence tomography to evaluate the postoperative structure of clear corneal incisions less than 4 mm in length has revealed a high incidence of early Descemet detachments and posterior wound gape. Posterior wound retraction also occurs in the majority of clear

corneal incisions after 3 years. The clinical relevance of these findings is still unknown, but it is hypothesized that they could lead to long-term refractive changes.[54] Clear corneal incisions with a length of 3.2 mm have been shown to induce 0.5 D of astigmatism, and this amount has not been shown to decrease with smaller wound sizes.[55,56] As mentioned previously, this can be advantageous when used to correct preexisting astigmatism but may be undesirable in other circumstances.

III. WOUND LOCATION

While wounds can be placed at any position theoretically, choice of location may be influenced by astigmatism considerations, preexisting ocular disease, and ergonomic comfort of the surgeon.

A. Astigmatism

The closer the incision is placed to the optical center of the cornea, the greater the degree of astigmatism induced.[12] Given the elliptical shape of the normal cornea, temporal incisions are generally further from the center and induce a smaller magnitude of astigmatism than superior incisions of equal size. This is true for both clear corneal and scleral tunnel incisions.[57-59] Wound location can also be selected so as to correct preexisting astigmatism.

B. Ocular Disease

Ocular disease may play an important role in determining not only whether the wound is placed in the cornea or sclera, but also the clock hour or quadrant chosen. For example, a temporal pterygium may lead to a choice of placing a superior or superotemporal wound, while a superior filtering bleb or superotemporal tube shunt may preclude placement of superior wounds.

C. Ergonomics

Ergonomic comfort of the surgeon is also important in planning the placement of the wound. For example, during phacoemulsification of the right eye, a right-handed surgeon has full temporal cornea access, but incisions in the superior cornea or sclera require the surgeon to sit at the head of the patient. In this position, a prominent brow or a globe positioned deep in the orbit may make surgical positioning and access difficult for the surgeon. Likewise, a high nose bridge can interfere with maneuverability of the second instrument. With the left eye, the surgeon has relatively improved access to the superotemporal globe, but a straight temporal incision requires the surgeon to be seated at the 4:30 position with spatial crowding from the patient's upper torso.

D. Endophthalmitis Risk

While several prospective and retrospective studies have reported an increased risk of postoperative endophthalmitis with temporal wound incisions,[8,9] others have found no statistically significant association between wound location and risk of endophthalmitis.[44,60,61]

IV. WOUND ARCHITECTURE

A. Incision Width

As techniques and technology have advanced in cataract surgery, surgeons have created smaller incisions. In order to remove the lens, the incision must be of sufficient size to accommodate the sleeve diameter of the phaco probe. The development of smaller probes has led to initial incisions less than 2 mm and as small as 0.9 mm, such as those used in bimanual phacoemulsification.[62]

The final wound dimension is determined by the size of the optic of the IOL to be inserted, or the size of the injector port when inserting foldable IOLs. Direct IOL insertion or insertion via an injector can stretch and permanently enlarge the incision, potentially resulting in loss of the designed self-sealing wound properties.[63,64] As lenses inserted through wounds of less than 2 mm become more widely accepted and studied, the final wound size necessary to perform cataract surgery with IOL implantation will continue to decrease.[65,66]

B. Incision Shape

The impact of incision shape on postoperative astigmatism is controversial. Some studies have revealed a significant change in postoperative astigmatism,[12,67,68] while others found no such difference.[69,70] Although the trend toward smaller, more astigmatism-neutral incisions has made wound-shape less relevant in routine phacoemulsification, incision shape is potentially important when shifts in postoperative astigmatism are desirable or when large incisions are unavoidable. Examples include the simultaneous correction of a preexisting astigmatism,[39] the conversion of an operation to an extracapsular cataract extraction, or the decision to insert a nonfoldable IOL.[67]

The 4 shapes described for scleral tunnel incisions are arcuate, straight, frown, and chevron. The arcuate incision follows a curved, circumlimbal trajectory that approximates the curvature of the adjacent limbus. The straight incision traces a simple linear trajectory in the direction tangential to the adjacent limbus. The frown incision follows a curved trajectory and can be thought of as an inverse-arcuate incision.[68] Lastly, the chevron is a modification of the arcuate incision that approximates the curvature of the adjacent limbus with 2 straight lines in a V formation.[71]

When an incision is made in the sclera, normal tension forces separate the 2 wound edges, causing gape. The curved incision allows the greatest degree of translational and rotational tissue movement,[12] and therefore induces the greatest magnitude of postoperative astigmatism.[67] The frown incision results in the least amount of tissue movement[12] and postoperative astigmatism.[68] In addition to the astigmatic benefit, the frown or chevron incision effectively shortens the length of the scleral tunnel, allowing less restriction to movement of surgical instrumentation without altering the chord length of the external incision.

C. Tunnel Length

Premature posterior or delayed anterior entry into the anterior chamber results in a tunnel that is too short or long, respectively, both of which can generate complications. A short tunnel can lead to poor control of anterior chamber depth and iris prolapse. Decreased tissue apposition and failure of the wound to self-seal may necessitate the use of sutures with potential postoperative astigmatic sequelae.[72] Maximum architectural stability is obtained in wounds 3.5 mm wide or less and of at least 2 mm in length.[73-75]

A long tunnel can decrease surgical instrument mobility in the anterior chamber due to oarlocking and impaired pivoting ability. The excessive manipulation of surgical instruments can tear the internal or external wound edges, induce scrolling or detachment of Descemet's membrane,[76,77] and create corneal striae, which in turn decreases intraoperative visibility and may damage corneal endothelium.[59] The endothelial cells can be further damaged by phaco-induced trauma as the probe tip enters the anterior chamber in closer proximity to the corneal endothelium[11] (see Figure 6-2).

V. WOUND CLOSURE

Both scleral tunnel and clear corneal incisions, when created properly, possess a self-sealing, valve-like tunnel design. If wound closure is felt to be inadequate, various techniques can be employed.

A. Sutures

Sutures may be used to provide additional support in scleral tunnel and clear corneal incisions. However, suture placement has been associated with increased amounts of surgically induced astigmatism, and well-constructed clear corneal incisions have been reported to have superior closure when compared to sutured corneal incisions.[78] Suture placement has not been found to decrease the rate of postoperative endophthalmitis,[8] and one study evaluating the incidence of postoperative hypotony found no difference between wounds closed with stromal hydration and those closed with sutures.[48]

B. Stromal Hydration

Corneal stromal hydration involves the forceful injection of fluid into the stroma adjacent to a clear corneal wound, causing stromal expansion and greater wound opposition. This technique has been shown to reduce the ingress of ocular surface fluid in the immediate postoperative period, but there is concern that wounds requiring hydration become inadequately sealed once the effect wears off.[47,79] The duration of the effect of hydration is a matter of debate, with articles reporting durations of 15 minutes to 1 week.[79,80]

C. Tissue Adhesives

A variety of synthetic and biologic tissue adhesives have been used for enhanced wound closure. Commonly used agents include cyanoacrylate-based and fibrin-based adhesives. The adjunctive use of cyanoacrylate-based adhesives has been shown to produce watertight scleral and clear corneal wounds whose resistance may be superior to sutured wounds.[81] Both fibrin-based and cyanoacrylate-based adhesives are reported to have a tensile strength comparable to sutures used in cataract surgery.[82]

The primary advantage of wound adhesives is enhanced wound closure whose effectiveness may exceed that of wound suturing. Disadvantages include an inconvenient preparation and application process, foreign body sensation, reactive conjunctival hyperemia, and, in the case of human fibrin glues, the theoretic risk of viral transmission.[83] Novel agents, including chondroitin sulfate aldehyde-, acrylic copolymer-, dendrimer-, and dendritic macromer-based tissue adhesives, may offer improved biocompatibility and a more favorable side effect profile.[81]

D. Other

Other proposed techniques for enhancing wound closure include increasing the target case-completion intraocular pressure, using peribulbar anesthesia with lid-taping instead of topical anesthesia, using methylcellulose-based viscosurgical devices rather than chondroitin sulfate or sodium hyaluronate, and internal wound tamponade by an air bubble in the anterior chamber.[48,84]

VI. CONCLUSION

The type, location, and architecture of the wound constructed each influence the surgical procedure, patient recovery, and visual outcome of phacoemulsification. While both scleral tunnel and clear corneal wounds may be used to successfully complete removal of the cataract, attention must be given to each individual patient and preexisting ocular disease, astigmatic profile, and facial anatomy. Wound architecture and surgical technique are also important in avoiding intraoperative complications, minimizing corneal endothelial damage, and proper wound closure. A thorough understanding of the advantages, disadvantages, and correct application of each element of wound construction is essential to the proper planning and ultimate visual outcome.

ACKNOWLEDGMENT

The authors would like to acknowledge Serena W. Tam for the design and illustration of the figures.

KEY POINTS

1. The 2 most common types of wounds for phacoemulsification are the scleral tunnel and clear corneal incisions.

2. Advantages of the scleral tunnel incision include conjunctival coverage and a greater vertical distance from the corneal endothelium to the phacoemulsification probe.

3. Advantages of the clear corneal incision include an undisturbed conjunctiva and the potential avoidance of a retrobulbar block.

4. Choice of wound location is influenced by astigmatic considerations, preexisting ocular disease states, and ergonomic comfort of the surgeon.

5. Incision characteristics such as width, shape, and tunnel length may all be modified, affecting astigmatic outcome, endothelial cell loss, and self-sealing properties of the wound.

REFERENCES

1. Leaming DV. Practice styles and preferences of ASCRS members—2003 survey. *J Cataract Refract Surg.* 2004;30(4):892-900.
2. *Analeyz, Inc.* 2010 survey practice styles and preferences of U.S. ASCRS members. Available at: www.analeyz.com/. Accessed 19.07.2012.
3. Virtanen P, Huha T. Pain in scleral pocket incision cataract surgery using topical and peribulbar anesthesia. *J Cataract Refract Surg.* 1998;24(12):1609-1613.
4. Patel BC, Clinch TE, Burns TA, et al. Prospective evaluation of topical versus retrobulbar anesthesia: a converting surgeon's experience. *J Cataract Refract Surg.* 1998;24(6):853-860.
5. Friedman DS, Bass EB, Lubomski LH, et al. Synthesis of the literature on the effectiveness of regional anesthesia for cataract surgery. *Ophthalmology.* 2001;108(3):519-529.
6. Boezaart A, Berry R, Nell M. Topical anesthesia versus retrobulbar block for cataract surgery: the patients' perspective. *J Clin Anesth.* 2000;12(1):58-60.
7. McGoldrick KE. Comment on topical anesthesia versus retrobulbar block for cataract surgery: the patients' perspective. *Surv Anesthesiol.* 2001;45(1):6-8.

8. Cooper BA, Holekamp NM, Bohigian G, Thompson PA. Case-control study of endophthalmitis after cataract surgery comparing scleral tunnel and clear corneal wounds. *Am J Ophthalmol.* 2003;136(2):300-305.

9. Nagaki Y, Hayasaka S, Kadoi C, et al. Bacterial endophthalmitis after small-incision cataract surgery: Effect of incision placement and intraocular lens type. *J Cataract Refract Surg.* 2003;29(1):20-26.

10. Bleckmann H, Vogt R. Experimental endothelial lesions by means of an ultrasound phacoemulsificator. *Graefes Arch Clin Exp Ophthalmol.* 1986;224(5):457-462.

11. Ogino K, Koda F, Miyata K. [Damage to cultured corneal endothelium caused by ultrasound during phacoemulsification]. *Nippon Ganka Gakkai Zasshi.* 1993;97(11):1286-1291.

12. Koch PS. Structural analysis of cataract incision construction. *J Cataract Refract Surg.* 1991;17(suppl):661-667.

13. Olsen T, Dam-Johansen M, Bek T, Hjortdal JO. Corneal versus scleral tunnel incision in cataract surgery: a randomized study. *J Cataract Refract Surg.* 1997;23(3):337-341.

14. Oshima Y, Tsujikawa K, Oh A, Harino S. Comparative study of intraocular lens implantation through 3.0 mm temporal clear corneal and superior scleral tunnel self-sealing incisions. *J Cataract Refract Surg.* 1997;23(3):347-353.

15. He Y, Zhu S, Chen M, Li D. Comparison of the keratometric corneal astigmatic power after phacoemulsification: clear temporal corneal incision versus superior scleral tunnel incision. *J Ophthalmol.* 2009;10621.

16. Hayashi K, Yoshida M, Hayashi H. Corneal shape changes after 2.0 mm or 3.0 mm clear corneal versus scleral tunnel incision cataract surgery. *Ophthalmology.* 2010;117(7):1313-1323.

17. Allan BD. Mechanism of iris prolapse: a qualitative analysis and implications for surgical technique. *J Cataract Refract Surg.* 1995;21(2):182-186.

18. Broadway DC, Grierson I, Hitchings RA. Local effects of previous conjunctival incisional surgery and the subsequent outcome of filtration surgery. *Am J Ophthalmol.* 1998;125(6):805-818.

19. Bellucci R. Anesthesia for cataract surgery. *Curr Opin Ophthalmol.* 1999;10(1):36-41.

20. Crandall AS. Anesthesia modalities for cataract surgery. *Curr Opin Ophthalmol.* 2001;12(1):9-11.

21. Navaleza JS, Pendse SJ, Blecher MH. Choosing anesthesia for cataract surgery. *Ophthalmol Clin North Am.* 2006;19(2):233-237.

22. Koch PS. Efficacy of lidocaine 2% jelly as a topical agent in cataract surgery. *J Cataract Refract Surg.* 1999;25(5):632-634.

23. Patel BC, Burns TA, Crandall A, et al. A comparison of topical and retrobulbar anesthesia for cataract surgery. *Ophthalmology.* 1996;103(8):1196-1203.

24. Langerman DW. Architectural design of a self-sealing corneal tunnel, single-hinge incision. *J Cataract Refract Surg.* 1994;20(1):84-88.

25. Jacobi FK, Dick HB, Bohle RM. Histological and ultrastructural study of corneal tunnel incisions using diamond and steel keratomes. *J Cataract Refract Surg.* 1998;24(4):498-502.

26. Claoue C, Lanigan C. Topical anaesthesia for cataract surgery. *Aust N Z J Ophthalmol.* 1997;25(4):265-268.

27. Konstantatos A. Anticoagulation and cataract surgery: a review of the current literature. *Anaesth Intensive Care.* 2001;29(1):11-18.

28. Modarres M, Parvaresh MM, Hashemi M, Peyman GA. Inadvertent globe perforation during retrobulbar injection in high myopes. *Int Ophthalmol.* 1997;21(4):179-185.

29. Cowley M, Campochiaro PA, Newman SA, Fogle JA. Retinal vascular occlusion without retrobulbar or optic nerve sheath hemorrhage after retrobulbar injection of lidocaine. *Ophthalmic Surg.* 1988;19(12):859-861.

30. Morgan CM, Schatz H, Vine AK, et al. Ocular complications associated with retrobulbar injections. *Ophthalmology.* 1988;95(5):660-665.

31. Hersch M, Baer G, Dieckert JP, et al. Optic nerve enlargement and central retinal-artery occlusion secondary to retrobulbar anesthesia. *Ann Ophthalmol.* 1989;21(5):195-197.
32. Johnson DA. Persistent vertical binocular diplopia after cataract surgery. *Am J Ophthalmol.* 2001;132(6):831-835.
33. Nicoll JM, Acharya PA, Ahlen K, et al. Central nervous system complications after 6000 retrobulbar blocks. *Anesth Analg.* 1987;66(12):1298-1302.
34. Gunja N, Varshney K. Brainstem anaesthesia after retrobulbar block: a rare cause of coma presenting to the emergency department. *Emerg Med Australas.* 2006;18(1):83-85.
35. Nielsen PJ. Immediate visual capability after cataract surgery: topical versus retrobulbar anesthesia. *J Cataract Refract Surg.* 1995;21(3):302-304.
36. Caprioli J, Park HJ, Kwon YH, Weitzman M. Temporal corneal phacoemulsification in filtered glaucoma patients. *Trans Am Ophthalmol Soc.* 1997;95:153-167; discussion 67-70.
37. Park HJ, Kwon YH, Weitzman M, Caprioli J. Temporal corneal phacoemulsification in patients with filtered glaucoma. *Arch Ophthalmol.* 1997;115(11):1375-1380.
38. Kershner RM. Clear corneal cataract surgery and the correction of myopia, hyperopia, and astigmatism. *Ophthalmology.* 1997;104(3):381-389.
39. Kaufmann C, Peter J, Ooi K, et al. Limbal relaxing incisions versus on-axis incisions to reduce corneal astigmatism at the time of cataract surgery. *J Cataract Refract Surg.* 2005;31(12):2261-2265.
40. Amesbury EC, Miller KM. Correction of astigmatism at the time of cataract surgery. *Curr Opin Ophthalmol.* 2009;20:19-24.
41. Freeman M, Kumar V, Ramanathan US, O'Neill E. Dehiscence of radial keratotomy incision during phacoemulsification. *Eye.* 2004;18(1):101-103.
42. McDonnell PJ, Taban M, Sarayba M, et al. Dynamic morphology of clear corneal cataract incisions. *Ophthalmology.* 2003;110(12):2342-2348.
43. Taban M, Sarayba MA, Ignacio TS, et al. Ingress of India ink into the anterior chamber through sutureless clear corneal cataract wounds. *Arch Ophthalmol.* 2005;123(5):643-648.
44. Colleaux KM, Hamilton WK. Effect of prophylactic antibiotics and incision type on the incidence of endophthalmitis after cataract surgery. *Can J Ophthalmol.* 2000;35(7):373-378.
45. Lundstrom M. Endophthalmitis and incision construction. *Curr Opin Ophthalmol.* 2006;17(1):68-71.
46. Monica ML, Long DA. Nine year safety with self-sealing corneal tunnel incision in clear corneal cataract surgery. *Ophthalmol.* 2005;112:985-986.
47. Francis IC, Roufas A, Figueira EC, et al. Endophthalmitis following cataract surgery: the sucking corneal wound. *J Cataract Refract Surg.* 2001;37:2235-2236.
48. Shingleton BJ, Rosenberg RB, Teixeira R, O'Donoghue MW. Evaluation of intraocular pressure in the immediate postoperative following phacoemulsification. *J Cataract Refract Surg.* 2007;33:1253-1257.
49. Ziakas NG, Georgiadis N. Conjunctival ballooning during scleral tunnel phacoemulsification. *J Cataract Refract Surg.* 2003;29(11):2046-2047.
50. Akura J, Funakoshi T, Kadonosono K, Saito M. Differences in incision shape based on the keratome bevel. *J Cataract Refract Surg.* 2001;27(5):761-765.
51. Grutzmacher RD, Oiland D, McKillop BR, Bunt-Milam AH. Donor corneal endothelial striae. *Am J Ophthalmol.* 1986;102(4):508-515.
52. Nartey IN, Ng W, Sherrard ES, Steele AD. Posterior corneal folds and endothelial cell damage in human donor eyes. *Br J Ophthalmol.* 1989;73(2):121-125.
53. Menapace R. Delayed iris prolapse with unsutured 5.1 mm clear corneal incisions. *J Cataract Refract Surg.* 1995;21(3):353-357.
54. Wang L, Dixit L, Weikert MP, et al. Healing changes in clear corneal cataract incisions evaluated using Fourier-domain optical coherence tomography. *J Cataract Refract Surg.* 2012; 38:660-665.
55. Gross RH, Miller KM. Corneal astigmatism after phacoemulsification and lens implantation through unsutured scleral and corneal tunnel incisions. *Am J Ophthalmol.* 1996;121:57-64.

56. Hill W. Expected effects of surgically induced astigmatism on AcrySof toric intraocular lens results. *J Cataract Refract Surg.* 2008;34:364-367.
57. Long DA, Monica ML. A prospective evaluation of corneal curvature changes with 3.0- to 3.5-mm corneal tunnel phacoemulsification. *Ophthalmology.* 1996;103(2):226-232.
58. Wirbelauer C, Anders N, Pham DT, Wollensak J. Effect of incision location on preoperative oblique astigmatism after scleral tunnel incision. *J Cataract Refract Surg.* 1997;23(3):365-371.
59. Oshika T, Tsuboi S, Yaguchi S, et al. Comparative study of intraocular lens implantation through 3.2- and 5.5-mm incisions. *Ophthalmology.* 1994;101(7):1183-1190.
60. Lundstrom M, Wejde G, Stenevi U, et al. Endophthalmitis after cataract surgery: a nationwide prospective study evaluating incidence in relation to incision type and location. *Ophthalmology.* 2007;114(5):866-870.
61. Miller JJ, Scott IU, Flynn HW, et al. Acute-onset endophthalmitis after cataract surgery (2000-2004): incidence, clinical settings, and visual acuity outcomes after treatment. *Am J Ophthalmol.* 2005;139:983-987.
62. Agarwal A, Agarwal A, Agarwal S, et al. Phakonit: phacoemulsification through a 0.9 mm corneal incision. *J Cataract Refract Surg.* 2001;27(10):1548-1552.
63. Steinert RF, Deacon J. Enlargement of incision width during phacoemulsification and folded intraocular lens implant surgery. *Ophthalmology.* 1996;103(2):220-225.
64. Kohnen T, Koch DD. Experimental and clinical evaluation of incision size and shape following forceps and injector implantation of a three-piece high-refractive-index silicone intraocular lens. *Graefes Arch Clin Exp Ophthalmol.* 1998;236(12):922-928.
65. Mencucci R, Ponchietti C, Nocentini L, et al. Scanning electron microscopic analysis of acrylic intraocular lenses for microincision cataract surgery. *J Cataract Refract Surg.* 2006;32(2):318-323.
66. Prakash P, Kasaby HE, Aggarwal RK, Humfrey S. Microincision bimanual phacoemulsification and Thinoptx implantation through a 1.70 mm incision. *Eye.* 2007;21:177-182.
67. Akura J, Kaneda S, Hatta S, Matsuura K. Controlling astigmatism in cataract surgery requiring relatively large self-sealing incisions. *J Cataract Refract Surg.* 2000;26(11):1650-1659.
68. Singer JA. Frown incision for minimizing induced astigmatism after small incision cataract surgery with rigid optic intraocular lens implantation. *J Cataract Refract Surg.* 1991;17(suppl):677-88.
69. Vass C, Menapace R, Rainer G. Corneal topographic changes after frown and straight sclerocorneal incisions. *J Cataract Refract Surg.* 1997;23(6):913-922.
70. Wollensak J, Pham DT, Seiler T. [Effect of incision form and tunnel length on induced astigmatism with the no-stitch technique]. *Ophthalmologe.* 1994;91(4):439-441.
71. Pallin SL. Chevron sutureless closure: a preliminary report. *J Cataract Refract Surg.* 1991;17(suppl):706-709.
72. Coombes A, Gartry D, eds. Cataract Surgery. London: BMJ Books, 2003:218.
73. Ernest PH, Fenzi R, Lavery KT, Sensoli A. Relative stability of clear corneal incisions in a cadaver eye model. *J Cataract Refract Surg.* 1995;21(1):39-42.
74. MacKool RJ, Russell RS. Strength of clear corneal incisions in cadaver eyes. *J Cataract Refract Surg.* 1996;22(6):721-725.
75. Fine IH, Hoffman RS, Packer M. Profile of clear corneal cataract incisions demonstrated by ocular coherence tomography. *J Cataract Refract Surg.* 2007;33:94-97.
76. Kim IS, Shin JC, Im CY, Kim EK. Three cases of Descemet's membrane detachment after cataract surgery. *Yonsei Med J.* 2005;46(5):719-723.
77. Nouri M, Pineda Jr R, Azar D. Descemet membrane tear after cataract surgery. *Semin Ophthalmol.* 2002;17(3-4):115-119.
78. May WN, Castro-Combs J, Kashiwabuchi RT, et al. Bacterial-sized particle inflow through sutured clear corneal incisions in a laboratory human model. *J Cataract Refract Surg.* 2011;37:1140-1146.

79. Vasavada AR, Praveen MR, Pandita D, et al. Effect of stromal hydration of clear corneal incisions: quantifying ingress of trypan blue into the anterior chamber after phacoemulsification. *J Cataract Refract Surg.* 2007;33:623-627.

80. Fukuda S, Kawana K, Yasuno Y, Oshika T. Wound architecture of clear corneal incision with or without stromal hydration observed with 3-dimensional optical coherence tomography. *Am J Ophthalmol.* 2011;151:413-419.

81. Kim T, Kharod BV. Tissue adhesives in corneal cataract incisions. *Curr Opin Ophthalmol.* 2007;18:39-43.

82. Shigemitsu T, Majima Y. The utilization of a biological adhesive for wound treatment: comparison of suture, self-sealing sutureless, and cyanoacrylate closure in the tensile strength test. *Int Ophthalmol.* 1996-1997;20(6):323-328.

83. Chan SM, Boisjoly H. Advances in the use of adhesives in ophthalmology. *Curr Opin Ophthalmol.* 2004;15:305-310.

84. Agarwal T, Singh D, Khokhar S, Panda A. Simple technique for sealing clear corneal wound leaks using a dynamic anterior chamber air bubble. *J Cataract Refract Surg.* 2011;37(9):1732.

7

ASTIGMATIC CONSIDERATIONS IN CATARACT SURGERY

Yuri S. Oleynikov, MD, PhD; Lynda Z. Kleiman, MD; and B. David Gorman, MD

I. INTRODUCTION

Contemporary cataract surgery has evolved from a procedure with the simple focus of removing an obstruction of the visual axis to a refractive procedure. Minimal spectacle dependence is expected by more and more patients. Control of astigmatism and proper intraocular lens (IOL) selection are imperative to a good refractive result. There are 2 astigmatic considerations in cataract surgery: control of astigmatism induced by the surgery and correction of preexisting astigmatism. Patient parameters and preference determine the refractive goal of the surgery. Emmetropia, monovision, mild residual astigmatism, or pseudoaccommodation should be discussed in detail prior to surgery.[1]

II. MINIMIZING ASTIGMATISM INDUCED BY CATARACT INCISIONS

A. General Principles

An incision bisects fibers within a tissue and results in relaxation of tension of those fibers due to separation of the wound edges by causing tissue gape. Tissue structure and internal distribution of tension determine resultant tissue deformation. The size, location, and architecture of a cataract incision determine its astigmatic effect. Larger and deeper incisions cause larger changes in corneal and scleral tissue. Experiments with various size incisions by Koch, Kuglen, and others showed that induced astigmatism is proportional to the cube of the incision length.[2] Incisions less than 3 mm produced clinically insignificant cylinder of <0.5 D.[3]

Henderson BA. *Essentials of Cataract Surgery, Second Edition (pp 69-79).*
© 2014 Taylor & Francis Group.

Figure 7-1. Scleral groove incisions for ECCE. (1) "Traditional" or "smile" incision. (2) Straight incision. (3) "Frown" incision.

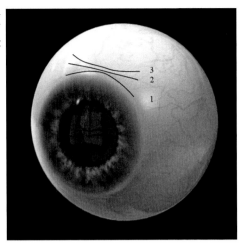

Sutures or tissue adhesive reverses tissue gape. Sutures with appropriate tension and location restore tissue architecture and correct induced astigmatism. Tight or improperly placed sutures compress, displace, and flatten tissue and cause central optical zone steepening in that meridian. Loose sutures leave the meridian flattened. Even properly sutured wounds relax over time, causing against-the-wound drift. The time during which the wound "drifts" depends on its size; the bigger the wound, the longer the duration. These changes overlap with the natural aging process in which the cornea drifts toward against-the-rule (ATR) astigmatism.

B. Classical Extracapsular Cataract Extraction Incisions

Historically, cataract incisions encompassed up to 180 degrees of the cornea. A classic extracapsular cataract extraction (ECCE) incision consists of a superior partial thickness scleral groove posterior to the limbus, a scleral tunnel, and an internal corneal "lip." The initial groove can curve parallel to the limbus ("traditional" or "smile"), be straight, or curve away from the limbus ("frown") (Figure 7-1). The latter is less prone to against-the-wound drift but makes surgery more technically challenging.[4] Longer tunnels provide more stability but may also lead to decreased mobility of instruments, or "oarlocking."

Curved "smile" incisions are the most common type of ECCE incisions. There are many ways to close these incisions. Suture material should be nonabsorbable. Sutures should induce 3 to 5 diopters (D) of with-the-rule (WTR) astigmatism because the incision typically drifts 1 to 3 D (up to 5 D) over several years. Astigmatism is managed by selective suture removal starting 1 month after surgery. Running "baseball," horizontal and vertical mattress, and

Masket variation sutures have been proposed to reduce surgically induced astigmatism. These techniques do not limit late ATR astigmatic drift. The vertical meridian can be relaxed in the presence of preexisting WTR astigmatism by leaving intentional wound gape. Each quarter millimeter of gape corrects 1 D of astigmatism up to 4 to 5 D.[1]

C. Clear Corneal Incisions

The advent of phacoemulsification and foldable IOLs and the introduction of smaller incisions decreased surgically induced astigmatism. Incisions of 3 mm or less induce less than 0.5 D, usually 0.2 to 0.4 D. Temporal scleral and corneal incisions caused no detectable astigmatism from postoperative day 1, while 3-mm superior incisions took less than 1 month to stabilize.[5,6] Nasal 3.5-mm corneal incisions induced slightly more astigmatism than temporal incisions. Temporal 1- and 2-plane clear cornea incisions induced the least astigmatism and were easy to perform, quickly becoming popular. Triplanar incisions with deep posterior grooves induce astigmatism and can be used to correct ATR astigmatism. Many surgeons place their incisions on the steep meridian to reduce preexisting astigmatism.[7] Another approach is to use astigmatically neutral temporal incisions and place additional incisions as described next.

Phacoemulsification burns can cause severe induced astigmatism. Heating collagen to above 60°C leads to its coagulation and local shrinkage,[8] leading to wound gape. The defect is difficult to correct because wound edges are disturbed and a watertight closure may cause high astigmatism. A wound burn should be watertight but tissue edges should not be approximated. Contemporary phaco machines minimize heat production but burns do occur, especially in sleeveless microincisional phaco.

III. TREATING PREEXISTING ASTIGMATISM AT THE TIME OF CATARACT SURGERY

Contemporary cataract incisions cause minimal astigmatism, which allows surgeons to focus on correction of preexisting astigmatism in the quest for emmetropia. Corneal biomechanics allow for predictable correction of regular astigmatism with minimal distortion and irregular astigmatism. The layers of the cornea consist of collagen fibrils extending from limbus to limbus with tension evenly distributed along the length of the fiber. In the midcentral corneal stroma, fibrils orient along horizontal and vertical meridians. The fibrils become thicker closer to the limbus and appear to be continuous with the sclera. Hundreds of sheets, or lamellae, of the fibers are regularly packed but are loosely connected to each other, allowing for sliding of the layers and redistribution of tension by bifurcating obliquely oriented fibrils and interspersing proteoglycans.[9] It is possible to manipulate these properties of the cornea to change its shape.

A. Effect of Incisions on Corneal Tissue

One can flatten the cornea in a steep meridian and reduce optical power by relaxing fibrils in that meridian with a perpendicular incision. The degree of flattening is proportional to the number of fibers cut and can be varied by depth of incision and its length. Due to interconnection of corneal fibers and redistribution of tension, incisions also will affect the meridian 90 degrees away. This is called coupling. The effect depends on the type and orientation of the incision.[10,11] An ideal incision has a coupling ratio of 1:1 (flattening of the incised meridian divided by steepening of the opposite meridian), resulting in a zero spherical shift. Indeed, it was found that 45- to 90-degree incisions in the 5- to 7-mm optical zone have those properties. Most incisions in younger individuals have a coupling ratio of less than 1 leading to small overall steepening. The keratometric coupling ratio increases with age and higher preoperative K's but data are limited and the effect is small.

Due to limited sliding of the fibrils, the effect of an incision is most pronounced near the incision. Consequently, the closer the incision is to the visual axis, the higher the effect of the incision on the visual properties of the eye. Incisions closer to the visual axis are also more likely to induce irregular astigmatism. The redistribution of fibril tension tends to smooth out such irregularities at more peripheral incisions. Because of corneal shape and structure, ATR astigmatism is more easily corrected by smaller incisions than WTR astigmatism.

B. Corneal and Limbal Relaxing Incisions

In the early 1980s, several surgeons investigated the use of corneal incisions for correction of astigmatism in cataract patients. Initially, so-called corneal relaxing incisions (CRIs) or astigmatic keratotomy (AK) were used—usually a pair of straight or arcuate clear cornea incisions between 5- and 7-mm optical zone to about 90% to 95% depth of the cornea. To correct greater astigmatism, a second pair of incisions was added peripherally to the first pair, but only 20% to 30% additional effect was achieved with higher irregular astigmatism. Arcuate incisions became more popular because it was believed they better preserved the 1:1 coupling ratio. These incisions were historically used in postkeratoplasty patients with high astigmatism. Their drawbacks included introduction of irregular astigmatism, glare, steepening of the cornea, fluctuations in refraction, and foreign body sensation.

Most cataract patients have moderate astigmatism of 0.5 to 3.0 D. Peripheral corneal relaxing incisions (PCRIs) or limbal relaxing incisions (LRIs) have become more popular than central CRIs for several reasons.

Risk of corneal perforation is reduced because they are performed in the thick peripheral cornea. Risk of irregular astigmatism is reduced because they are located far from the visual axis. Peripheral incisions cause minimal foreign body sensation and glare and allow faster visual recovery. Extensive experimentation resulted in multiple nomograms that take into account age, axis, amount of astigmatism, and specifics of technique. Some nomograms define incisions in millimeter length, but most commonly degrees of arc are used to compensate for variability in corneal diameter.[1,12] Several nomograms are widely used today—Donnenfeld and Nichamin nomograms for LRIs and Lindstrom nomogram for CRI in 5- to 7-mm optical zone. An online LRI calculation tool utilizing Donnenfeld and NAPA (Nichamin Age and Pachymetry Adjusted) nomograms is also available at http://www.lricalculator.com/. Other nomograms in use include Gills,[13] Wang,[14] and Cristobal.[15]

The incision or multiple incisions are placed on the steep meridian and the length is varied based on the amount of necessary correction. Dr. Osher's approach keeps the length of the incisions constant at 3 mm and varies the distance from the visual axis.[16] Another technique called paired clear corneal incision in which the cataract incision is placed on the steep meridian and a second identical penetrating incision is placed opposite the first is rarely used because it compromises anterior chamber stability and sterility.[17]

C. Surgical Technique of Corneal Relaxing Incisions or Limbal Relaxing Incisions

Patient selection and education are important in avoiding unrealistic expectations and unhappy patients. The goal is to minimize astigmatism and prevent overcorrections. Choosing the proper axis is very important. Although LRIs are less sensitive to off-axis shift than CRIs/AK, improper placement of the incisions can make vision worse and may be difficult to correct. The most common serious error is being 90 degrees away from the proper axis. Clear written preoperative plans should be reverified before surgery. It is helpful to find an iris or scleral landmark close to the proper axis and document it in the office.

Keratometry, corneal topography, and manifest refraction are taken into account and the axis is selected preoperatively if measurements agree. It is wise to delay astigmatism correction until after cataract surgery if the axis and magnitude cannot be reliably determined. The patient is seated (the same position as when taking preoperative measurements) and the steep axis is marked with an indelible pen. Alternatively, intraoperative keratometry may be performed during surgery with a Placido-disk keratoscope and the steep axis marked. The incisions can be placed before or after cataract extraction. Performing LRI at normal IOP with live keratoscopy before cataract extraction helps confirm that all of the astigmatism has been removed. But if one of the incisions is leaking, this may complicate cataract extraction itself. Placing incisions at the end of surgery minimizes that risk and allows for unanticipated complications in the cataract procedure, such as whether the cataract incision was enlarged or sutures were placed, and thus the incisions can be modified or withheld.

After the axis is marked and verified, the length of the incision is marked with the help of an arcuate or radial keratotomy (RK) marker. A fixation ring is often used. A front-cutting calibrated adjustable blade or a preset 600-μm blade is inserted perpendicularly to the corneal surface 0.5 mm central to the anterior border of the surgical limbus and an incision is performed with a fluid motion. An LRI generally should not overlap with a clear corneal incision as it may destabilize it, although the main incision can be placed through an LRI in some cases of ATR astigmatism.

If any small vessels are cut, the bleeding is allowed to stop spontaneously. The incision is reopened and irrigated and the depth is checked with balanced salt solution (BSS) on a cannula. Microperforations are rare with a 600-mm setting. A large perforation may occur if the blade is incorrectly set or calibrated. Large perforations associated with anterior chamber collapse should be sutured and sutures removed 1 to 2 weeks postoperatively. Various devices are available for blade support and globe stabilization but are not commonly used.

LRIs can also be performed at the slit lamp on some patients for mild-to-moderate astigmatism to augment previous incisions or for primary incisions. Lidocaine gel allows for adequate anesthesia and speculum is needed for proper exposure. The technique is very similar to OR LRIs but extra care needs to be taken with blade calibration to avoid perforation. Should perforation occur, limiting eye rubbing with a shield and placing a bandage contact lens will allow the incision to be sealed quickly.

The technique is similar for CRIs in the 5- to 7-mm optical zone. The visual axis is marked by corneal reflex while the patient is looking at the microscope light, the optical zone is marked concentric to it, and the arc is marked on the steep meridian. A pachymeter is used to determine corneal thickness at the incision site, and a variable blade is set at 90% to 95% of the thickness. The eye is stabilized with a ring or forceps and the incisions performed similarly to LRI. Precision is more important given the thinner cornea and the proximity to the visual axis, and good wrist and arm support is helpful. The incisions are irrigated and checked for proper depth.

Recently, another option has become available for LRI during cataract surgery—femtosecond arcuate incisions. Initially available on Intralase (Abbott Medical Optics [AMO]) for AK after penetrating keratoplasty, this technology is available now on femtosecond cataract surgery platforms, such as LenSx (Alcon), LensAR (LensAR Inc), Victus (Bausch & Lomb),

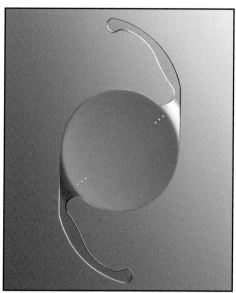

Figure 7-2. AcrySof toric IOL. (Reprinted with permission from Alcon Laboratories, Inc.)

and OptiMedica. The technique is dependent on the laser system used and nomograms are being fine tuned. Incision position can be adjusted closer to visual axis or further toward the limbus and offer highly precise and clean incision. Live optical coherence tomography (OCT) corneal pachymetry measurement allows for proper selected depth (80% to 90%) and minimizes perforations. Just as in femtosecond LASIK flap creation, the incision needs to be opened with a secondary instrument to break residual collagen bridges and achieve full effect. This can be done at the end of surgery under a Placido ring keratoscope or intraoperative aberrometry, such as ORA System (WaveTec Vision, http://getorasystem.com/). ORA System aberrometer is attached to the microscope and collects a reflected beam wavefront much like eximer wavefront system aberrometer. The eye is usually filled with BSS (or, sometimes, viscoelastic) to normal intraocular pressure, and measurement is made aphakic or pseudophakic to confirm lens power and LRI placement. Femtosecond incisions can be opened in stages under live control to minimize actual measured astigmatism.

D. Toric Intraocular Lenses and Excimer Laser Correction

There are several alternative approaches to astigmatism correction in the setting of cataract surgery. Foldable and nonfoldable toric IOLs are available. STAAR Surgical's silicone toric IOL has a spherical posterior surface, toric anterior surface, and a plate haptic design (Figure 7-2).

Figure 7-3. AMO TECNIS Toric IOL. (Reprinted with permission from Abbott Medical Optics.)

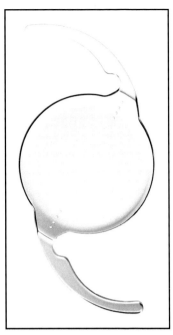

They are available in 2 and 3.5 D toric power for correction of 1.5 and 2.25 D of corneal astigmatism. The lens is placed in the bag through an astigmatically neutral 3-mm corneal wound and rotated into position after viscoelastic removal. Two lenses may be sutured together and placed in the bag to provide up to 4.3 D of correction.[18] Use of these lenses is limited by postoperative rotation. Rotation of 10 degrees decreases correction by one third, 20 degrees by two thirds, and >30 degrees increases cylinder. Several studies showed that up to 18% of lenses rotate more than 30 degrees, and 7% >40 degrees, leading to more than 10% reoperation rate.[19,20] Plate design IOLs may dislocate posteriorly after yttrium-aluminum-garnet (YAG) capsulotomy.

Another widely used toric lens is based on the popular acrylic Alcon AcrySof SA60 platform. The Food and Drug Administration (FDA) approved smaller power T3-T5 IOLs of up to 3 D in IOL plane on September 14, 2005. In May 2011, FDA also approved higher astigmatism models of AcrySof Toric lens T6-T9 for up to 6 D in the IOL plane, translating into 4.11 D in the corneal plane (Figure 7-3) in regular and aspheric IQ models. Preliminary results from Alcon suggested that this model may demonstrate better stability. The material of this lens has certain adhesiveness for the capsular material, which allows the lens to remain where it was surgically placed.

Typically, the steep axis of astigmatism and/or the horizontal axis are marked preoperatively at the slit lamp. Lens power and model are determined with an online calculator at http://www.acrysoftoriccalculator.com based on preexisting corneal astigmatism. After cataract extraction is complete, the toric lens is inserted into the capsular bag and rotated clockwise to place IOL markings 10 to 15 degrees before the steep axis. Viscoelastic is then removed from under the lens for improved adhesion, the rest of the viscoelastic is removed, and the lens is brought to perfect alignment with the steep axis via final rotation. Intraoperative aberrometry (ORA Systems) can be performed at this point to confirm full correction. The lens can still be adjusted clockwise at this point but with some difficulty. The final result is very sensitive to proper alignment and requires a meticulous technique.

Toric lenses can also be combined with relaxing incisions to treat high astigmatism that exceeds available IOL power. Using an AcrySof toric IOL in keratoconus or posttransplant patients who are not good candidates for LRI/AK can result in excellent uncorrected vision postoperatively.

The newest FDA approved toric IOL in the United States is the AMO TEC-NIS Toric (Abbott Medical Optics; see Figure 7-3). It is a one piece acrylic IOL with a wave-front designed aspheric optic and a frosted, continuous 360 degree posterior square edge. The IOL has a 6mm optic and 13 mm haptic to haptic diameter. The lens is available from +5 to +34 D, with 0.5-D increments. The TECNIS toric corrects from 1.00 to 4.00 D in the IOL plane.

Future IOLs may include a novel light-adjustable lens (LAL), a silicone IOL under development from Calhoun Vision. This lens can be implanted in a usual fashion and then adjusted in the early postoperative period with low intensity ultraviolet light to provide desired correction. It can also be used with wavefront data to correct total optical error of the eye or for temporary multifocal correction that can be erased if a patient is unsatisfied.

Many surgeons also often use excimer laser after cataract surgery is done and healing is complete. Photorefractive keratectomy (PRK) is often the procedure of choice given relatively small corrections needed, absence of pressure on the eye during the procedure, and age of the patients. Results are good and excellent precision can be obtained.

IV. CONCLUSION

Cataract surgery has evolved so that it is possible to minimize postoperative refractive error. Patient expectations have increased as a result. Cataract surgeons must be familiar with many refractive tools and techniques. No single approach is best for all patients, and careful planning and attention to detail are essential. Novel technologies will continue to make refractive cataract surgery even more rewarding.

KEY POINTS

1. Cataract surgery has evolved into a refractive procedure with the goal of eliminating or significantly reducing the need for spectacle dependence.

2. One must consider not only the astigmatism induced by the cataract incision itself, but also the correction of preexisting astigmatism.

3. Incision length, depth, and distance from the visual axis all affect astigmatism.

4. LRIs are commonly used to correct preexisting astigmatism, and published nomograms are helpful in tailoring a surgical approach.

5. Toric IOLs and excimer laser ablation are alternative approaches to correcting astigmatism in the patient for refractive cataract surgery. No single approach is best suited for all patients.

REFERENCES

1. Lindstrom RL, Osher RH, Wang L. Control of astigmatism in the cataract patient. In: Steinert RF, ed. *Cataract Surgery: Technique, Complications, Management*. Philadelphia: WB Saunders; 2004:253-266.

2. Armeniades CD, Boriek A, Knolle Jr GE. Effect of incision length, location, and shape on local corneoscleral deformation during cataract surgery. *J Cataract Refract Surg*. 1990;16(1):83-87.

3. Samuelson SW, Koch DD, Kuglen CC. Determination of maximal incision length for true small-incision surgery. *Ophthalmic Surg*. 1991;22(4):204-207.

4. Spaeth G. *Ophthalmic Surgery: Principles and Practice*. 3rd ed. Philadelphia: WB Saunders; 2003.

5. Merriam JC, Zheng L, Merriam JE, Zaider M, Lindstrom B. The effect of incisions for cataract on corneal curvature. *Ophthalmology*. 2003;110(9):1807-1813.

6. Merriam JC, Zheng L, Urbanowicz J, Zaider M. Change on the horizontal and vertical meridians of the cornea after cataract surgery. *Trans Am Ophthalmol Soc*. 2001;99:187-195; discussion 195-187.

7. Tejedor J, Murube J. Choosing the location of corneal incision based on pre-existing astigmatism in phacoemulsification. *Am J Ophthalmol*. 2005;139(5):767-776.

8. Sporl E, Genth U, Schmalfuss K, Seiler T. Thermomechanical behavior of the cornea. *Ger J Ophthalmol*. 1996;5(6):322-327.

9. Tasman WM. *Duane's Ophthalmology 2006*. Philadelphia: Lippincott Williams & Wilkins; 2006.

10. Weiss JS, ed. *Refractive Surgery*. San Francisco, CA: American Academy of Ophthalmology; 2005.

11. Gills JP, Rowsey JJ. Managing coupling in secondary astigmatic keratotomy. *Int Ophthalmol Clin*. 2003;43(3):29-41.

12. Nichamin LD. Management of astigmatism in conjunction with lens surgery. In: Tasman WM, ed. *Duane's Ophthalmology 2006*. Philadelphia: Lippincott Williams & Wilkins; 2006.

13. Gills JP. *Nomogram for Limbal Relaxing Incisions with Cataract Surgery*. Tapron Springs, FL: St. Luke's Cataract and Laser Institute; 1999, available at: http://www.stlukeseye.com.

14. Wang L, Misra M, Koch DD. Peripheral corneal relaxing incisions combined with cataract surgery. *J Cataract Refract Surg.* 2003;29:712–722.

15. Cristóbal JA, del Buey MA, Ascaso FJ, Lanchares E, Calvo B, Doblaré M. Effect of limbal relaxing incisions during phacoemulsification surgery based on nomogram review and numerical simulation. *Cornea.* 2009;28(9):1042-1049.

16. Osher RH. Transverse astigmatic keratotomy combined with cataract surgery. *Ophthalmol Clin North Am.* 1992;5:717-725.

17. Ben Simon GJ, Desatnik H. Correction of pre-existing astigmatism during cataract surgery: comparison between the effects of opposite clear corneal incisions and a single clear corneal incision. *Graefes Arch Clin Exp Ophthalmol.* 2005;243(4):321-326.

18. Gills JP. Treating astigmatism at the time of cataract surgery. *Curr Opin Ophthalmol.* 2002;13(1):2-6.

19. Leyland M, Zinicola E, Bloom P, Lee N. Prospective evaluation of a plate haptic toric intraocular lens. *Eye.* 2001;15(Pt 2):202-205.

20. Sun XY, Vicary D, Montgomery P, Griffiths M. Toric intraocular lenses for correcting astigmatism in 130 eyes. *Ophthalmology.* 2000;107(9):1776-1781; discussion 1781-1772.

8

OPHTHALMIC VISCOSURGICAL DEVICES

Kathryn Bollinger, MD, PhD and Scott D. Smith, MD, MPH

I. INTRODUCTION

Viscoelastic substances play an essential role in intraocular surgery.[1-3] They are used in phacoemulsification cataract surgery to protect the corneal endothelium from mechanical damage and to deepen the anterior chamber, providing space for surgical manipulation. These substances, however, have a wide array of functions including injection at the pupil-anterior capsule junction to break synechiae in small-pupil cataract surgery and placement underneath nuclear fragments to prevent loss in the event of posterior capsule rupture.[3-6] In addition, viscoelastic substances are used to minimize further trauma to the zonules in cases of zonular dehiscence and to increase control during insertion of foldable intraocular lenses. Because of the myriad of important functions that viscoelastic substances serve in intraocular surgery they have been renamed ophthalmic viscosurgical devices (OVDs).[7]

II. HISTORICAL PERSPECTIVE

A number of surgical techniques were originally developed to protect the corneal endothelium and provide room for manipulation of intraocular tissues.[1-6] Initially, balanced salt solution and air were used but both were quickly lost from the anterior chamber during procedural movements. Sodium hyaluronate (Healon) was the first viscoelastic substance introduced commercially and was used in human intraocular surgery starting in 1979. Amvisc, released in 1983, is also a sodium hyaluronate product but is slightly less viscous than Healon. Methylcellulose (Methocel) was originally used in 1979 to coat implants prior to introduction into the anterior chamber. This OVD has since been mainly replaced by other substances because it requires

Henderson BA. *Essentials of Cataract Surgery, Second Edition (pp 81-85).*
© 2014 Taylor & Francis Group.

increased infusion pressure and use of a large-bore cannula for injection. Viscoat, a combination of chondroitin sulfate and sodium hyaluronate, was developed by Cooper Vision-Cilco and has traditionally provided useful tissue coating but is less effective at maintaining space and separating tissue because of its low viscosity.

III. RHEOLOGY

The clinical applications for the different OVDs are determined in large part by their rheologic properties, including viscosity, pseudoplasticity, viscoelasticity, and coatability.[1,8] Rheology is the study of the relationship between the deformation of physical bodies and the forces generated within them. In this regard, OVDs have some properties of fluids and some of solids and vary among each other with respect to many of these characteristics.

A. Viscosity

The viscosity of a solution is defined as its resistance to flow. This property is determined mainly by a composite of molecular weight and concentration; substances with high molecular weight and high concentration will have the highest viscosity. This is an important property of OVDs because high-viscosity solutions will be difficult to displace from the anterior chamber and will move tissues more effectively than those of low viscosity.

B. Pseudoplasticity

Substances have the property of pseudoplasticity when their viscosity changes with shear rate. Shear is the friction that occurs when a plate is made to move in relation to another plate with a solution between them. Shear rate is the speed at which the plate is moved in relation to the second plate. OVDs such as chondroitin sulfate do not have the property of pseudoplasticity; their viscosity is constant regardless of how fast the plate is moving. Substances such as sodium hyaluronate and methylcellulose, however, do show pseudoplasticity. Therefore, the faster the plate is moving, or the higher the shear rate, the lower the viscosity for these OVDs. This behavior is important in intraocular surgery because a substance with greater pseudoplasticity will move more easily through a small cannula as flow continues but will also more readily extrude from the anterior chamber during the turbulence of phacoemulsification.

C. Viscoelasticity

Elasticity is the ability of a material to return to its original shape after deformation. Substances without elasticity such as balanced salt solution will be forced into an adjoining space or out of the wound when the cornea is deformed by outside pressure. In contrast, all OVDs will promote reformation of corneal shape following stress such as occurs with corneal retraction or insertion or withdrawal of instrumentation. Therefore, anterior chamber volume will be maintained despite manipulation to varying degrees depending on the viscoelasticity of the OVD. Viscoelasticity also allows for ocular tissue protection from high frequency mechanical deformations that occur secondary to phacoemulsification vibrations or irrigating streams. The amount of viscoelasticity that a particular OVD displays is dependent on its viscosity, molecular length, and configuration.

D. Coatability

The coating ability of an OVD is determined mainly by surface tension and contact angle. Surface tension relates to the forces acting at the interface between a viscoelastic substance and a tissue or surgical instrument. The contact angle is the angle that a drop of substance forms with a flat surface. Lower surface tension and lower contact angle result in superior coatability. Substances that contain chondroitin sulfate such as Viscoat tend to show better coatability and are used, for example, to coat an implant prior to placement into the eye. Sodium hyaluronate tends to have less coatability.

IV. COHESIVE VERSUS DISPERSIVE

In general, ophthalmic surgeons group OVDs into 2 classes: cohesive and dispersive.[1-4,8] Cohesive OVDs contain long chains of sodium hyaluronate molecules and include Healon, Provisc, and Amvisc. They are high molecular weight, high-viscosity substances that tend to maintain space well when there is minimal movement within the anterior chamber. However, during conditions of turbulence (phacoemulsification) or other surgical manipulation, the long-chained cohesive OVDs tend to entangle and come out of the eye as a bolus. This results in suboptimal tissue protection during surgery. However, this type of OVD is easily removed from the eye at the end of the surgery and therefore presents little risk for unintentional retainment and postsurgical intraocular pressure (IOP) spikes.

Dispersive OVDs such as Viscoat, a combination of short-chained chondroitin sulfate and sodium hyaluronate, are low-viscosity, low molecular weight substances that also display low surface tension. This combination of properties allows these OVDs to separate and disperse in the anterior chamber thereby providing excellent coating and protection for the corneal endothelium during phacoemulsification. Because of their molecular structure, dispersive OVDs are also less likely to conglomerate and extrude from the eye than the cohesive substances. However, this property makes the dispersive OVDs more difficult to aspirate from the anterior chamber at the end of a procedure and this results in an increased risk for postoperative IOP spikes.

V. NEW OPHTHALMIC VISCOSURGICAL DEVICES

A new formulation of sodium hyaluronate has been recently introduced called Healon 5. This OVD has both a high molecular weight and high concentration and is inherently different in its physical properties when compared with both cohesive and dispersive substances.[9] Healon 5 has been termed *viscoadaptive* because it displays a combination of behaviors during intraocular surgery.[9,10] Because of its high molecular weight and concentration, this OVD is highly retentive and maintains the anterior chamber shape during surgical manipulation better than cohesive substances such as traditional Healon. However, Healon 5 can also be fractured and compartmentalized and therefore coats the endothelium similar to dispersive substances. Healon 5 must be fully aspirated from the anterior chamber at the end of a procedure because, if left behind, it may cause IOP spikes with greater frequency than the other OVDs.[11,12]

The appearance of a new OVD, DisCo Visc, has established another category for viscoelastic substances. DisCo Visc (hyaluronic acid 1% and chondroitin sulfate 4%) is classified as a higher viscosity dispersive OVD.[13] This substance has an intermediate to high viscosity but is still highly dispersive. DisCo Visc behaves like a cohesive OVD with respect to ease of removal from the anterior chamber. In addition, it provides endothelial protection similar to a dispersive substance. Therefore, this OVD has rheological characteristics that make it suitable for the entire surgical procedure.

VI. THE IDEAL OPHTHALMIC VISCOSURGICAL DEVICE

The ideal OVD is biocompatible within the eye, maintains space during surgical manipulation, and coats and protects intraocular tissues. It should also be easily removed from the anterior chamber at the end of a procedure and should have little effect on IOP. In addition, the ideal OVD should be low cost. These attributes are not entirely met by the OVDs currently available, but new developments and improvements continue to be made.

KEY POINTS

1. OVDs protect the corneal endothelium and provide space for surgical manipulation. Therefore, they play an essential role in cataract surgery.

2. OVDs are used in special surgical situations such as injection underneath nuclear fragments in the event of posterior capsule rupture.

3. Cohesive OVDs such as Healon and Provisc maintain space well but show poor endothelial coatability.

4. Dispersive OVDs provide excellent endothelial coating but are more difficult to aspirate from the anterior chamber at the end of a procedure.

5. New OVDs such as Healon 5 and DisCo Visc display a combination of cohesive and dispersive properties and may, therefore, have a wider range of uses than traditional viscoelastics.

REFERENCES

1. Liesegang T. Viscoelastic substances in ophthalmology. *Surv Ophthalmol.* 1990;34(4): 268-294.

2. Lane SS, Lindstrom RL. Viscoelastic agents: formulation, clinical applications, and complications. *Semin Ophthalmol.* 1992;7(4):253-260.

3. Tognetto D, Cecchini P, Ravalico G. Survey of ophthalmic viscosurgical devices. *Curr Opin Ophthalmol.* 2004;15:29-32.

4. Bissen-Miyajima H. Ophthalmic viscosurgical devices. *Curr Opin Ophthalmol.* 2008;19: 50-54.

5. Colvard D, Kandavel R. Viscoelastic solutions to challenging surgeries. *Rev Ophthalmol.* 2006;13(3):1-3.

6. Arshinoff SA. Dispersive-cohesive viscoelastic soft shell technique. *J Cataract Refract Surg.* 1999;25(2):167-173.

7. Arshinoff SA. New terminology: ophthalmic viscosurgical devices. *J Cataract Refract Surg.* 2000;26:627-628.

8. Arshinoff SA. The physical properties of ophthalmic viscoelastics in cataract surgery. *Ophthalmic Pract.* 1991;9:81-86.

9. Dick HB, Krummenauer F, Augustin AJ, Pakula T, Pfeiffer N. Healon5 viscoadaptive formulation: comparison to Healon and Healon GV. *J Cataract Refract Surg.* 2001;27(2):320-326.

10. Mammalis N. OVDs. Viscosurgical, viscoelastic, and viscoadaptive. What does this mean? *J Cataract Refract Surg.* 2002;28(9):1497-1498.

11. Dada T, Muralidhar R, Jhanji V. Intraocular pressure rise after use of Healon 5 during extracapsular cataract surgery. *Can J Ophthalmol.* 2007;42(2):338.

12. Modi SS. Safety, efficacy, and intraoperative characteristics of DisCoVisc and Healon ophthalmic viscosurgical devices for cataract surgery. *Clin Ophthalmol.* 2011;5:1381-1389.

13. Arshinoff SA, Jafari M. New classification of ophthalmic viscosurgical devices. *J Cataract Refract Surg.* 2005;11:2167-2171.

9

CAPSULORRHEXIS

Kevin M. Miller, MD

I. INTRODUCTION

A number of important technical advances facilitated the evolution from extracapsular cataract extraction with manual expression of the lens nucleus to small incision phacoemulsification. Lens removal by ultrasonic phacoemulsification was the main advancement, but other developments such as viscoelastics, foldable intraocular lenses (IOLs), and capsulorrhexis were also important. Viscoelastics, interchangeably known as ophthalmic viscosurgical devices (OVDs), coat and protect the corneal endothelium, iris, and lens capsule during surgery while maintaining space for the critical steps of surgery such as IOL implantation. Foldable IOLs allow the cataract incision to remain as small as the phacoemulsification needle. Capsulorrhexis ensures centration of the IOL within the capsular bag as the bag fibroses and contracts around the lens postoperatively. Arguably, other advances such as sutureless incision closure and topical anesthesia also played important roles in the evolution to small incision cataract surgery.

This chapter will review the rationale for capsulorrhexis, describe my method for performing it, and present solutions on how to avoid and handle problems. Special situations will also be discussed such as surgery in infants and children, posterior capsulorrhexis, optic capture, bimanual phacoemulsification, and the use of capsule stains. The reader should note that the accepted spelling of the word *capsulorrhexis* has evolved from one "r" to 2 rs. Older literature should be searched using the spelling *capsulorhexis*.

Henderson BA. *Essentials of Cataract Surgery, Second Edition (pp 87-100).*
© 2014 Taylor & Francis Group.

II. HISTORICAL OVERVIEW OF CAPSULORRHEXIS

The first IOL manufactured in the laboratory phase of foldable IOL development had a silicone plate-haptic design. The STAAR Surgical model AA4203 is the commercial version of this early lens. As a side note, the first foldable IOL actually sold in the United States was the Advanced Medical Optics SI18NB. This lens is a 3-piece foldable silicone lens with Prolene haptics. Plate-haptic IOLs were attractive to the early designers because they could be implanted through very small incisions. However, plate-haptic IOLs had to be implanted and remain inside the capsular bag because of their short overall length. If implanted in the ciliary sulcus, these IOLs would uniformly decenter. The dilemma facing the developers of the new foldable plate-haptic lens technology was how to confine the IOL to the capsular bag when the predominant anterior capsule opening at that time was a can-opener capsulotomy.[1]

In the days when extracapsular surgery with manual expression of the nucleus was the norm, surgeons were often polled as to where they thought they placed the IOL. Invariably, most surgeons felt they placed the optic and both haptics inside the capsular bag, even though they performed a can-opener capsulotomy. Ninety percent or more of the time the surgeons would be sure the lens was in the capsular bag. Many of these eyes were subsequently autopsied and a different perspective emerged. Pathologists found that one or both haptics were in the ciliary sulcus 50% of the time. Is it possible to reconcile these 2 perspectives or explain what happens to an IOL to change its position after implantation? The answer is yes. As the capsular bag contracts around an IOL after surgery, one of the haptics often pops out when there is a can-opener capsulotomy in the anterior capsule. One or more of the radial relaxing incisions in the anterior capsule splits open as the capsule fibroses. With plate haptic lenses, it is critical that they remain confined to the capsular bag for all time. The continuous tear of a capsulorrhexis ensures that any IOL implanted within the confines of the capsular bag will remain there forever.

III. HOW TO PERFORM A CAPSULORRHEXIS

This section describes my technique for performing a manual capsulorrhexis. Throughout the chapter, I will use the term *capsulorrhexis* instead of *anterior capsulorrhexis*, but these two are interchangeable. Posterior capsulorrhexis is described in Section VIII on p. 96. My capsulorrhexis technique is suitable for most types of cataracts.

- It is important to fill the anterior chamber with plenty of OVD. I inject enough that the anterior dome of the lens is flattened and OVD begins spilling out of the incision.
- The capsulotomy is begun by puncturing the anterior capsule with a bent 30-gauge needle. Either the surgeon or a scrub technician can

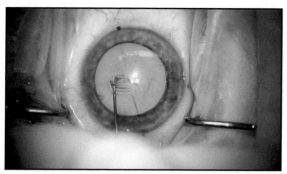

Figure 9-1. The capsule puncture and initial tear are best accomplished using a 30-gauge bent needle.

bend the needle using a needle holder. Prebent needles are available commercially, but I do not generally like the gauge or design of the needles currently available. I find that a 30-gauge needle gives maximum maneuverability inside the eye and excellent cutting power (Figure 9-1). Larger needles can be used, but the larger the gauge, the more trouble the surgeon will have avoiding contact with the corneal endothelium. Some surgeons like to use sharp-tipped capsulorrhexis forceps to make the initial capsule puncture. I find that the tips dull after a few uses.

- I prefer to make the initial puncture small and central. I am right-handed, so I start the puncture just right of center and slice the needle through the capsule to just left of center so that the initial tear is approximately 3 to 3.5 mm in length. The needle should be pushed in only as far as necessary to cut the capsule. Pushing too far in will stir up the cortex and force it up into the viscoelastic, obscuring the surgeon's view. This problem is particularly evident with milky white cortical cataracts. With the needle on the far left side of the tear, the capsule is elevated and pulled toward the incision, creating an edge that flops over toward the incision. A bent needle is much better for pulling the capsule toward the incision than pushing it away from the incision. The capsule flap should be left high in the OVD so that it can be grasped easily (Figure 9-2). It should not be pushed onto the capsule where it will be harder to engage.

- Next, the capsule flap is grasped with capsulorrhexis forceps. Many different types of capsulorrhexis forceps are available. Direct-action Utrata forceps are popular. I now prefer cross-action Inamura forceps (Figure 9-3). They work nicely through sub 2.4-mm incisions. It is important to keep the capsulorrhexis forceps in the middle of the phacoemulsification incision at all times so that the eye remains centered in the field of the microscope and the OVD remains inside the eye. The capsule should be torn with a shearing motion (ie, the capsule

Figure 9-2. The capsule is flapped over toward the incision, making it is easy to grasp.

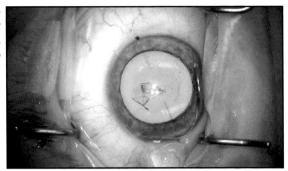

Figure 9-3. Capsulorrhexis forceps are used to complete the tear.

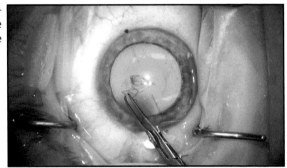

should be folded over and pulled tangentially in a spiral fashion until the desired diameter is reached). The tear beneath the incision is the hardest to make (Figure 9-4).

- After achieving the desired diameter, it is important to tear tangentially all the way around (Figure 9-5), maintaining a constant distance from the pupil margin. The distance to maintain depends on the diameter of the pupil. With most IOLs, it is appropriate to make the capsulorrhexis 0.5 to 1 mm smaller than the diameter of the optic. For a 6-mm optic, I make the capsulorrhexis 5 to 5.5 mm in diameter. The surgeon should regrasp the capsule whenever necessary. As a right-handed surgeon, I tear the capsulorrhexis in the counterclockwise direction. It might be easier for left-handed surgeons to tear in the clockwise direction.

- I usually find it necessary to regrasp the capsule flap 4 or 5 times to tear it all the way around. The surgeon should not be embarrassed to let go and regrasp. When letting go, the capsulorrhexis forceps should be released high up in the middle of the anterior chamber so the capsule will be easier to regrasp. When regrasping, never do so close to the cut edge. If the eye suddenly moves, the capsulorrhexis may

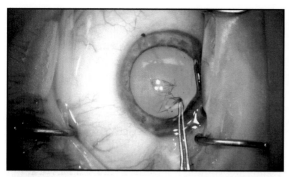

Figure 9-4. The hardest part of the capsulorrhexis is the turn beneath the incision.

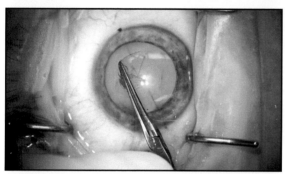

Figure 9-5. Optimal control is achieved when a shearing tear is utilized. The torn capsule is pulled tangentially all the way around, regrasping as necessary, and maintaining a constant distance from the pupil.

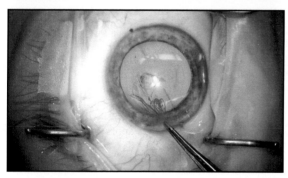

Figure 9-6. The goal of the capsulorrhexis step is a circular tear that is a little smaller than the diameter of the optic that will be implanted.

quickly radialize. Always grasp 1 to 3 mm upstream from the cut edge. The importance of tearing tangentially all the way around cannot be overemphasized. The capsulorrhexis is completed on the left side of the pupil in the surgeon's view (Figure 9-6). For a left-handed surgeon, the capsulorrhexis is completed on the right side of the pupil. I like to pull the capsule out of the eye using the capsulorrhexis forceps, but it is not entirely necessary. If left in, it will come out during the hydrodissection or phacoemulsification step.

IV. PITFALLS AND HOW TO AVOID THEM

The hardest part of cataract surgery for the beginning surgeon is making a consistently good capsulorrhexis. Frequent practice is important for improving. For those who have access, the Eyesi Surgical simulator for cataract (VRmagic Holding AG) is an excellent surgical simulator for practicing capsulorrhexis. In this section, I will review a few common capsulorrhexis pitfalls and offer my advice for dealing with them.

- A capsulorrhexis can always be made larger, but it can never be made smaller. It is important to make the initial capsule puncture and tear small and central, and then spiral it out to the desired diameter. If the initial capsule tear goes wide, the entire capsulorrhexis will be larger than necessary. A capsulorrhexis that overlaps the edge of the optic for 360 degrees is optimal for retarding posterior capsule opacification. Tight adhesion of the anterior and posterior capsule leaflets impedes migration of lens epithelial cells behind the optic. A capsulorrhexis that overlaps the optic 360 degrees also makes it safer when it comes time to make a circular Nd:YAG laser posterior capsulotomy opening. When the anterior capsulotomy goes wide of the optic, vitreous will occasionally migrate around the edge of the optic into the anterior chamber.

- The most common problem experienced by beginning surgeons is outward radialization of the capsulorrhexis. The trick is to recognize the impending problem before the tear extends too far peripherally. The common beginner mistake is to pull the flap radially in toward the center of the pupil when the radialization begins to happen, as though one were swinging a rock in the circle at the end of a rope. Pulling the capsule flap centrally converts the shearing tear into a ripping tear. Ripping is inherently less controlled. The capsule tends to run radially outward when it is ripped.[2]

- The first thing a surgeon should do when the capsulorrhexis begins to extend peripherally is stop and inject more OVD to flatten the anterior dome of the lens. Then the capsule should be flopped over so that it aligns with the tangent of the intended circle. Sometimes it is necessary to tear the capsule outwardly a little bit before it can be brought around. If the capsulorrhexis goes out beneath the pupil, the surgeon can continue the tear as long as he or she has a sense of where it is going. Sometimes it is useful to introduce a Kuglen iris push-pull hook to push the pupil back and visualize the tear as it is being redirected. If control cannot be achieved at the tear site, the surgeon should stop. Indiscriminate pulling on the capsule flap will cause the tear to go posteriorly through the zonules and around the backside of the lens. Capsulorrhexis rescue techniques described in Section

VI (p. 94) should be used at this point. Alternatively, the surgeon can puncture the capsule again with a 30-gauge needle and tear it in the reverse direction. The 2 tears can be joined at the point where the initial tear went wide.

- Another common problem is difficulty visualizing the capsule. This occurs most often when a tear proceeds over an area where white cortical material is present. The key here is good focus and magnification. Before capsule stains were available, all surgeons had to confront this problem head-on. It helps to avoid stirring up the cortex. The surgeon should not press down on the capsule when the cortex is milky because this will stir cortical lens material into the OVD. Using capsulorrhexis forceps after the initial capsule puncture instead of a bent needle puts less pressure on the capsule. The more the capsule is depressed, the more cortex that will be expressed. If the OVD becomes mixed with cortex and the view degrades, an irrigation-aspiration probe can be inserted and the contaminated viscoelastic material removed. More OVD can be injected to improve visibility and the tear can continue under high magnification. If the surgeon anticipates visibility problems at the outset, he or she should stain the capsule before it is punctured.

- A final problem for beginning surgeons has to do with ergonomics. Many surgeons like to hold the capsulorrhexis forceps with one hand. I prefer maneuvering them with 2 hands. I use my right hand to grasp the forceps; I keep my left index finger on the instrument just outside the incision. I find I have more control if I pivot the forceps inside the eye around my index finger. It is also important, as I mentioned earlier, to stay at the center of the phacoemulsification incision and not up against the edge or roof of the tunnel. The beginning surgeon is usually so interested in what is happening at the tip of the forceps that no attention is paid to what is happening to the eye as a whole. Often the eye is badly rotated, full of corneal striae, and virtually out of the field of the microscope. Staying wound neutral throughout the procedure is important for maximizing visibility.

V. SPECIAL CONSIDERATION IN INFANTS AND CHILDREN

Infants and children have soft lenses and elastic capsules. They also have little scleral rigidity. When an incision is made into the pediatric eye, the anterior chamber shallows, putting additional stress on the anterior capsule. When the capsule of an infant or child is punctured, it often radializes immediately.[3]

- It is important to fill completely, or even overfill, the anterior chamber of an infant's eye with OVD before the capsule is punctured. Highly retentive cohesive viscoelastics are particularly useful for flattening the dome of the anterior lens capsule. It is best to have little or no convexity in the anterior capsule of an infant. The capsulorrhexis tends to run off the surface of the dome very quickly and it can radialize before the surgeon has a chance to gain control.

- It is important to make the initial capsulotomy small and central and to spiral it out to a very small diameter. I generally shoot for an initial size of 3 to 3.5 mm in infants. It never stays this small; it always goes wider. If the initial tear is extended to 4 or 4.5 mm, it will be very difficult to maintain that diameter as the capsulorrhexis proceeds.

- Whenever it is evident that the capsulorrhexis is going wide, the surgeon should stop and inject more viscoelastic to flatten the dome of the lens again. It may be necessary to do this several times before the capsulorrhexis is completed. There is no problem making a capsulotomy 3 mm in diameter, removing the cataract, and going back to enlarge the capsulotomy secondarily. Much greater control will be achieved once the bulk of the lens is removed from the capsule.

- The general problem of capsule elasticity, posterior pressure, and tendency for radialization may continue into teenage and early adult years. Increasing scleral rigidity and lens rigidity and decreasing capsule elasticity combine to make the capsulorrhexis easier with time and increasing age.

VI. CAPSULORRHEXIS RESCUE

The capsulorrhexis does not always proceed the way the surgeon wants. Sometimes intralenticular pressure makes it run wide. This is particularly common in the white intumescent cataract, which produces the Argentinian flag sign. Intralenticular pressure is also common in the infant eye. Less commonly, posterior pressure from a tight lid speculum, a Valsalva maneuver, a sudden uncontrolled pull on the flap, or an inadequate OVD fill of the anterior chamber can cause the capsulorrhexis to run wide.

When the surgeon sees that the capsulorrhexis is beginning to run wide, he or she should immediately stop and assess the situation. Are any of the causative factors listed above at play? If yes, they should be addressed. It never hurts to inject additional amounts of highly cohesive OVD to flatten the dome of the anterior capsule. If the tear has not gone too far out, flapping it over and pulling tangentially in a shearing fashion should allow the surgeon to regain control.

If this does not work, a technique espoused by Brian Little should be tried next. His technique is to inject OVD to completely fill the anterior chamber,

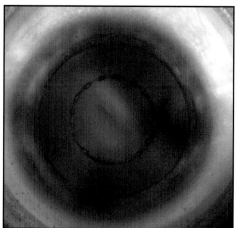

Figure 9-7. A femtosecond laser can make a capsulorrhexis that is predictably sized and positioned.

unfold and flatten the capsular flap, grasp the flap near the root of the tear, and put traction on the flap in the capsular plane—backward first, then centrally, but never anteriorly.[4] As the tear circles back around, the usual technique can be resumed.

VII. FEMTOSECOND LASER CAPSULORRHEXIS

Problems with capsulorrhexis size, circularity, and placement have been solved in large measure by femtosecond laser technology, although new problems have arisen. A femtosecond laser creates a tiny gas bubble at each location where it is fired. A cylinder pattern is applied at the desired diameter starting some distance inside the lens and finishing some distance anterior to the lens capsule, thereby compensating for any tilt of the lens relative to the laser interface. A small amount of tissue coagulation may also occur as strain gauge testing of capsulorrhexis strength demonstrates that openings made by femtosecond lasers withstand a greater amount of mechanical stretching than those made by continuous tear techniques (Figure 9-7).

Seldom is the anterior capsule freely floating in the anterior chamber after a femtosecond laser creates it. It is usually tethered to the anterior lens cortex. In some cases, there are "postage stamp" tags where the laser did not completely amputate the capsule. In some of these, the skip areas may be the result of the patient interface device. Rigid curved interfaces may cause endothelial folds that interfere with imaging and laser energy delivery. Even with liquid optic interfaces, skip lesions can develop if subtle corneal opacities block laser light delivery to a portion of the capsule. The surgeon should remove the amputated capsule cautiously. Tags can be resistant to tearing in the usual sense and radial run away tears may extend posteriorly.

Because femtosecond lasers facilitate the predictability of capsulorrhexis size and location, they may improve effective lens position calculations. Additionally, they may reduce the rate of posterior capsule opacification since 360-degree optic overlap of square edge lenses has been shown to reduce the posterior migration of lens epithelial cells. Lastly, they may enable the widespread adoption of accommodating lenses that are dependent on the geometry of the capsulorrhexis, such as the Synchrony dual optic intraocular lens (Visiogen, Abbott Medical Optics).

VIII. POSTERIOR CAPSULORRHEXIS

Posterior capsules in infants and children often cloud quickly after cataract surgery. Nd:YAG lasers that shoot straight down are not widely available for performing posterior capsulotomies on patients who are supine on an operating table. Therefore, many surgeons prefer to open the pediatric posterior capsule, and even perform a limited anterior vitrectomy, at the time of cataract surgery.

A. Advantages

A posterior capsulorrhexis has all the advantages of an anterior capsulorrhexis. An IOL can be implanted in the capsular bag if there are well-constructed, continuous anterior and posterior capsulotomies. In addition to providing optimum long-term centration of the IOL, there is no chance of uveitis developing because of haptic erosion into vascular tissue in the ciliary sulcus.

B. Technique

Performing a good posterior capsulorrhexis is trickier than performing a good anterior capsulorrhexis because the capsular bag is floppy at the time it is done. There is no lens material to provide counter-traction. The technique for creating a posterior capsulorrhexis depends on whether a pars planavitrectomy was previously performed and whether a plaque is present on the capsule, but the basics are similar from case to case. A straight 30-gauge needle is used to puncture the capsule centrally, and viscoelastic is injected between the capsule and the anterior hyaloid, if it is still present. This causes the posterior capsule to dome forward. Capsulorrhexis forceps are then used to grasp the capsule and tear it in a circular fashion. The surgeon should attempt to tear the capsule tangentially, as is the case with the anterior capsule, but this can be difficult. The posterior capsulorrhexis should be kept relatively small initially because it tends to radialize. When a posterior capsule plaque is present, the surgeon should tear around the plaque if it is not too large. It is difficult to tear through a plaque. If a plaque extends beyond the diameter of the desired capsulorrhexis, I may use Vannas or retinal scissors to cut through it rather than tear around it.

I often perform a posterior capsulorrhexis if a patient has a history of a pars plana vitrectomy and develops a dense central posterior capsule plaque. In such eyes, there is little concern over vitreous loss and the plaque may impair visual recovery for a long time before a laser capsulotomy can be performed safely. Any remaining anterior cortical gel can be removed quickly after the posterior capsulorrhexis has been made. The risks of cystoid macular edema and retinal tear or detachment usually associated with inadvertent posterior capsule rupture should be relatively low in the setting of a previous pars planavitrectomy.

IX. OPTIC CAPTURE

It is possible to capture the optic of an IOL, if necessary, in a good capsulorrhexis.[5] For instance, if the posterior capsule is completely blown open, the surgeon can place the haptics of the lens in the ciliary sulcus and capture the optic posteriorly through the capsulorrhexis. This might be desirable, for instance, if the diameter of the haptics on the IOL is insufficient for proper sulcus fixation. There are many ways to capture an optic. Both haptics can be placed in the ciliary sulcus and the optic can be pushed through both the anterior and posterior capsulorrhexis openings. This is often done in pediatric eyes to retard lens epithelial cell migration over the anterior hyaloid. Alternatively, the haptics can be placed inside the capsular bag and the optic can be captured anterior to the capsulorrhexis. In all cases, the capsulorrhexis must be smaller than the optic for the optic to remain captured. The primary benefit of optic capture is that it ensures centration of the optic when things are not perfect. A disadvantage is that the capsule opening tends to stretch in the direction in which the haptics insert into the optic and narrow in the other direction. The capsule opening then takes on an oval or marquise shape with a short diameter in one meridian that may cause glare symptoms at night.

X. CAPSULORRHEXIS IN BIMANUAL PHACOEMULSIFICATION

Standard capsulorrhexis forceps, especially Utrata forceps, are too large to manipulate through an incision that is less than 2-mm wide. Special capsulorrhexis forceps have been developed for smaller incisions such as those used in bimanual or sleeveless phacoemulsification. These instruments have a circular shaft and a spring-loaded mechanism that allows the user to pinch the handles at the proximal end of the device to open and close small forceps at the distal end. These forceps are elegant for making a capsulorrhexis through a sub 2-mm incision, but they are more difficult to use than standard capsulorrhexis forceps.

XI. CAPSULE STAINING

A. Indications

Good visualization is critical for performing each step of the capsulorrhexis. I use higher magnification and excellent focus to give the best visualization of the capsule. If the cortex is white or a nucleus is densely brunescent, staining the capsule will facilitate visualization.[6] I find it useful to stain the capsule when I implant additional devices in the capsular bag such as Morcher artificial iris segments (Morcher GmbH). Trypan blue is the most common capsule dye in use at this time. Methylene blue should not be used, as it is toxic to the corneal endothelium. Indocyanine green does not stain the capsule as well as trypan blue.

B. Technique

Staining the anterior capsule is a simple procedure. A large air bubble is injected into the anterior chamber after the paracentesis is created and before OVD is injected. The capsule stain is injected through the air bubble onto the anterior lens surface. I find it helpful to rub or paint the dye into the capsule using the injection cannula; this increases the staining effect. Balanced salt solution is then injected to wash out most of the dye. OVD is injected next to increase the space available so that the capsulorrhexis can be performed in the usual fashion. The surgeon will note improved contrast between the capsule and underlying lens material once the capsule is punctured with the bent 30-gauge needle, making it easier to visualize the edge of the capsulorrhexis. The capsule will be a little more brittle as it is torn because of the trypan blue (Figure 9-8).

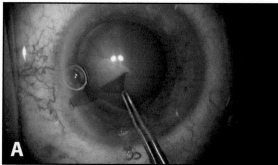

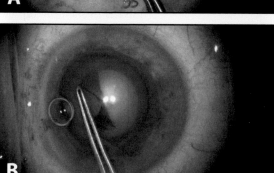

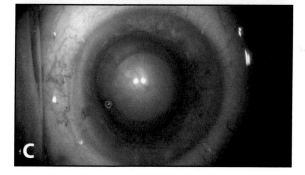

Figures 9-8. Trypan blue may be used to enhance contrast in the setting of a mature cortical or dense brunescent cataract. In this example, the patient had a white cataract and associated zonular rupture with lens indentation or "coloboma" from remote eye trauma.

Key Points

1. The primary benefit of a capsulorrhexis is that it confines the IOL to the capsular bag as the capsule fibroses and contracts around the lens.

2. Start the capsulorrhexis by making the initial puncture with a bent 30-gauge needle and flopping the tear toward the incision so that it can be grasped using capsulorrhexis forceps.

3. Always pull tangentially when tearing the capsulorrhexis to maintain optimum control.

4. If you start to lose control, inject more viscoelastic material and begin tearing tangentially again. If the capsulorrhexis extends beneath the pupil margin, repuncture the capsule and tear it in the reverse direction or use the Brian Little capsulorrhexis rescue technique.

5. It takes practice to become good at creating a uniformly consistent capsulorrhexis.

References

1. Gimbel HV, Neuhann T. Continuous curvilinear capsulorhexis. *J Cataract Refract Surg.* 1991;17:110-111.

2. Seibel BS. *Phacodynamics: Mastering the Tools and Techniques of Phacoemulsification Surgery.* 4th ed. Thorofare, NJ: SLACK Incorporated; 2005.

3. Gimbel HV, Basti S. Optimal capsulorhexis technique in pediatric eyes. *J Cataract Refract Surg.* 1996;22:3-4.

4. Little BC, Smith SH, Packer M. Little capsulorhexis tear-out rescue. *J Cataract Refract Surg.* 2006;32:1420-1422.

5. Gimbel HV, DeBroff BM. Intraocular lens optic capture. *J Cataract Refract Surg.* 2004;30:200-206.

6. Jacobs DS, Cox TA, Wagoner MD, Ariyasu RG, Karp CL. American Academy of Ophthalmology; Ophthalmic Technology Assessment Committee Anterior Segment Panel. Capsule staining as an adjunct to cataract surgery: a report from the American Academy of Ophthalmology. *Ophthalmology.* 2006;113:707-713.

10

HYDRODISSECTION AND HYDRODELINEATION

Eydie Miller-Ellis, MD

I. INTRODUCTION

Hydrodissection and hydrodelineation are sandwiched between the more glamorous phacoemulsification steps of capsulorrhexis and nucleus removal. Hydrodissection and hydrodelineation separate the nucleus from the surrounding cortex and are essential for safe nuclear rotation during phacoemulsification and nuclear delivery during standard extracapsular cataract extraction.

The goal is first to shear the attachments between the lens capsule and its surrounding cortex (hydrodissection) and then to separate the epinuclear bowl from its attachment to the lens nucleus (hydrodelineation). Successful completion of these steps will result in a lens nucleus that can be freely rotated during nucleus sculpture and division (thus minimizing stress on the zonule), an epinuclear bowl that protects the lens capsule during nucleus removal, and a cortex that can be more easily removed. Hydrodissection also loosens the nucleus and facilitates nuclear expression in standard extracapsular cataract extraction.

Hydrodissection is the great facilitator of cataract surgery. It is low-tech in terms of the instruments needed to complete this maneuver, thus it is an underappreciated step. Hydrodelineation, although not essential, is desirable because it separates the harder nucleus from the softer, adherent epinucleus. The resultant epinuclear bowl helps protect the lens capsule from instrument trauma as the nucleus is manipulated.

Henderson BA. *Essentials of Cataract Surgery, Second Edition (pp 101-105).*
© 2014 Taylor & Francis Group.

II. INSTRUMENTS

The instruments needed to complete this step are very simple: a 25- to 30-gauge cannula and a 3-cc syringe.

A. Cannula

The 25- to 30-gauge cannula is typically angled or curved to facilitate placement under the anterior lens capsule. The tip may be flattened to allow it to slip under the capsule more easily. A J-tip cannula may be used to hydrodissect the subincisional cortex.

B. Syringe

A 3-cc syringe is the ideal size for intraocular use. It can be handled easily with one hand and has good tactile feedback during the injection. A tuberculin syringe (1 cc) does not allow enough injection force or fluid volume to achieve optimal hydrodissection. A 5 or 10-cc syringe may result in greater force with injection but less control during the maneuver.[1]

III. TECHNIQUE

A. Preparation

If the anterior chamber (AC) is still filled with viscoelastic from the preceding capsulorrhexis, partially empty the AC to make room for the increased fluid volume that will occur with this step. If a very dispersive/retentive viscoelastic such as Healon 5 (Advanced Medical Optics) is used, tracks should be made in the material with the hydrodissection cannula to make a pathway for the balanced salt solution (BSS) to exit the eye. Otherwise, the expanded fluid volume in the AC can lead to blowout of the lens capsule or lens during this maneuver.

B. Hydrodissection

The hydrodissection cannula is placed on a 3-cc syringe filled with BSS. The tip of the cannula is then passed beneath the anterior lens capsule a sufficient distance to allow a forward wave of fluid during injection. Otherwise there is backflow into the AC and ineffective hydrodissection. Fluid must be injected with sufficient force to shear adhesions between the lens capsule and cortex. Repeat this maneuver 2 to 3 times at different locations to ensure complete dissection. Using the heel of the hydrodissection cannula, gentle depression of the nucleus after irrigating the BSS can be helpful to propagate the fluid wave completely and prevent capsular blowout.

HELPFUL HINTS

1. Use your nondominant hand to stabilize the syringe and your dominant hand for injection. This helps maintain control of the syringe while the plunger is being depressed. The nondominant hand serves as a fulcrum and support while the dominant hand performs this maneuver.

2. After the fluid wave is complete, the lens nucleus shifts anteriorly due to the increased fluid volume between the nucleus and the capsule bag. Gently press on the anterior lens surface with the hydrodissection cannula to decompress the fluid from behind the lens, thus making space for additional hydrodissection.

C. Hydrodelineation

For hydrodelineation, the cannula tip is placed into the edge of the epinucleus. The fluid must be injected with more force than during hydrodissection because the epinuclear-nuclear adhesion is stronger than the cortex-epinuclear adhesion. The fluid wave results in the appearance of a "golden ring," which indicates successful epinuclear separation.

D. Potential Complications

The most feared complication of hydrodissection is damage to the lens capsule. Mechanical trauma from the cannula itself can occur if the cannula is placed too forcefully and peripherally under the anterior capsule and causes mechanical disruption of the capsule. In addition, if the capsulorrhexis is small and the nucleus itself blocks egress of the injected fluid from the capsule bag, the fluid can build up behind the nucleus, distend the capsule, and result in a posterior capsular rupture. This is more common with a large dense nucleus. This "intracapsular capsular block syndrome"[2,3] can be avoided by tilting the nucleus with the cannula tip to allow egress of the injected fluid and by ensuring that the capsulorrhexis is at least 5 mm in diameter.

A lens with a fibrotic posterior subcapsular plaque is also at higher risk of posterior capsule rupture during hydrodissection because the capsule may be weak at the area of fibrosis and prone to tearing at the interface. Slow, limited hydrodissection may be more prudent in this case. In addition, concentrating more on hydrodelineation will allow mobilization of the lens while still protecting the capsule.

The cannula may also be inadvertently placed above the anterior capsule.[4] The fluid will then be injected at the lens zonule and track back to the vitreous. This vitreous hydration increases posterior pressure and shallows the AC. If this occurs, decompress the AC and wait 5 to 10 minutes for the eye to re-equilibrate. Hydrodissection can usually be continued, but the AC remains shallow and the vitreous may need to be decompressed in some cases.

E. Special Technique: Cortical Cleavage Hydrodissection

1. Cortical cleavage hydrodissection

Fine described a technique called *cortical cleavage hydrodissection*,[5] the purpose of which is to cleave the cortex from the lens capsule during hydrodissection so that more will remain attached to the epinucleus. Thus, cortex will be removed along with the epinuclear bowl and the amount of cortex remaining is minimized, thus decreasing the time needed for cortical cleanup. To achieve this, the cannula tip is used to tent up the anterior capsule and advanced so that the injection occurs near the lens equator. Care must be taken not to inject any fluid until the cannula tip is in position under the anterior capsule. After the injection, decompress the nucleus prior to initiating the next fluid wave.

2. Posterior polar cataracts

There may be a congenital absence of the central pole of the posterior capsule in posterior polar cataracts. Hydrodissection is often not recommended in these cases, and only gentle hydrodelineation is performed. Minimal ultrasound energy is used for nucleus removal, and viscodissection is used to mobilize the epinucleus and cortex,[6] which helps prevent posterior capsular rupture and potential dislocation of the lens onto the vitreous cavity.

IV. CONCLUSION

Hydrodissection is an essential step in safe phacoemulsification. The ability to freely rotate the nucleus is crucial to minimizing zonular stress during nucleus removal. As with all steps in cataract surgery, successful completion of each step facilitates the completion of the next.

KEY POINTS

1. Keep the cannula tip beneath the anterior capsule while injecting fluid.
2. Apply slow, constant pressure on the syringe so that the fluid wave will propagate.
3. Watch for a complete fluid wave to ensure adequate hydrodissection.
4. Watch for the "golden ring" sign as confirmation of hydrodelineation.
5. Confirm rotation of the lens before proceeding to phacoemulsification.

REFERENCES

1. Chang DF. Six tips on hydrodissection technique. *Cataract and Refractive Surgery Today.* Available at: http://www.crstoday.com. Accessed 05.03. 07.
2. Miyake K. Intraoperative capsular block syndrome: the condition causes a dropped nucleus. *Cataract and Refractive Surgery Today.* Available at: http://www.crstoday. com. Accessed 05.03. 07.
3. Ota I, Miyake S, Miyake K. Dislocation of the lens nucleus into the vitreous cavity after standard hydrodissection. *Am J Ophthalmol.* 1996;121:706-708.
4. Fishkind WJ. Avoiding and managing complications from hydrodissection. *Cataract and Refractive Surgery Today.* Available at: http://www.crstoday.com. Accessed 05.03.07.
5. Fine III. Cortical cleavage hydrodissection. *J Cataract Refract Surg.* 1992;18(5):508-512.
6. Fine IH, Packer M, Hoffman RS. Management of posterior polar cataract. *J Cataract Refract Surg.* 2003;29(1):16-19.

11

FLUIDICS/PUMPS

John D. Au, MD and Roger H. S. Langston, MD

I. INTRODUCTION

Small incision cataract surgery requires the flow of fluid through the eye in order to dissipate the heat created by the phaco needle, to remove the emulsified nucleus, to strip the residual cortical material, and to remove the viscoelastics. The flow must be controlled well enough to maintain the anterior chamber and avoid damage to the delicate structures of the eye. In this closed system, the movement of the fluid is modulated by varying height of the infusion bottle, the aspiration flow rate, and the vacuum settings of the pump (Figure 11-1). Modern phacoemulsification machines allow for fixed or linear control of most of these parameters as well as other features such as surge control, automatic attenuation of phaco power under low flow conditions, and variable rise times. Other factors that affect the movement of material through this system include the nature of the material in the anterior chamber and the lines and the amount of occlusion at the phaco or irrigation/aspiration (I/A) tip. The use of burst and pulsed modes of phaco power also can influence flow.

II. INFLOW

Infusion of fluid into the eye can be created by a programmable pump, but it is often a gravity feed system in which the pressure is created by a difference between the bottle height and the patient's eye (not the bottle height above the machine although this ideally should be the same). Infusion flow needs only to be high enough to match current and anticipated outflow.

Bottle height and inflow must be adjusted as outflow is altered by changes in the machine settings or by surgical maneuvers, otherwise an unstable

Henderson BA. *Essentials of Cataract Surgery, Second Edition (pp 107-115)*.
© 2014 Taylor & Francis Group.

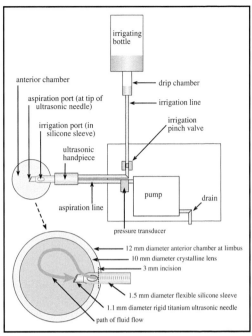

anterior chamber will result. The bottle height will usually need to be higher
with higher aspiration rates and with incisions that are less competent
(leaky). Air pump or forced infusion systems, founded on systems such as
the Alcon ACCURUS, utilize air generated by a pump to actively push fluid
into the eye independent of bottle height. The advantages are a more constant
intraoperative anterior chamber volume and minimal surge.

Inflow tubing is usually wider in diameter and softer than outflow tubing
as compliance is less of an issue on the inflow side and the softer tubing
improves ergonomics. On the outflow side tubing needs to be more rigid (less
compliant) to minimize surge[1] (see following text).

III. OUTFLOW

Control of outflow is multifactorial and influenced by several factors at the
same time. These include incision architecture, phacoemulsification and I/A
tip and port size, pump type, tubing size and compliance, vacuum, venting,
and aspiration settings.

Incision width should be standardized for the phaco tip and I/A instrument used. The incision should not be watertight. Consequently some flow
around the instrument is inevitable, and for the most part is useful in helping
to avoid wound burns and prevent heating of the phaco needle. If the incision
is too large, it may result in damage to the eye tissues from excessive flow

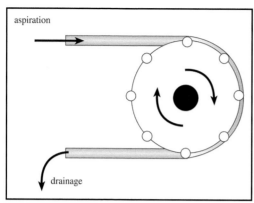

aspiration

drainage

Figure 11-2. Peristaltic pump. (Reprinted with permission from Seibel BS. *Phacodynamics: Mastering the Tools and Techniques of Phacoemulsification Surgery.* 4th ed. Thorofare, NJ: SLACK Incorporated; 2005.)

and difficulty in maintaining a stable anterior chamber. If it is too narrow (tight) and/or too long, it may lead to crimping of the infusion sleeve as the instrument is manipulated, impairing inflow and causing an unstable anterior chamber or thermal damage.

Most of the fluid exiting the eye is removed by the phaco machine pump. Two major types of pump are in common use in phaco systems: flow pumps (peristaltic) and vacuum pumps (Venturi). Hybrid pumps with features of both systems could be considered to be a third type.

Peristaltic pumps (Figure 11-2), a type of flow pump, control fluid movement through the outflow line by the action of a series of rollers that move along the flexible outflow tubing, forcing fluid through the system. This also creates a relative vacuum at the aspiration port when it is partially or completely occluded. The flow rate is controlled by the speed of the rollers, as is the rise time (the interval between occlusion and reaching maximum vacuum). It should be noted that flow and aspiration with the pump system are essentially the same. The vacuum level is determined by how long the rollers run when the line is occluded. The advantage of this system is that vacuum and flow (aspiration) can be independently controlled. In this type of pump, vacuum is used primarily to hold the material at the tip of the hand piece (like glue). Flow (aspiration rate) is adjusted to modify the speed at which material is swept toward the tip (like a magnet). Partial occlusion reduces flow through the system.[2]

A common form of vacuum pump (Figure 11-3) is based on the Venturi principle: the flow of gas or liquid across a port creates a vacuum proportional to the rate of flow. The vacuum is then utilized in these pumps to create a fluid flow. Decreasing the vacuum decreases the pump flow. Vacuum level and aspiration flow rates are *not* independently controlled. The rise time depends on vacuum level and varies inversely with it. Vacuum pumps characteristically have a rapid rise time.

Figure 11-3. Vacuum pump. (Reprinted with permission from Seibel BS. *Phacodynamics: Mastering the Tools and Techniques of Phacoemulsification Surgery.* 4th ed. Thorofare, NJ: SLACK Incorporated; 2005.)

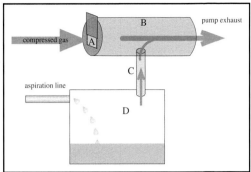

In a Venturi pump, the direct linear control of vacuum allows indirect linear control of aspiration rate as long as the aspiration port is not occluded. Unlike a flow pump, in vacuum pumps, bottle height and inflow will influence outflow unless the aspiration port is occluded.[2]

Hybrid pump systems such as Allergan's SOVEREIGN and Bausch and Lomb's CONCENTRIX pumps can be digitally programmed to behave like a peristaltic or a vacuum pump with the goal of adding flexibility for the surgeon.

IV. SETTINGS

The fluidic systems for phaco units are designed to be effective and safe with the use of hand pieces and tubing of various configurations, and the companies who manufacture them have recommended settings of their machines. Nonetheless, surgeons have the opportunity and responsibility to adjust these settings in order to maximize the efficiency and safety of the procedure for various surgical circumstances. Understanding the nuances of this subject is gained chiefly through surgical experience. However, some principles are basic.

Inflow should be adequate to maintain the anterior chamber even as the outflow through the incisions and the pump varies. The bottle height will usually need to be higher with higher aspiration flow rates and with larger, leakier incisions. However, if the incision is very large, as in converting a phaco case to an extracapsular extraction for example, the bottle height will need to be lowered in order to reduce flow and reduce the risk of iris prolapse and other complications. The high inflow pressures used in contemporary phaco surgery are only acceptable with a controlled outflow system.

Some phaco experts have advocated very low flow rates, inflow and outflow, in order to slow the pace of events in the anterior chamber, especially for beginning phaco surgeons. This makes sense as higher flow rates speed up movement of nuclear material, and potentially of iris and capsule; however, when reducing flow it is important to maintain sufficient flow to cool the phaco tip and prevent incision burns. Bottle height will have to be raised (elevated) with the higher flow rates associated with quadrant removal or phaco chop techniques. Bottle height should be evaluated hydrodynamically with the pump running and the port unoccluded so that adequate inflow will match outflow. Consideration should also be given for the effects of surge (see below).

Sculpting of the nucleus (low aspiration, low vacuum in a peristaltic system) can be done with very little vacuum as the nuclear material is stabilized by the zonules and capsule. Vacuum is not needed to hold the nuclear material at the phaco tip. The aspiration rate needs only be adequate for removing the nuclear material and cooling (approximately 20 cc per minute is usually adequate).

When manipulating nuclear fragments or quadrants, vacuum and aspiration (flow) usually have to be higher, especially with dense cataracts, in order to counter the tendency of the longitudinal ultrasound energy to push material away from the tip. Baseline settings of 30 cc per minute flow and 200 mm Hg vacuum are a reasonable starting point. Torsional phaco tips, such as Alcon's OZiL, decrease tip occlusion time and repulsion associated with traditional longitudinal ultrasound. This, in turn, decreases the need for higher flow and vacuum settings, and therefore reduces the risk of surge.[3,4]

For chopping, a similar aspiration flow rate with a vacuum of 300 mm Hg is a compromise between an acceptable rapid rise time and a safety margin against surge. The higher vacuum level may be needed in order to grasp and manipulate the nucleus. Surge, or postocclusion surge, occurs when a fragment that is occluding the port is suddenly aspirated at high vacuum levels usually as the fragment is phacoemulsified. Surge is due in large measure to the compliance of the plastic tubing within the pump. As the vacuum pressure increases, the tubing partially collapses. The tubing then snaps open when the vacuum is released, causing a sudden surge of fluid into the line. This causes a partial collapse of the anterior chamber and a sudden forward movement of the posterior capsule. Surge effects can be minimized by using lower vacuum, lower aspiration rates, and higher infusion bottle height. Some phaco needles also have an aspiration bypass port to allow slight flow when the tip is occluded. Such bypass systems, such as that found on the Alcon phaco needles, incorporate small holes in the shaft of the phaco tip to provide this alternate fluid pathway during tip occlusion, thereby decreasing surge. Manufacturers also utilize more rigid (less compliant) tubing in aspiration lines. The inherent resistance to flow of aspirated material in the line also probably modulates surge, especially with smaller hose tubing. Microprocessors are also now available to modify surge by sensing the restoration of flow after occlusion and immediately lowering vacuum by slowing or reversing the pump. When utilizing equipment with such surge-control features, vacuum levels in excess of 500 mm Hg may be safely used.

Scroll pumps put the pump directly in the aspiration flow path and therefore can utilize tubing with the minimum compliance needed for hand piece control, hence decreasing surge potential.

Vacuum pumps can also utilize relatively noncompliant tubing, but unless the machine has a preset available to alter rise time, and several do, the rise time is usually very rapid and with occlusion break the flow is high, and therefore so is the risk of surge.

I/A of residual cortex can be accomplished with modest aspiration flow rates as the instrument tip can generally be placed near the cortical material to be aspirated. This, in addition to whatever surge control has been built into the machine by the manufacturer, reduces surge risk. Linear vacuum with a high limit is used so that the cortex can be stripped into the center of the anterior chamber where vacuum is utilized to pull it through the 0.2- or 0.3-mm aspiration port.

Rise time is the interval between occlusion of the phaco or I/A tip and attainment of maximum preset vacuum. In a peristaltic or flow system, this is governed by the flow rate setting. Even though there is no flow when the tip is occluded, the aspiration flow rate setting governs the speed of the pump. Doubling the flow rate halves the rise time. In some systems, for example the Alcon's Infinity, the rise time can be altered by a preset in which the machine senses an increase in pressure in the inflow line and increases vacuum (indicating occlusion) and then changes the speed of the pump, up or down as predecided by the surgeon. Increasing the pump speed increases the risk of surge.

V. FOOT PEDAL CONTROL OF FLUIDICS

Most foot pedals (Figure 11-4) can be set up for fixed and/or linear control of surgical functions—aspiration, vacuum, and power. There is usually slight resistance, when moving from one position to the next. Commonly in phaco mode there are 4 positions. Position 0, when the pedal is not depressed, is set for no irrigation, no aspiration, and no power. Position 1, initial depression, is set for irrigation (at a rate determined by the bottle height and incision leakage) without aspiration or phaco. When manipulating nuclear material, as rotation of the nucleus in "divide and conquer" techniques, it is important to be in position 1 so that the inflow maintains the anterior chamber and capsular bag architecture. Position 2, further foot pedal depression, is set for irrigation plus aspiration at a fixed rate and no phaco. The rate of aspiration will be influenced by the amount of occlusion of the aspiration port. Position 3, still further foot pedal depression, adds phaco power at either a fixed level or with linear control by further depression of the foot pedal. Additional phaco variations include pulsed phaco or burst mode. Pulse mode delivers

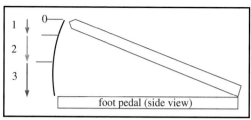

foot pedal (side view)

Figure 11-4. Foot pedal control. (Reprinted with permission from Seibel BS. *Phacodynamics: Mastering the Tools and Techniques of Phacoemulsification Surgery.* 4th ed. Thorofare, NJ: SLACK Incorporated; 2005.)

phaco power in regular "on" and "off" time intervals, linearly controlled by foot pedal position. In burst mode, stable power strokes are delivered with varying time intervals. The frequency of bursts increases proportional to foot pedal depression, such that with maximal depression, continuous phaco is delivered. Also available is the addition of sonic vibrations such as with Alcon Ozil.

Phaco power indirectly affects fluidics. Phaco power breaks up nuclear material and allows it to be aspirated. It also tends to push nuclear material away from the tip. Therefore phaco, in general, tends to increase flow through the system. Lowering phaco power tends to allow aspiration flow to pull material toward the tip partially or completely occluding it and thereby reducing or stopping flow. Pulsed phaco appears to even out flow rates as the case proceeds. Vacuum is ordinarily a preset in phaco mode and varies with the amount of occlusion and rise time.

In I/A mode, gravity feed irrigation is on in positions 1, 2, and 3 and the flow rate is determined by the bottle height. Both vacuum and aspiration are activated in positions 2 and 3 and both can be fixed or linear. If fixed vacuum is chosen, occlusion will result in a rise in vacuum to that set level. If linear vacuum is selected, the vacuum can be raised to whatever maximum is chosen by further depressing the foot pedal. Fixed aspiration provides for a fixed aspiration flow rate in pedal positions 2 and 3. Linear aspiration control provides for linear control of aspiration flow rate proportional to the foot pedal position. Combining linear aspiration and linear vacuum creates a Venturi-like system.

Occasionally during a procedure unwanted material will be aspirated, occluding the tip of the phaco or I/A hand piece. Phaco machines are designed with a venting system so that returning to position 0 will break the vacuum. In the Alcon Infinity, there is a reflux preset, that limits reflux pressure to the current infusion pressure plus a specified additional amount. This can be used to release capsule, iris, or lens material. Reflux is usually a factory set default and is foot pedal controlled.

VI. AUDIBLE SIGNALS

- Vacuum tone: Pitch varies relative to the amount of vacuum. The volume can be reduced but cannot be turned off.
- Occlusion tones: Intermittent beeping indicates that vacuum is at or near its preset limit and aspiration flow is reduced or stopped to avoid exceeding this limit. Continued phaco with no aspiration flow may result in thermal injury, especially if the corneal incision is tight.
- Phaco occlusion tone: High-pitched double beep that cannot be turned off.
- I/A occlusion tone: Lower single beep that can be turned off. Voice messages indicate mode changes.

VII. TROUBLE SHOOTING

A. Problem: Inadequate Infusion With Unstable Anterior Chamber

Possible causes include the following:
(a) Bottle was not vented.
(b) Bottle is empty.
(c) Height of bottle relative to patient's eye is too low.
(d) Infusion line is kinked.
(e) The fitting to the hand piece is loose.
(f) The incision is too tight.
(g) Manipulation of the hand piece is compressing the infusion sleeve.
(h) There is too much viscoelastic in the anterior chamber.
(i) Outflow has increased.

B. Problem: Cannot Attract and Hold Nuclear Material at the Phaco Tip

Possible causes include the following:
(a) Too much phaco power is pushing the material away, or creating too large a space in the nuclear fragment to allow occlusion. Therefore, use less phaco power.
(b) The vacuum setting is too low—unlikely unless it is very low. Except in Venturi-type systems, raising vacuum has little effect on aspiration flow rate. Enough vacuum is necessary to maintain occlusion.
(c) Aspiration flow rate is set too low. Possible but consider option (a) first.

C. Problem: Inadequate Aspiration

Possible causes include the following:

(a) There is a leak in the aspiration line.

(b) There is air in the aspiration line.

(c) The hand piece is clogged.

(d) The flow rate or vacuum setting is too low—consider options (a), (b), and (c) before changing settings that usually work for you.

Finally, quoting from the manual that comes with Alcon's Infinity phaco machine, "Good clinical practice dictates testing for adequate irrigation, aspiration flow, reflux and operation as applicable for each hand piece prior to entering the eye."[5]

KEY POINTS

1. Flow (aspiration rate) and vacuum are controlled independently in a peristaltic pump system.

2. Aspiration flow rate and vacuum are not independent in a vacuum pump system (Venturi).

3. Unlike flow pumps, bottle height and inflow in vacuum pumps will influence outflow unless the aspiration port is occluded.

4. Inflow should be adequate to maintain the anterior chamber volume even as the outflow through the incisions and the pump varies.

5. Surge effects can be minimized by using lower vacuum, lower aspiration rates, and higher infusion bottle height.

REFERENCES

1. Steinert RF. *Cataract Surgery: Expert Consult.* 3rd ed. Saunders, Philadelphia, PA; 2009: 75-92.

2. Seibel BS. *Phacodynamics: Mastering the Tools and Techniques of Phacoemulsification Surgery.* 4th ed. Slack Incorporated, Thorofare, NJ; 2005:2-81.

3. Allen D. The OZil Torsional Phacoemulsification Technology: an overview and study results. *Cataract and Refractive Surgery Today.* 2006:4-6.

4. Miyoshi T, Yoshida H. Emulsification action of longitudinal and torsional ultrasound tips and the effects on treatment of the nucleus during phacoemulsification. *J Cataract Refract Surg* 2010;36:1201-1206.

5. Alcon Laboratories, Inc. *INFINITI Vision System Operator's Manual.* Irvine, CA: Author; 2004.

12

MAXIMIZING EFFICIENCY WITH PHACOEMULSIFICATION SETTINGS

Saraswathy Ramanathan, MD

I. INTRODUCTION

Efficiency is usually the last priority to a beginning cataract surgeon. The immediate goal is to remove the cataract and to "stay out of trouble" while doing it. However, there are ways even for the beginning surgeon to optimize the potential for removing the cataract and at the same time to minimize the overall time spent in the eye. Attention to the actual settings that one chooses to remove the nucleus and epinucleus can actually make phacoemulsification easier and facilitate both learning and efficiency.

II. DEFINITIONS

A. Efficiency

The term *efficiency* must be defined. For the purposes of this chapter, I will use efficiency to mean complete nuclear and epinuclear removal using minimal ultrasound power and minimal overall time in the eye. One might believe that the most important factor in maximizing efficiency with settings is the ultrasound power. Surprisingly, this is not the case. It is not the ultrasound power that is most important, but rather the aspiration flow rate and the vacuum that impact efficiency the most.

B. Aspiration Flow Rate

By aspiration flow rate, or simply "aspiration," I mean the rate at which fluid and particles come to the ultrasound tip. Higher aspiration means faster flow and faster movement of nuclear and epinuclear pieces to the tip.

Henderson BA. *Essentials of Cataract Surgery, Second Edition (pp 117-123)*. © 2014 Taylor & Francis Group.

C. Ultrasound Power

Once the nucleus is at the tip, ultrasound power is responsible for emulsifying it into a small enough piece to fit through the tip and travel through the bore of the ultrasound handle. The surgeon must choose a power level that is just enough to break up the nuclear fragment into small enough chunks to be vacuumed through the tip. The surgeon must also choose between longitudinal ultrasound power and torsional ultrasound. Longitudinal ultrasound delivers an axial cutting force that will tend to push the nuclear piece away from the tip and create a "tunnel-like" cavity into the tissue, much like a jackhammer. Torsional ultrasound, on the other hand, is produced by side-to-side oscillation of the phaco tip, and therefore delivers the ultrasound force to a larger region of tissue.

D. Vacuum

Once the ultrasound has "handled" the nuclear fragment, it is the vacuum that determines how quickly the fluid or particle will make its way through the tip. Softer nuclear and epinuclear pieces need less vacuum to pull the tissue through the ultrasound tip. Harder and denser nuclei need higher vacuum levels to draw them through the tip. Vacuum rise occurs when the ultrasound hand piece tip is occluded. Maximum vacuum is generated when the tip is completely occluded. This occlusion may occur with any tissue or substance (eg, nucleus, epinucleus, viscoelastic, iris, and vitreous), but for the purposes of this discussion, occlusion with the nucleus or epinucleus is assumed.

Aspiration and vacuum are integrally related as the flow rate determines how readily a piece will flow to the tip and the vacuum determines how easily the piece will climb up and through the ultrasound hand piece. As a result, aspiration and vacuum are generally titrated up and down together. The 3 parameters (aspiration, ultrasound power, and vacuum) all work together to create "followability" or the way in which successive nuclear fragments smoothly move from their starting positions to the tip, get emulsified at the tip, and then are removed through the hand piece.

E. Fixed Versus Variable Parameters

Each main parameter (ultrasound, aspiration, and vacuum) can be selected as either fixed or variable. If the parameter is fixed, then it will appear at that designated level throughout the excursion of the foot pedal position. For example, if aspiration is set fixed at 33 cc/min, then as soon as the surgeon depresses the phaco foot pedal into position 2, an aspiration flow rate of 33 cc/min will be created in the eye. Similarly, if a fixed vacuum limit of 400 is chosen, then as soon as complete occlusion of the tip occurs, the vacuum limit of 400 is enforced and any "excess" vacuum is vented.

Variable settings allow the particular parameter to increase in a linear fashion throughout the foot pedal position. For example, when the aspiration is set on 35 cc/min and is variable, the surgeon will depress the foot pedal into position 2 and get some aspiration, but will not reach the full 35 cc/min until the foot pedal is at the "bottom" of position 2. Likewise, if ultrasound is set on 60% and variable, the full 60% power will not be attained until the foot pedal is fully depressed.

The purpose of fixed versus variable settings is to give the surgeon maximum control of the speed and efficiency of tissue removal. In general, the more parameters on fixed settings, the faster things happen. On the other hand, for the beginning surgeon, variable settings may allow the surgical steps to occur at a slower, more "controlled" pace. In addition, for eyes with some sort of compromise (especially weak zonules, pseudoexfoliation, and history of trauma), variable parameters give the surgeon finer control over forces generated within the eye.

III. BASIC PHACOEMULSIFICATION SETTINGS

Every surgeon will develop his or her own settings for all parts of the phacoemulsification. Table 12-1 is a sample of parameters used for the beginning surgeon. Settings for irrigation and aspiration of cortex are outside the scope of this chapter's discussion and will be covered elsewhere.

A. Sculpting

All parameters (ultrasound, vacuum, and aspiration) are usually kept at mid-range during the sculpting phase of the phacoemulsification. Since at this point the nucleus is one large piece, high levels of aspiration will cause excessive movement of the piece toward the tip. Instead, the settings during sculpting are focused on emulsifying moderate amounts of nucleus and efficiently moving those pieces through the hub of the phacoemulsification tip. Aspiration is set just high enough to engage the nucleus and keep it at the tip. Ultrasound is set just high enough to emulsify the tissue so that the tip can continue moving across the nucleus. Vacuum is adjusted just high enough to keep the tissue that has been emulsified moving through the hand piece.

B. Chopping

During the chopping phase, success depends upon the nucleus being held tightly onto the tip. For that reason, the vacuum limit must be relatively high. On a machine with a peristaltic pump, the aspiration flow rate will drive the maximum vacuum level (achieved only when there is full occlusion), and so the aspiration limit must be set relatively high as well. Table 12-1 summarizes the parameters typically used by surgeons who are transitioning to chopping techniques.

TABLE 12-1. TYPICAL PHACO SETTINGS FOR THE BEGINNING SURGEON								
	Ultra-sound		Power		Aspi-ration	Vacuum	Pulse Rate	Burst Width
	Longi-tudinal	% time on	Tor-sional	% time on				
Sculpt	0		100		22 mL/min	90 mm Hg		
Chop	65	40	0	0	35 mL/min	42 mm Hg	2 pps	
Section removal	0 to 40		80 to 100		35 mL/min	380 mm Hg		100 ms
Epinucleus	0		100		33 mL/min	330 mm Hg		
pps = pulses per second; ms = milliseconds								

C. Nuclear Section Removal

For purposes of this discussion, I will use the term *section* to refer to any nuclear section, whether it is a small chopped section, a quadrant, or even a heminucleus. The beginning surgeon will likely be performing a divide-and-conquer technique, so the "section" being removed would be a quadrant. In a chopping technique, the "section" would likely be smaller than a quadrant. Regardless of the size of the piece, the principles (with respect to phacoemulsification settings) of section removal are similar.

Since sections are fairly large and the goal during section removal is to bring the section to the tip and hold it there, aspiration flow rate must be relatively high. High vacuum will quickly remove these fragments from the eye once they are emulsified (and possibly chopped into small fragments).

The surgeon has 3 choices as far as section removal is concerned: continuous, burst, and pulse. All will have similar parameters and similar settings for aspiration, ultrasound power, and vacuum. However, the 3 modalities differ significantly in terms of how the parameters are controlled by the surgeon. In continuous mode, the ultrasound power is delivered without interruption, as long as the surgeon keeps the foot pedal in position 3. As the foot is depressed lower in position 3, the power increases until the maximum preset limit is reached. In burst and pulse modes, the ultrasound power is delivered to the eye in discrete "packets" of energy. These packets are more or less controlled by the surgeon (depending on the mode).

1. Pulse

In pulse mode, the packet of energy is determined by the ultrasound power, which is delivered for a predetermined duration. The surgeon may choose the rate of delivery of these packets by manipulating the pulse rate. The higher the pulse rate, the more rapidly the ultrasound packets are delivered. The lower the pulse rate, the less frequently the packets are delivered. Therefore, when the surgeon depresses the foot pedal enough to generate irrigation, aspiration, and ultrasound ("position 3"), full aspiration flow rate and pulse rate are generated.

2. Burst

Similar to pulse mode, a packet of ultrasound energy (the surgeon determines the power level) is delivered in burst mode. However, in this mode, the surgeon also sets the *duration* of the ultrasound packet, or burst width. As the burst width is increased, a longer ultrasound packet is delivered to the eye. In addition, the surgeon directly controls the frequency with which ultrasound packets are delivered to the eye by increasing his or her pressure on the foot pedal. In position 3, both vacuum and packet frequency increase as the foot is depressed lower until maximum vacuum and continuous phacoemulsification are achieved.

3. The difference between pulse and burst modes

Although the actual settings may not appear to be very different in pulse versus burst mode, the 2 modalities result in a fairly different surgical experience. Pulse mode allows for efficient but slightly slower removal of the nucleus. One reason that the surgery proceeds more slowly is that the vacuum often cannot build to its maximum level. Maximum vacuum requires occlusion of the tip. Since the pulse rate delivers specified pulses of ultrasound energy to the section at the tip, these pulses often push the piece off the tip. The advantage of this is that the piece keeps moving on the tip. As the piece bounces at the tip, there is less likelihood of vacuum surge as the last bit of nucleus is removed. The disadvantage is that occlusion is disrupted and vacuum fails to build. For the beginning surgeon, pulse mode is often the preferred method for removing nuclear sections since overall efficiency is still quite high, and yet, the removal of tissue progresses in a slightly slower, more controlled fashion. In addition, there are fewer variables with pulse mode that need to be directly managed. For the more experienced surgeon, the increased speed and efficiency of burst becomes highly desirable.

4. Specific uses of burst and pulse

Burst is usually the preferred method of nuclear section removal when conditions are optimal. "Optimal conditions" imply that the nucleus is of average density and that all steps in the surgery prior to section removal have proceeded smoothly. If any of these steps have been compromised, pulse is recommended. Specific examples of instances in which pulse might be preferred to burst are the following:

- Small capsulorrhexis
- Anterior capsular tear
- Zonular weakness
- Very dense nucleus
- Sharp section edges
- Shelved sections

The surgeon may elect to switch to burst once the initial sections have been removed and there is more room to maneuver the remaining sections. If there is any compromise of the capsule or zonules, then the surgeon will likely use pulse exclusively especially once any vitreous has been properly addressed.

D. Epinucleus Removal

If there is an epinuclear plate, it can be efficiently and safely removed using settings that use ultrasound, aspiration, and vacuum all at low to moderate levels. Table 12-1 shows typical settings for epinucleus removal. The goal during epinucleus removal is to bring the epinuclear tissue to the tip and evacuate it, but to leave the posterior capsule intact. For this reason, more aspiration and vacuum are needed than in the sculpting phase, but less than in section removal or chop. Often, removal of epinucleus is aided by viscodissection so that aspiration and vacuum can work even more efficiently.

IV. CONCLUSION

Using basic principles, even the beginning surgeon can manipulate settings to his or her advantage in phacoemulsification. If these principles are used at the start of the learning curve, the surgeon will quickly progress to removing the cataract safely and with maximum efficiency.

KEY POINTS

1. Aspiration flow rate determines how quickly fluid and materials come to the tip.
2. Vacuum occurs only when the tip is occluded and helps to remove material at the tip.
3. Use the pulse setting when you want slower, more controlled nuclear removal.
4. Use burst mode for maximum speed and efficiency.
5. Use the epinuclear setting for epinucleus removal.

SUGGESTED READINGS

Badoza D, Fernandez Mendy J, Ganly M. Phacoemulsification using the burst mode. *J Cataract Refract Surg.* 2003;29(6):1101-1105.

Corydon L, Krag S, Thim K. One-handed phacoemulsification with low settings. *J Cataract Refract Surg.* 1997;23(8):1143-1148.

Packer M, Fishkind WJ, Fine IH, Seibel BS, Hoffman RS. The physics of phaco: a review. *J Cataract Refract Surg.* 2005;31(2):424-431.

Steinert RF, ed. *Cataract Surgery: Techniques, Complications, Management.* Philadelphia, PA: WB Saunders; 2004.

Yow L, Basti S. Physical and mechanical principles of phacoemulsification and their clinical relevance. *Indian J Ophthalmol.* 1997;45(4):241-249.

13

PHACOEMULSIFICATION
NONCHOPPING TECHNIQUES

Talia Kolin, MD and Mario A. Meallet, MD

I. INTRODUCTION

Nonchopping phacoemulsification techniques, also known as nuclear-fracturing techniques, have facilitated cataract surgery immensely, allowing for safer and more efficient means of nucleus removal. The fundamental principle underlying all nuclear-fracturing techniques is the creation of "breaks" to divide the lens into smaller fragments for controlled removal through a small incision.

Gimbel was the first to propose a structured approach with the "divide-and-conquer" nucleofractis phaco technique.[1] This method involves the creation of 2 deep grooves in the nucleus that intersect centrally and are then cracked into 4 quadrants. These smaller sections of lens can be brought away from the capsule into a "safe zone" for emulsification and removal. Other interesting fracturing techniques include chip and flip, down slope sculpting, and phaco sweep. By using these methods, phacoemulsification can be performed safely and successfully on nearly all types of cataracts.

II. KEY POINTS IN
DIVIDE-AND-CONQUER TECHNIQUE

A. Phaco Settings

The initial nuclear groove formation requires the use of a moderate degree of phaco energy with low aspiration and vacuum settings. Quadrant removal requires higher aspiration and vacuum settings to allow the phaco tip to engage the lens fragments. (The surgeon should always confirm the settings prior to entering the eye.)

Henderson BA. *Essentials of Cataract Surgery, Second Edition* (pp 125-134).
© 2014 Taylor & Francis Group.

B. Grooving Technique

Goal: Deep sculpting to facilitate cracking
The goal is to create a sulcus that is 90% of the depth of the lens. The sulcus depth is the most important aspect for facilitating a complete crack at the base of the lens. Groove length is not as important and should not extend into the far lens periphery. A good rule of thumb is to limit the length of the groove to the length of the capsulorrhexis.

C. Cracking Technique and Bisection of the Two Halves

Goal: Nucleofractis of the nuclear plate and rim and the remaining nuclear material
It is important to achieve a complete separation of the posterior nucleus. A complete crack of the periphery is not as important (leaving a portion of the cortex and epinucleus intact is not problematic). The phaco tip and second instrument must be positioned deep in the groove, and the second instrument is rotated to simulate a paddle-like movement while the phaco tip is moved in the opposite direction to create a crack. The grooving of the 2 halves requires a motion that is more posterior to anterior in nature. Far peripheral grooves are not necessary. Cracking of the posterior aspect of the lens is more important than cracking the periphery.

D. Quadrant Removal

Goal: Rotation, reposition, and removal of nucleus
Engage the quadrants in the region of the nucleus (the middle portion of the cataract). Occlude the tip and pull the fragment centrally. Once the phaco tip and nuclear fragment are positioned centrally and at the level of the iris, the quadrant can be safely removed.

III. PHACO SETTINGS

Creation of the initial sulcus is best achieved using a moderate degree of phacoemulsification energy with low aspiration and vacuum settings. The nucleus should not move during the sculpting phase. If it does, more power is needed to smoothly groove the nucleus. This includes not completely occluding the phaco tip while grooving. Become familiar with the type of machine that is used in your operating room. The most commonly used machines are those that are based on peristaltic technology, and the typical settings for initial grooving with these machines are a phaco power setting of 20% to 60%, vacuum of 60 mm Hg, and aspiration setting of 25 to 30 mm Hg. There is no aspiration action with Venturi-based machines, and phaco power setting of 20% to 60% and vacuum of 150 mm Hg. These settings prevent the phaco tip from engaging the lens material with significant vacuum, thus allowing the phaco tip to move smoothly through the groove without causing significant lens movement.

Typical settings for quadrant removal are phaco power setting of 20% to 60%, vacuum of 350 mm Hg, and aspiration of 25 mm Hg for the peristaltic machines and phaco power setting of 20% to 60% and vacuum of 350 mm Hg for Venturi-based machines. The phaco power can be increased or decreased depending on the ease of cutting. Phaco power greater than 60% is only rarely required and should be used only no significant motion by the most experienced surgeons and only when absolutely necessary. Vacuum settings for the divide-and-conquer technique are generally lower than for chopping techniques because the desired effect in the former is to engage the fragments and draw them into a central location where they can be safely phacoemulsified.

IV. GROOVING TECHNIQUE

In creating the initial lens sulcus, the depth of the groove is of the utmost importance because this will allow the surgeon to ideally position the phaco tip and second instrument to crack the base of the lens. In general, the groove does not need to extend into the periphery, maintaining the peripheral rim keeps the bag distended and the posterior capsule on stretch. A useful guide is to use the extent of the capsulorrhexis to gauge the length of the groove.

The sweeping arcuate movement of grooving should simulate the posterior curvature of the nucleus. Familiarity with the dimensions of the lens will provide the surgeon with a level of confidence that the posterior capsule is not at risk during this phase of the case. The average lens has a diameter of 9 mm and a thickness of 4.5 mm centrally. The rationale for limiting the length of the initial groove is that the lens thickness and the proximity of the posterior capsule decrease in the periphery. How do these dimensions compare to the length of the phaco tip? A useful guideline is to create a groove that is 1.5 phaco tips wide and 3 deep. The standard phaco tip is 1.2 mm in diameter, thus yielding a groove that is 1.8 mm × 3.6 mm centrally. In making smooth passes, there should be no ridges or step-offs in the groove. Widening the groove to 1.5 times the width of the thinner portion of the phaco tip will create adequate space to accommodate the phaco tip and second instrument for cracking. The goal of grooving should be to achieve 90% depth centrally with a length of approximately 6 mm (Figure 13-1). The power should be adjusted so that the nucleus is being sculpted and not rocked. There can be significant nuclear movement during the grooving step.

In soft lenses, the Y sign can be used to indicate that the groove is of adequate depth and that the nucleus is ready to be cracked. The Y sign has been described by Kurian et al and is used to describe the posterior embryonal

Figure 13-1. A short, deep groove of approximately 6-mm length is illustrated. Note the groove does not extend beyond the edge of the 6-mm capsulorrhexis. The groove is of 90% depth centrally and the width is twice that of the 1.2-mm phaco tip.

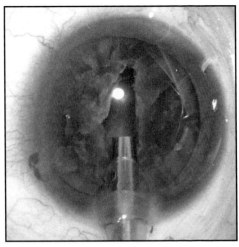

Y suture that can be visualized at the center of the trench and can be used as an endpoint for grooving.[6]

V. CRACKING TECHNIQUE

Achieving a consistent, even crack of the posterior cataract is an important piece in mastering the divide-and-conquer technique. A complete posterior crack reflects that the entire nuclear component of the lens has been thoroughly bisected. Extension of the crack into the far periphery is not nearly as vital because the peripheral cortex and epinucleus can be easily divided with a second instrument during quadrant removal. The second instrument is inserted through a paracentesis site that is positioned 2 to 3 clock hours from the main wound site.

The position of the phaco tip and the second instrument in the deepest central portion of the groove is critical. It is often easiest to position the phaco tip first and then place the second instrument immediately adjacent to it (Figure 13-2). It is critical to place the instruments deep in the groove prior to cracking the lens. The second instrument is manipulated with a spinning motion between the thumb and index finger, which will result in a paddle-like movement of the second instrument within the eye, with no movement or distortion of the paracentesis (Figure 13-3). The movement is one of spinning, not pulling. Pulling causes distortion of the cornea and also displaces the eye, significantly diminishing the surgeon's view. Pushing and pulling at the paracentesis or the wound can also create an increase in vitreous pressure, causing collapse of the anterior chamber and potential rupture of the posterior capsule.

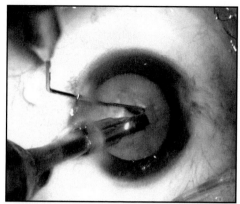

Figure 13-2. The phaco tip is positioned deep in the central part of the groove. The second instrument is then positioned adjacent to the phaco tip deep in the groove.

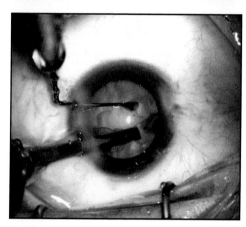

Figure 13-3. With a paddle-like movement of the second instrument and an opposite motion of the phaco tip, a central crack is achieved.

The initial crack in the technique described here is performed after formation of the initial groove. An alternative is to create a "maltese-cross" configuration by creating grooves at 90 degrees from the initial sulcus (Figure 13-4A). However, this technique can prove more difficult because the lateral walls have less surface area for opposition of the instruments when attempting to crack. Another alternative to the separation movement of the instruments as described here is to use a criss-cross action in separating the halves (Figure 13-4B). This technique is effective but can be more difficult to master because the phaco tip can obstruct the movement of the second instrument.

Once the posterior crack is visualized, it can be carefully extended subincisionally by moving the phaco tip and second instrument toward the subincisional portion of the groove and again performing the separation to ensure that the posterior crack is complete. As Koch stated, "The densely packed dry nucleus cracks easily. The looser, more hydrated cataract resists

Figure 13-4. (A) Maltese-cross formation by grooving in 2 opposite 90-degree meridians. (B) Cracking by criss-cross movements of the phaco tip and the second instrument.

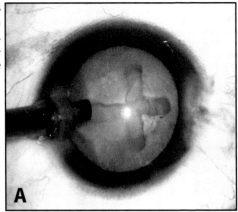

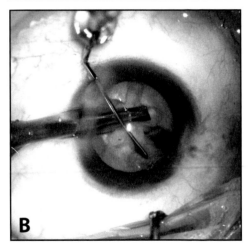

cracking."[2] If the posterior plate does not crack, the best approach is to carefully shave the plate to make it thinner and to attempt cracking once more.[2]

VI. BISECTION OF THE TWO HALVES

The final step in cracking requires bisection of the 2 halves. The required motion is one of posterior to anterior grooving of the halves followed by the orientation of the phaco tip and second instrument deep in the sulcus to separate the 2 quadrants (Figure 13-5). This step can be quite challenging because the grooves are shorter and shallower than the initial groove. In addition, the 2 instruments must fit into a tighter space and the separation movement must be oriented posteriorly to achieve cracking of the posterior portion of the cataract.

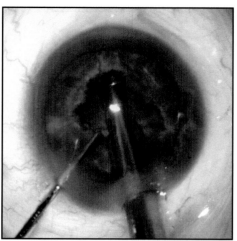

Figure 13-5. The grooving of the heminucleus consists of a posterior-to-anterior motion. The crack is achieved by positioning the instruments into the groove and separating.

Ideally, 4 equal quadrants are produced. However, this is not always possible and, not infrequently, the surgeon is faced with 3 unequal pieces. This scenario does not preclude advancing to quadrant removal, which can still be performed safely and efficiently with less-than-perfect segmentation of the nucleus (discussed further next). In this circumstance, however, chopping techniques become desirable because these pieces are very amenable to manipulation with the phaco tip and chopper.

VII. QUADRANT REMOVAL

The preferred method of quadrant removal is to present the posterior edge of the fragment to the phaco tip by gently lifting the fragment with the second instrument and engaging the piece with higher vacuum and higher flow rates and drawing it into the pupillary center (Figure 13-6). The phaco tip is used to impale the fragment, the vacuum is then allowed to increase, and the piece is drawn into the papillary plane. The second instrument remains under the segments being emulsified in order to protect the posterior capsule. By using the second instrument to coax the fragments toward the anterior chamber, the phaco tip is kept at a safe distance from the posterior capsule. "Fishing" for these pieces with the phaco tip is a risky maneuver that is certain to result in capsular rupture.

If the surgeon is faced with unequal segments, the more prudent approach is to remove the smaller pieces first. The smaller pieces are much easier to engage, and once they have been removed, a greater "working space" exists for removal of the larger portions. Often the remaining fragment is a full half that was unable to divide further. It is not unusual for experienced surgeons

Figure 13-6. Quadrant removal is easily achieved once all 4 grooves have been completed and all cracks have been successfully performed.

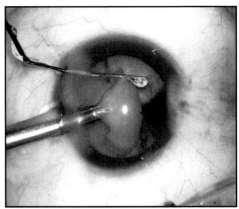

to prolapse a large fragment into the anterior chamber and carefully perform removal, often with the assistance of a chopper. The result will be favorable as long as care is taken to complete the bulk of the work in the pupillary space and avoid contact with the endothelium. Judicious use of a viscodispersive agent can help protect the endothelium in the latter maneuver.

Quadrant removal for beginning surgeons is often made difficult by the inability to establish sufficient vacuum to draw the pieces into the pupillary center. The dexterity to approach the lens fragment, to deliver a single millisecond pulse of phaco power to firmly engage the piece, and then to return to foot position 2 and allow vacuum to build takes many months to master. One method of avoiding frustration during this period is to use viscoelastic to float the pieces into the pupillary plane and safely perform removal. However, these types of tricks should be seen as temporizing measures that should be used until the appropriate technique has been mastered.

VIII. ALTERNATE APPROACHES TO NONCHOPPING

There are many variations to the nonchopping technique, including chip and flip, down slope sculpting, and phaco sweep. Familiarity with many different techniques enables the surgeon to select the most efficient method of extraction for each individual lens. Fine introduced the "chip and flip" technique for lens removal. Central sculpting of the nucleus is performed after hydrodelineation and hydrodissection until only a thin nuclear plate remains. A second instrument is then introduced through the side-port incision to move the inferior lens edge toward the center of the capsular bag. The pieces of the rim are then removed at the 5:00 to 6:00 positions. The nucleus is rotated, and the rim continues to be removed at the 6:00 position. Once the entire rim is removed, the second instrument is used to elevate the remaining nuclear plate anteriorly. The plate can then be emulsified safely. The epinucleus is then engaged and removed with aspiration alone.[3]

Gimbel's down slope sculpting technique involved sculpting the upper central aspect of the nucleus. This is a useful technique for patients with small pupils. Sculpting is done after gently moving the lens inferiorly with a second instrument. Sculpting can then be performed parallel to the posterior capsule. This method of sculpting minimizes the chance of rupturing the posterior capsule. Once the groove is sufficiently deep, the instruments are placed deep within the lens and a fracture is made. The remaining nucleus can then be removed with the divide-and-conquer technique previously described.[4]

The phaco sweep is a modification that Gimbel made to the down slope technique. A central groove is formed in this approach, followed by sculpting lateral to the initial groove. The result is a horizontal shelf that can be easily cracked. This is accomplished by stabilizing the upper portion of the lens with the phaco tip and using the second instrument to push against the inferior wall. The remainder of the lens can then be removed as described previously.[5]

IX. Conclusion

Nonchopping phacoemulsification techniques allow efficient removal of cataracts. The divide-and-conquer technique described is an organized and systematic approach to lens removal. It involves groove formation and cracking followed by quadrant removal. This technique, when mastered, can be nucleofractis successfully to remove most types of cataracts.

Key Points

1. Create a nuclear groove that is 90% of the depth of the lens. The sulcus depth is the most important aspect for facilitating a complete crack at the base of the lens.

2. Groove length is not as important as groove depth and should not extend into the far lens periphery. A good rule of thumb is to limit the length of the groove to the length of the capsulorrhexis.

3. Cracking of the posterior aspect of the lens is more important than cracking the periphery.

4. In general, create a groove that is 1.5 phaco tips wide and 3 deep.

5. If the surgeon is faced with unequal segments, the more prudent approach is to remove the smaller pieces first.

REFERENCES

1. Gimbel HV. Divide and conquer nucleofractis phacoemulsification: development and variations. *J Cataract Refract Surg.* 1991;17:281-291.
2. Koch PS, Katzen LE. Stop and chop phacoemulsification. *J Cataract Refract Surg.* 1994;20:566-570.
3. Fine IH. The chip and flip phacoemulsification technique. *J Cataract Refract Surg.* 1991;17:366-371.
4. Gimbel HV. Down slope sculpting. *J Cataract Refract Surg.* 1992;18:614-618.
5. Gimbel HV, Chin PK. Phaco sweep. *J Cataract Refract Surg.* 1995;21:493-496.
6. Kurian M, Das S, Umarani B, Naqappa S, Shetty R, Shetty BK. Y sign: clinical indicator to stop trencing and start cracking. *J Cataract Refract Surg.* 2013:39:493-496.

14

PHACO CHOP TECHNIQUES

David F. Chang, MD

I. INTRODUCTION

All chopping techniques rely on the principle of lens "disassembly," in which the firm nucleus is divided into smaller maneuverable pieces.[1-8] As a result the 10-mm wide nucleus can be removed through a 5-mm diameter capsulorrhexis, and the majority of the nucleus is emulsified near the center of the pupil at a safe distance from the iris, posterior capsule, and corneal endothelium.

II. CHOPPING PREREQUISITES

The *capsulorrhexis* preserves the bag-like anatomy of the capsule.[9] It provides secure fixation and centration of the intraocular lens (IOL), and its continuous edge renders the capsular bag much more resistant to tearing during nuclear emulsification.[9-12] *Hydrodissection* separates the nucleus from the capsule and cortex so that it can spin within the capsular bag.[13] It also loosens the capsular-cortical attachments, which facilitates cortical cleanup.[14,15]

The *hydrodelineation* wave cleaves a thin epinuclear shell apart from the firm endonucleus, reducing the dimensions of the central mass that must be chopped, fragmented, and emulsified. In addition, the bulk of the epinuclear shell blocks the exposed posterior capsule from trampolining toward the phaco tip as the final endonuclear fragments are emulsified.

III. CLASSIFICATION OF CHOPPING TECHNIQUES

Since Kunihiro Nagahara first introduced the concept of phaco chop in 1993, many different chopping variations have been described.[4,6-8] This diverse array of modifications can be confusing to transitioning surgeons. For

Henderson BA. *Essentials of Cataract Surgery, Second Edition (pp 135-148).*
© 2014 Taylor & Francis Group.

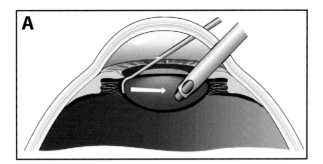

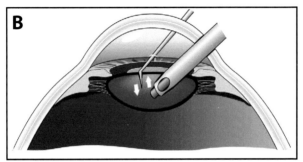

Figure 14-1. Instrument positioning in horizontal chop (A) and vertical chop (B). (Reprinted with permission from Chang DF. *Phaco Chop and Advanced Phaco Techniques: Strategies for Complicated Cataracts.* 2nd ed. Thorofare, NJ: SLACK Incorporated; 2013.)

simplification, this author first proposed that all chopping methods be conceptually divided into 2 general categories: horizontal and vertical.[6] Both share the same benefit of fragmenting the nucleus manually but accomplish this objective in different ways. The classic Nagahara technique exemplifies *horizontal* chopping because the instrument tips move toward each other in the horizontal plane during the chop (Figure 14-1A). In *vertical* chopping, the 2 instrument tips move toward each other in the vertical plane in order to create the fracture (Figure 14-1B).

IV. PHACO PRECHOP

Takayuki Akahoshi and Jochen Kammann pioneered methods of prechopping the nucleus prior to insertion and use of the phaco tip. In the case of a denser lens, one manual instrument must generally hook the equator (as with horizontal chopping) so that the penetrating and chopping forces are not transmitted directly to the capsular bag and zonules.

One potential problem with prechop techniques is that there is no phaco tip to aspirate the lens debris liberated after the initial chop. This may impair visibility for subsequent steps. Another problem is that prechop techniques and instrumentation are designed to create 4 nuclear quadrants. For denser and larger nuclei, it is more desirable to create multiple smaller pieces. With dense nuclei it is also difficult to judge how deeply the splitting instrument has penetrated. Over-penetration risks posterior capsule perforation. Finally, prechopping requires additional steps and instrumentation that are avoided when the phaco tip itself is utilized for the chopping technique. By prechopping and softening the nucleus the femtosecond laser further reduces the amount of ultrasound or manual instrument energy needed to remove the lens. As would be expected, the denser the nucleus the greater the reduction in ultrasound energy and time afforded by femtosecond laser nucleotomy is.[16]

V. STOP AND CHOP

Paul Koch's "stop and chop" method is a hybrid of divide-and-conquer and horizontal chopping. A deep, central groove is first sculpted in order to crack the nucleus in half. One then *stops* the divide-and-conquer method, and *chops* the heminuclei.[3] Although this method utilizes some horizontal chopping, this author coined the term *nonstop chop* to differentiate and designate pure chopping techniques that eliminate all sculpting.[6]

The advantage of "stop and chop" is that it avoids the difficult first chop. As a result, one only chops across the radius, rather than the full diameter of the nucleus. Second, unlike with the initial nonstop chop, the phaco tip can be positioned within the trough up against the side of the heminucleus that is to be cleaved. Finally, the presence of the trough facilitates removal of the first fragment because it is not tightly wedged inside the capsular bag. While chopping the heminuclei does reduce total ultrasound energy, the majority of sculpting during divide-and-conquer is used to create the first groove. Thus, "stop and chop" does not provide the full benefits of nonstop chopping listed next.

VI. PURE CHOPPING TECHNIQUES

There are 5 important advantages to phaco chop:
1. Reduction in energy delivery
2. Reduction in stress on the zonules and capsular bag
3. Supracapsular emulsification
4. Decreased reliance on the red reflex
5. Greater reliance on the chopper than the phaco tip

A. Reduction in Energy Delivery

Pure chopping techniques eliminate lens sculpting. Ultrasound energy is not required to subdivide the nucleus and is reserved for the phaco-assisted aspiration of mobile fragments.[7,17-20] The marked reduction in phaco power and energy is particularly important for brunescent nuclei where the risk of endothelial cell loss and wound burn is higher.

B. Reduction in Stress on the Zonules and Capsular Bag

The capsular bag fixates the nucleus during sculpting, which risks zonular trauma when dealing with a bulky brunescent nucleus. Unlike a soft nucleus that absorbs pressure like a pillow, a large firm nucleus directly transmits any instrument forces, such as sculpting, rotation, and cracking directly to the capsular bag and zonules. With chopping it is the phaco tip that braces and immobilizes the nucleus against the incoming mechanical force of the chopper (see Figure 14-1). The manual forces, generated by one instrument pushing against the other, replace the need for ultrasound energy to fragment the nucleus. In addition, these manual forces are directed centripetally inward away from the zonules, rather than outward toward the capsule. This significant difference in zonular stress is readily appreciated when both chopping and sculpting are compared from the Miyake-Apple viewpoint in cadaver eyes.

C. Supracapsular Emulsification

Chopping provides many of the same advantages of supracapsular phaco techniques.[5] With phaco chop, virtually all of the emulsification is reserved for phaco-assisted aspiration of small fragments that have been elevated out of the capsular bag. This allows the emulsification to be performed centrally in the pupillary plane at a safe distance from the iris, posterior capsule, and endothelium. The phaco tip does not need to travel outside the central 2 to 3 mm zone of the pupil, which decreases the chance of incising the iris or capsulorrhexis edge in eyes with poor mydriasis. However, unlike with other supracapsular techniques, the all-or-none prerequisite of prolapsing the entire nucleus anteriorly out of the capsular bag and through the capsulorrhexis is avoided.

D. Decreased Reliance on the Red Reflex

The increasingly brighter red reflex at the base of the trough allows us to judge the depth of the phaco tip during sculpting. During chopping the maneuvers performed with the instruments are more kinesthetic and tactile. Because it is not necessary to visualize the exact depth of the phaco tip, chopping is advantageous with a poor or absent red reflex, such as with small pupils and cortical or mature nuclear cataracts.

E. Greater Reliance on the Chopper Than the Phaco Tip

Finally, with phaco chop, it is the chopper that executes the most important maneuvers. The phaco tip remains relatively immobile in the center of the pupil, providing an exit conduit for the fragmented lens material. Compared to the phaco tip, the chopper provides much greater maneuverability and freedom of motion. This is advantageous if the nucleus fails to rotate for any reason (eg, extremely loose zonules, unsuccessful hydrodissection, or the need to avoid hydrodissection, such as with polar cataracts). In these situations, sequential chops can be made without rotating the nucleus by simply repositioning the chopper in different equatorial locations and chopping toward the centrally impaled phaco tip. In addition to the improved efficiency of chopping techniques, safety is enhanced by these aforementioned attributes of reduced ultrasound power, reduced zonular stress, decreased reliance on the red reflex, and the supracapsular and central location of emulsification. These features universal to both horizontal and vertical chopping make them optimal techniques for difficult and complicated cases. The improved ability to handle brunescent nuclei, white cataracts, loose zonules, posterior polar cataracts, crowded anterior chambers, capsulorrhexis tears, and small pupils should be the primary motivation for a divide-and-conquer surgeon to transition to phaco chop.[4,6,21,22]

VII. HORIZONTAL PHACO CHOP

Nagahara's original technique is the classic horizontal chopping method. All subsequent variations make use of the same principle whereby the chopper hooks the endonucleus inside the capsular bag and chops centrally toward the fixating phaco tip in the horizontal plane. The horizontal chopping technique relies upon compressive force to fracture the nucleus. This exploits natural fracture planes in the lens created by the lamellar orientation of the lens fibers. The key first step is to hook the nuclear equator with the chopper tip within the epinuclear space of the peripheral capsular bag prior to initiating the horizontally directed chop (Figure 14-1A and 14-2A).[6]

A. Initial Placement of the Chopper Tip

Hydrodelineation is particularly important for horizontal chopping because it decreases the diameter of the endonucleus that must be peripherally hooked and divided by the chopper.[6] In addition, the separated soft epinucleus provides a working zone for the chopper where it can be manipulated peripheral to the endonuclear equator without overly distending or tearing the capsular bag.

Prior to placing the chopper, the central anterior epinucleus should be aspirated with the phaco tip. This allows one to better visualize and estimate the

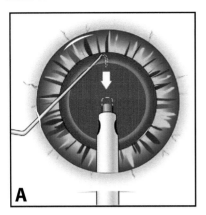

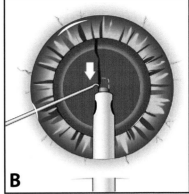

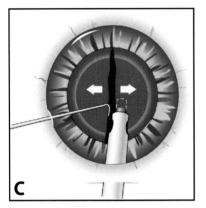

Figure 14-2. In horizontal chop, the chopper hooks the nuclear equator (A) and chops directly toward the phaco tip (B). Upon contact, sideways separation of the tips (C) pries the 2 heminuclei apart. (Reprinted with permission from Chang DF. *Phaco Chop and Advanced Phaco Techniques: Strategies for Complicated Cataracts.* 2nd ed. Thorofare, NJ: SLACK Incorporated; 2013.)

size of the endonucleus and the amount of separation between the endonucleus and the surrounding capsular bag. The chopper tip touches the central anterior endonucleus and maintains contact as it passes peripherally beneath the opposing capsulorrhexis edge. This ensures that the tip stays inside the bag as it descends and hooks the endonucleus peripherally. Although some surgeons tilt the chopper tip sideways to reduce its profile as it passes underneath the capsular edge, this is generally unnecessary unless the capsulorrhexis diameter is small. The elongated horizontal chopper tip can be kept in an upright and vertical orientation because the capsulorrhexis will stretch like an elastic waistband without tearing.

Once it reaches the epi/endonuclear junction, the chopper tip should be vertically oriented as it descends into the epinuclear space alongside the edge of the endonucleus (see Figure 14-1A and 14-2A). The smaller the endonucleus, the larger the epinucleus, and the easier this step will be. Slightly nudging the nucleus with the chopper confirms that it is alongside the equator and that it is within, rather than outside, the bag. Trypan blue capsular dye improves visualization of the anterior capsule for this step and is a useful teaching adjunct.[23,24] Another helpful measure for transitioning surgeons is to inject a dispersive ophthalmic viscosurgical device (OVD), such as Viscoat, beneath the nasal capsulorrhexis edge. This further separates the anterior capsule from the endonucleus and displaces any overlying cortex and epinucleus to afford optimal visualization of these anatomic relationships.

B. Executing the First Chop

Next, one must deeply impale the nucleus with the phaco tip. The phaco tip should be directed vertically downward and positioned as proximally as possible in order to maximize the amount of nucleus located in the path of the chopper (see Figure 14-1A). If the depth of the phaco tip is too shallow, sufficient compression of the central nucleus cannot occur. Once impaled, the phaco tip holds and stabilizes the nucleus with vacuum in foot pedal position 2.

The chopper tip is pulled directly toward the phaco tip, and upon contact, the 2 tips are moved directly apart from each other (Figure 14-2B). This separating motion occurs along an axis perpendicular to the chopping path, and propagates the fracture across the remaining nucleus located behind the phaco tip (Figure 14-2C). The denser and bulkier the endonucleus, the further the hemisections must be separated in order to cleave the remaining nuclear attachments. Thanks to the elasticity of the capsulorrhexis, a wide momentary separation of large nuclear hemisections will not tear the capsular bag.

In order for the initial chop to succeed, a substantial amount of the central endonucleus must lie within the path of the chopper. Particularly if the anterior epinucleus has not been removed, it is easy to misjudge the depth of the 2 instrument tips. If the phaco tip is too superficial or too central, or the chopper tip is not kept deep enough throughout the chop, the nucleus will not fracture.[6] Instead, the chopper will only score or scratch the anterior surface. The larger and denser the nucleus is, the more difficult proper positioning of the 2 instrument tips becomes. Fear of perforating the posterior capsule creates a counterproductive, but natural tendency to elevate the chopper tip during the chop.

The ergonomics and tactile "feel" of the horizontal chop will vary significantly as one advances along the spectrum of nuclear density. A soft nucleus has the consistency of soft ice cream and no resistance is felt as the chopper is moved. With a medium density nucleus, the chopper encounters slight resistance, indicating that some compression is taking place. This resistance becomes much greater when chopping a dense nucleus, where the compressive force is followed by a sudden snap as the initial split occurs. To develop sufficient compressive force, one must move the chopper tip directly toward the phaco tip until they touch before commencing the sideways separating motion. Veering the chopper tip to the left as it approaches the phaco tip prevents the instruments from touching. However, this limits the compressive force and causes the nucleus to swivel and turn.

C. Removing the First Chopped Fragment

Upon completion of the initial chop the nucleus should be bisected in half. After rotating the bisected nucleus 30 to 45 degrees in a clockwise direction, the opposite heminucleus is impaled with the phaco tip in a central location. Repeating the same steps of hooking the equator and chopping toward the phaco tip creates a small, pie-shaped fragment. The strong holding force afforded by high vacuum facilitates elevation of this first piece out of the bag. Insufficient holding force may be the result of inadequate vacuum settings or failure to completely occlude the tip. Single burst mode can enhance the phaco tip's purchase of a firm nuclear piece by better preserving the initial seal around the opening.

Every subsequent chop is a repetition of these steps, and each wedge-shaped piece is emulsified as soon as it is created. Once half of the capsular bag is vacated, the phaco tip can impale and carry the remaining heminucleus toward the center of the pupil. This allows the horizontal chopper tip to be positioned alongside the outer edge under direct visualization and without having to pass it beneath the anterior capsule.

One advantage of horizontal chopping is that larger nuclear pieces can be subdivided into smaller and smaller fragments. The size of the pieces should be kept proportional to the size of the phaco tip opening. Poor followability and excessive chatter of firm fragments engaged by the phaco tip may indicate that they are too large. Because of their greater overall dimensions, brunescent nuclei will need to be chopped many more times than soft nuclei.

VIII. VERTICAL PHACO CHOP

Hideharu Fukasaku's "phaco snap and split" and Vladimir Pfeifer's "phaco crack" (renamed "phaco quick chop" by David Dillman) are examples of *vertical* chopping because when the chop is first initiated, the instruments move toward each other in the vertical plane (see Figure 14-1B).[4,6,8] Whereas the horizontal chopper moves inward from the periphery toward the phaco tip, the vertical chopper is used like a spike or blade from above to incise downward into the nucleus just anterior to the centrally impaled phaco tip (Figure 14-3A). Depressing the sharp spiked tip downward, while simultaneously lifting the nucleus slightly upward imparts a shearing force that fractures the nucleus (see Figure 14-1B). This contrasts with the compressive force produced by horizontal chopping. After initiating a partial thickness split, the embedded instrument tips are used to pry the 2 hemisections apart (Figure 14-3B). Just as with horizontal chopping, this sideways

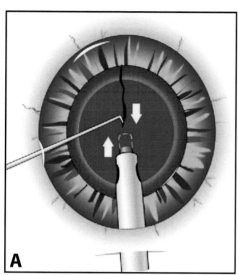

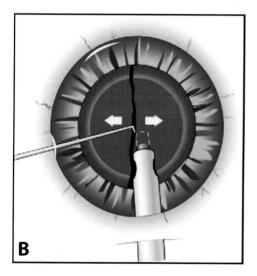

Figure 14-3. In vertical chop, the sharp-tipped chopper incises the nucleus just anterior to the centrally impaled phaco tip (A). Sideways separation of the 2 hemisections extends the fracture through the remainder of the nucleus (B). (Reprinted with permission from Chang DF. *Phaco Chop and Advanced Phaco Techniques: Strategies for Complicated Cataracts.* 2nd ed. Thorofare, NJ: SLACK Incorporated; 2013.)

separation of the instrument tips extends the fracture deeper and deeper until the remainder of the nucleus is cleaved in half.

Whereas the depth of the chopper tip is key for horizontal chopping, adequate depth of the phaco tip is the most crucial factor in vertical chop.[6] This is because the centrally impaled phaco tip must completely immobilize the nucleus against the incoming sharp chopper tip in order to generate enough shearing force to fracture it. Slightly elevating the impaled phaco tip also prevents the descending chopper tip from pushing a firm nucleus against the posterior capsule. The need for a strong purchase is also why high vacuum and single burst mode are more critical for vertical than for horizontal chop.

Much like a chisel with a block of ice, the vertical chopper tip can be used to cleave the nucleus into multiple pieces of variable size. The vertically chopped edges may appear sharp, like pieces of broken glass, because there is none of the crushing force that characterizes horizontal chop involved. The sharp vertical chopper tip generally stays central to the capsulorrhexis. Thus, in contrast to horizontal chopping, it is always visualized and does not pass underneath the anterior capsule or behind the iris. For each of the 2 different chopping techniques, one should position the more important instrument first. For horizontal chop, this means hooking the nucleus with the chopper tip first. With vertical chop, the nucleus should first be impaled with the phaco tip.

IX. COMPARING HORIZONTAL AND VERTICAL CHOP—WHICH TECHNIQUE?

Although the author uses both techniques with equal frequency, they employ different mechanisms that have complimentary advantages and disadvantages. It is worth learning and utilizing both variations for this reason. Vertical chopping requires a nucleus that is brittle enough to be snapped in half. A lack of firmness explains the difficulty of performing vertical chop or divide-and-conquer techniques in soft nuclei. The ability of the chopper tip to easily slice through a soft nucleus instead of fracturing it makes horizontal chopping an excellent method for these cases.

Horizontal chopping is more advantageous for eyes with deeper-than-average anterior chambers, where the phaco tip must approach the nucleus from an extremely steep angle.

In such eyes, one must take measures to prevent or reverse lens-iris diaphragm retro-displacement syndrome (LIDRS). The momentary pupillary block can be reversed or prevented by lifting the pupil edge off of the anterior capsule, so that irrigation fluid can flow into the posterior chamber.

Horizontal chop is also this author's preference for weak zonule cases, such as traumatic cataracts. Because of the inwardly directed, compressive instrument forces, horizontal chop produces the least amount of nucleus movement or tilt. Finally, horizontal chop is more effective for subdividing smaller, mobile nuclear fragments—particularly if they are brunescent. Because small mobile pieces are hard to fixate adequately, attempting to vertically shear such fragments with a chopper will often dislodge the small piece instead. Trapping and then crushing the fragment between the horizontal chopper and the phaco tip will immobilize and divide it most effectively.

The limitation of horizontal chopping is in its relative inability to transect thicker, brunescent nuclei. Indeed, horizontal chopping should never be utilized in the absence of an epinuclear shell since there will be insufficient space in the peripheral bag to accommodate the chopper. Frequently, the horizontally directed path of the chopper is not deep enough to sever the leathery posterior plate of an ultra-brunescent nucleus. If this occurs, the partially chopped pieces will still be connected at their apex, like the petals of a flower. In such cases, it is best to try injecting a dispersive OVD through one of the incomplete cracks in the posterior plate to distance it from the posterior capsule. Since a dispersive OVD resists aspiration, the surgeon can attempt to carefully phaco through the remaining connecting bridges that have been visco-elevated away from the posterior capsule.

Because vertical chop is more consistently able to fracture the leathery posterior plate, it is well suited for denser nuclei.[6] In horizontal chop, this propagating fracture continues horizontally toward the surgeon, but it will not tend to advance further and further posteriorly. In contrast, with vertical chop, as the 2 halves are pried apart, the advancing fracture propagates downward in the vertical plane until it eventually transects the posterior-most layer. With an ultra-brunescent lens, the vertical chopper should approach the embedded phaco tip more diagonally. This provides more of a horizontal vector that pushes the nucleus against the phaco tip, while the vertical vector initiates the downward fracture. This "diagonal" chop therefore combines the mechanical advantages of both strategies. With denser nuclei, one should also begin by sculpting a small, deep pit centrally.[25,26] By entering at the base of the pit, the phaco tip can impale more deeply than would have been possible without this preliminary de-bulking. Retracting the irrigation sleeve further maximizes penetration of the phaco tip.

A. Comparison of Horizontal and Vertical Choppers

Horizontal choppers feature an elongated, but blunt-ended tip. A tip length of 1.5 to 2.0 mm length is necessary in order to transect thicker nuclei, and the inner cutting surface of the shaft may be sharpened for this purpose of incising denser lens material. The very end of the tip is always dull to diminish the risk of posterior capsule perforation. The author prefers the curved shape of an elongated microfinger because it can wrap snuggly around the lens equator without distending or stretching the peripheral fornices of the capsular bag (see Figure 14-1A).[6] The microfinger design also allows one to cup the nucleus equator so that it cannot slip away as the compression begins. Vertical choppers feature a shorter tip that has a sharpened point in order to penetrate denser nuclei (see Figure 14-1B). If the tip is too dull, it will tend to knock the nucleus off of the phaco tip rather than incising into it. In contrast to horizontal choppers, the length of the vertical chopper tip is less important since it never encompasses one side of the nuclear segment.

The 3-dimensional motions required of the chopper are much simpler with vertical chop. Compared to horizontal chop, the chopper tip is not placed as peripherally and simply incises downward into the nuclear mass. The tip is kept vertically oriented and is always visible until it descends into the nucleus. In contrast, the horizontal chopper tip is much longer, must execute a far more difficult set of motions, must pass underneath the capsulorrhexis, and must be blindly positioned behind the peripheral iris before initiating the chop. The side-port incision should always serve as the motionless fulcrum for the chopper shaft. In order to avoid displacing or distorting the side-port incision, somewhat counterintuitive movements must be made with the horizontal chopper in particular.

X. CONCLUSION

Horizontal and vertical chopping are variations that rely upon different mechanisms to provide complementary advantages and common benefits. The author utilizes both chopping techniques routinely depending on the nuclear density.[6] With dense lenses, one may employ both techniques during the same case, and the Chang double-ended combination chopper (Katena Products, Inc) was designed to provide both a horizontal and a vertical chopper on a single instrument (see Figures 14-1 to 14-3). This also allows the surgeon using a sharp vertical chopper to easily switch to the blunt-tipped horizontal chopper for epinuclear manipulation and removal. The Seibel vertical chopper tip has the profile of a rounded blade with no sharp point that could contact the posterior capsule. For this reason, transitioning surgeons often prefer the Chang horizontal/Seibel vertical chopper as their first combination chopper.

KEY POINTS

1. Phaco chop improves safety by limiting ultrasound energy and reducing stress on the capsule and zonules.

2. To fracture the nucleus, horizontal chopping utilizes compressive forces, while vertical chopping relies upon shearing forces.

3. With horizontal chop, the chopper passes beneath the capsulorrhexis edge and hooks the nuclear equator, while the phaco tip is embedded just within the proximal capsulorrhexis edge to encompass as much nucleus as possible in the chopper's path.

4. With vertical chop, chopper stays central to the capsulorrhexis and incises just in front of the phaco tip, which is deeply embedded in the center of the nucleus to maximize fixation.

5. Using horizontal chop to subdivide mobile fragments into progressively smaller pieces reduces chatter and particle turbulence.

REFERENCES

1. Shepherd JR. In situ fracture. *J Cataract Refract Surg.* 1990;16:436-440.
2. Gimbel HV. Divide and conquer nucleofractis phacoemulsification: development and variations. *J Cataract Refract Surg.* 1991;17:281-291.
3. Koch PS, Katzen LE. Stop and chop phacoemulsification. *J Cataract Refract Surg.* 1994;20:566-570.
4. Vasavada AR, Desai, JP. Stop, chop, chop, and stuff. *J Cataract Refract Surg.* 1996;22:526-529.
5. Maloney WF, Dillman DM, Nichamin LD. Supracapsular phacoemulsification: a capsule-free posterior chamber approach. *J Cataract Refract Surg.* 1997;23:323-328.
6. Chang DF. Converting to phaco chop: why and how. *Ophthalmic Practice.* 1999;17(4):202-210.
7. Fine IH, Packer M, Hoffman RS. Use of power modulations in phacoemulsification. Choo-choo chop and flip phacoemulsification. *J Cataract Refract Surg.* 2001;27:188-197.
8. Arshinoff SA. Phaco slice and separate. *J Cataract Refract Surg.* 1999;25:474-478.
9. Gimbel HV, Neuhann T. Development, advantages, and methods of the continuous circular capsulorrhexis technique. *J Cataract Refract Surg.* 1990;16:31-37.
10. Assia EI, Legler UF, Merrill C, et al. Clinicopathologic study of the effect of radial tears and loop fixation on intraocular lens decentration. *Ophthalmology.* 1993;100:153-158.
11. Assia EI, Legler UF, Apple DJ. The capsular bag after short- and long-term fixation of intraocular lenses. *Ophthalmology.* 1995;102:1151-1157.
12. Ram J, Apple DJ, Peng Q, et al. Update on fixation of rigid and foldable posterior chamber intraocular lenses. Part I: Elimination of fixation-induced decentration to achieve precise optical correction and visual rehabilitation. *Ophthalmology.* 1999;106:883-890.
13. Fine IH. Cortical cleaving hydrodissection. *J Cataract Refract Surg.* 1992;18:508-512.
14. Peng Q, Apple DJ, Visessook N, et al. Surgical prevention of posterior capsule opacification. Part 2: Enhancement of cortical clean up by focusing on hydrodissection. *J Cataract Refract Surg.* 2000;26:188-197.

15. Vasavada AR, Singh R, Apple DJ, et al. Effect of hydrodissection on intraoperative performance: Randomized study. *J Cataract Refract Surg.* 2002;28:1623-1628.
16. Uy HS, Edwards K, Curtis N. Femtosecond phacoemulsification: the business and the medicine. *Curr Opin Ophthalmol.* 2012;23:33-39. Review.
17. Pirazzoli G, D'Eliseo D, Ziosi M, Acciarri R. Effects of phacoemulsification time on the corneal endothelium using phacofracture and phaco chop techniques. *J Cataract Refract Surg.* 1996;22:967-969.
18. DeBry P, Olson RJ, Crandall, AS. Comparison of energy required for phaco-chop and divide and conquer phacoemulsification. *J Cataract Refract Surg.* 1998;24:689-692.
19. Ram J, Wesendahl TA, Auffarth GU, Apple DJ. Evaluation of in situ fracture versus phaco chop techniques. *J Cataract Refract Surg.* 1998;24:1464-1468.
20. Wong T, Hingorani M, Lee V. Phacoemulsification time and power requirements in phaco chop and divide and conquer nucleofractis techniques. *J Cataract Refract Surg.* 2000;26:1374-1378.
21. Chang DF. Chapter 31: prevention pearls and damage control. In: Fishkind W, ed. *Complications in Phacoemulsification.* New York, NY: Thieme; 2002.
22. Chang DF. *Phaco Chop and Advanced Phaco Techniques: Strategies for Complicated Cataracts.* 2nd ed. Thorofare, NJ: SLACK Incorporated; 2013.
23. Horiguchi M, Miyake K, Ohta I, Ito Y. Staining of the lens capsule for circular continuous capsulorrhexis in eyes with white cataract. *Arch Ophthalmol.* 1998;116:535-537.
24. Melles G, de Waard P, Pameyer J, Beekhuis W. Trypan blue capsule staining to visualize the capsulorrhexis in cataract surgery. *J Cataract Refract Surg.* 1999;25:7-9.
25. Vasavada AR, Singh R. Step-by-step chop in situ and separation of very dense cataracts. *J Cataract Refract Surg.* 1998;24:156-159.
26. Vanathi M, Vajpayee RB, Tandon R, et al. Crater-and-chop technique for phacoemsulsification of hard cataracts. *J Cataract Refract Surg.* 2001;27:659-661.

15

IRRIGATION AND ASPIRATION

Wuqaas M. Munir, MD and Carol L. Karp, MD

I. INTRODUCTION

Removal of residual cortical material following phacoemulsification can at times be challenging and can lead to posterior capsular rupture. Understanding the principles and techniques of irrigation and aspiration (I/A) will enable the surgeon to use a structured approach and allow for safe and efficient evacuation of residual cortex.

II. CORTEX ANATOMY

During cataract surgery, lens cortex can be encountered surgically in 2 layers: supranuclear cortex and peripheral cortex. Surgically, cortex exhibits a high degree of "followability."[1] Cortical material flows to the I/A tip easily and is likewise able to be aspirated without difficulty. The same is not true of more solid, stiff nuclear material.

- Epinucleus, or supranuclear cortex, refers to the soft, continuous region of cortex surrounding the nucleus.[1] Hydrodelineation will often produce this epinuclear shell.[2] Careful manipulation of the epinucleus can allow for its removal as a single bowl.

- Peripheral cortex, as the name implies, is located beneath the anterior capsule, into the equatorial region, and lines the posterior capsule.[1] Peripheral cortex tends to have a more fibrous texture. Under the anterior capsule and in the equator, intralenticular cells retain a pseudofibrous metaplastic capability. These cells are also involved in thickening of the anterior lens capsule, which leads to firm attachments of the cortex to the capsule in these locations.[3] Intralenticular cell attachments are not present adjacent to the posterior capsule. This

Henderson BA. *Essentials of Cataract Surgery, Second Edition (pp 149-156).*
© 2014 Taylor & Francis Group.

differential property is important to consider during aspiration of cortical fibers, as peripheral cortex requires a stripping action from the equatorial and anterior lens capsule in order to achieve a meticulous cortical cleanup.

III. INSTRUMENTATION

Although a variety of hand piece configurations are available, most aspiration instruments use a 0.3-mm side-ported orifice. This size allows for efficient aspiration, while minimizing inadvertent lens capsule entrapment. Cortical aspiration can be performed using a coaxial or a bimanual technique.

A. Coaxial Versus Bimanual

Both irrigation and aspiration of the I/A instrument typically coexist on a coaxial hand piece with an outer irrigating sleeve surrounding a central aspirating port. Since most cataract surgeons still employ coaxial phacoemulsification, coaxial I/A remains a popular choice. However, subincisional cortical cleanup can sometimes be difficult.

Bimanual I/A separates the I/A portions into separate hand pieces.[4] These smaller hand pieces fit through smaller wounds, including paracentesis ports. The hand pieces can be inserted interchangeably, allowing access to all subincisional locations (Figure 15-1). In addition, the irrigating hand piece can be directed to control fluid inflow away from suspect areas such as capsular tears. The use of smaller incisions also allows for better control of fluid inflow and outflow, providing improved anterior chamber stability.

One small disadvantage to most bimanual techniques is that they require a second paracentesis port, since the main wound is often too large to maintain adequate seal with insertion of a small diameter bimanual instrument. An alternative option is to use a standard coaxial hand piece for irrigation through the main wound, with the smaller bimanual hand piece for aspiration through the paracentesis. The larger diameter coaxial hand piece provides the high flow needed to maintain the anterior chamber and obviates the need for additional incisions. As an alternative to automated bimanual systems, nonautomated bimanual I/A instrumentation can also be used with similar advantages (Simcoe I/A). These manually controlled I/A devices provide a very controlled cortical cleanup and are especially useful in the setting of a posterior capsular rupture.

B. Soft Versus Metal Sleeve

Traditional coaxial I/A hand pieces consist of a metal irrigating sleeve with a central metal aspirating port. However, given the smaller diameter of I/A versus phacoemulsification hand pieces, these metal sleeves allow for wound gape and subsequent anterior chamber instability. Newer silicone soft sleeves

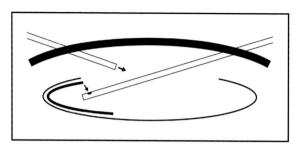

Figure 15-1. Bimanual irrigation and aspiration provides easier access to subincisional cortex.

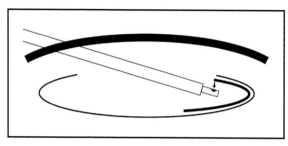

Figure 15-2. A straight aspiration tip is most suitable for reaching cortex away from the incision.

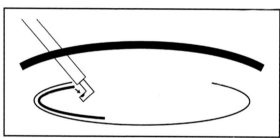

Figure 15-3. A 90-degree angled tip can assist in removing subincisional cortical material.

are available that provide for tighter wound seals and more stable anterior chamber maintenance. These benefits of chamber maintenance extend also to viscoelastic removal and may improve intraocular lens (IOL) rotational stability.

C. Irrigation and Aspiration Tips

Coaxial I/A hand pieces come in a variety of tip angles, with a side aspiration port. A straight tip allows for easy access to cortical material 180 degrees from the main incision (Figure 15-2). However, subincisional cortex can be difficult to reach with this tip. A 90-degree tip, conversely, provides for more facile subincisional cortex removal (Figure 15-3) but can be a hindrance when approaching cortical material opposite the incision. Intermediate tips, such as at 45 degrees or "banana" shaped, can be helpful for all-purpose use. For capsular vacuuming, roughened tips or silicone tips can be used to enhance

TABLE 15-1. EXAMPLE SETTINGS FOR IRRIGATION AND ASPIRATION MODES			
	Cortex Removal	Capsular Vacuum	Viscoelastic Removal
Aspiration (mL)	40	10	50
Vacuum (mm Hg)	650	10	650
Bottle height (cm)	100	100	100

posterior capsule polishing. Some surgeons are using silicone tips for all parts of the cortical removal. In addition, disposable tips may reduce the likelihood of debris retention and clogging as can be present in reusable metal tips.

D. Settings

Most surgeons adapt their I/A settings based on situational and personal preference (Table 15-1). For cortical I/A, high vacuum settings allow for ease in epinuclear removal and cortical stripping. Capsular vacuum settings, however, demand much lower vacuum and aspiration rates. While capsule may still be incarcerated at these low settings, the safety margin is greatly enhanced when working near the posterior capsule with this mode. Removal of viscoelastic is usually under both high vacuum and aspiration rate settings to promote adequate irrigation of the anterior chamber.

IV. TECHNIQUE

The I/A hand piece is classically used for cortex removal. However, there are a number of other circumstances in which the I/A hand piece is used in cataract surgery, and the techniques of I/A can be approached in a stepwise fashion.

A. Wounds and Hydrodissection

Like most steps in successful cataract surgery, efficient I/A depends upon the steps that precede it. A properly constructed incision is vital to maintaining a tight wound, especially when using metal-sleeved coaxial I/A. Hydrodissection is essentially the first step in cortical removal. Well executed cortical cleaving hydrodissection can sometimes eliminate the need for the I/A by allowing for nearly full cortex removal during phacoemulsification.[2]

B. Epinucleus and Nuclear Chips

Following phacoemulsification of the nucleus, a residual epinuclear bowl may sometimes remain. Often, this epinucleus is freely mobile secondary to prior hydrodissection. If attachments still exist, it is beneficial to maintain the integrity of the entire bowl. Using the I/A hand piece, this epinuclear shell can be gently relieved from its capsular attachments by approaching the sub-anterior capsule rim with the I/A aspirating port facing up, applying gentle aspiration until occlusion is achieved. The cortical material is then teased toward the pupillary center and then released. This procedure is repeated for the entire circumference of the epinucleus, making sure not to aspirate any material at this point. By maintaining the epinuclear bowl until all of attachments are released, the epinuclear rim can be used as a protective shell against capsular entrapment in the I/A port. Once the epinucleus is free, it can be brought into the anterior chamber for aspiration. Alternatively, the I/A tip can be introduced underneath the bowl with the aspirating tip up to allow for safe removal.

Occasionally, small nuclear remnants are left following phacoemulsification that are often too stiff to be aspirated using the I/A alone. A second instrument can be inserted through the paracentesis and used to gently push the material into the I/A side port once occlusion is achieved.

C. Cortical Stripping

The mainstay of I/A-assisted cortical removal, cortical stripping, requires deliberate technique to avoid capsular complications. Peripheral cortical fibers may be present as interspersed wisps or as confluent cortex. To reach peripheral cortex to the left of the incision, the hand piece should be positioned along the right edge of the wound. The reverse position with the hand piece at the left edge of the wound is employed to reach cortex to the right of the incision. Some surgeons prefer to remove the more challenging subincisional cortex first, while others remove subincisional cortex at the end of cortical cleanup.

Introducing the I/A tip with the side port facing up, the subanterior capsular region is approached, taking care to maintain distance from the posterior capsule as well as the anterior capsule edge. Gentle aspiration is then applied to engage cortical fibers. If occlusion is not reached or inadequate quantity of cortex is grasped, the tip can be reintroduced under the anterior capsule and toward the equator if necessary. Once the port is full of cortical material, occlusion is achieved, and vacuum begins to rise, the tip is withdrawn toward the pupil, maintaining occlusion through continued aspiration. As the anterior capsular edge is cleared, more vigorous aspiration can be applied, allowing the I/A vacuum to strip the cortical fibers. Alternatively, with cortical material filling the port, manual stripping of the cortex can be performed with gentle rotation of the tip toward the pupillary center, followed by aspiration once the cortex is free of attachments.

This technique is repeated for the full circumference of the capsular bag. In order for I/A-assisted cortical stripping to be successful, proper occlusion with cortical material is necessary. Often, large arcs of cortex can be incorporated

Figure 15-4. Capsular polish entails carefully placing the aspiration tip down toward the posterior capsular plaque and gently prying the cortical fibers from the capsule.

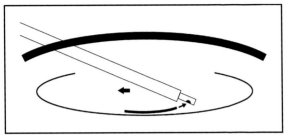

by repeated engagement of the subanterior capsular cortical fibers along a sweeping arc, until all peripheral cortical fibers have been removed.

D. Capsular Polish

On occasion, a resilient posterior cortical plaque may remain. Posterior subcapsular cataracts often present such a challenge. This plaque may be approached with a variety of methods. First, to reduce the likelihood of posterior capsular rupture, the I/A settings should be adjusted for capsular vacuuming (see Table 15-1), reducing vacuum and aspiration rate for greater safety near the capsule. The I/A tip can then be brought with the side port perpendicular to, or carefully facing down toward, the posterior cortical material. A gentle sweeping motion can be used to catch the edge of the plaque and pry the fibers from the capsule (Figure 15-4). To assist in a scraping technique, a studded tip may be used to provide greater friction against the fibrotic cortical fibers. If an edge can be lifted, viscoelastic may also be injected under this edge to help "viscodissect" the plaque.[5]

Caution must be exercised in removing resilient posterior capsular plaques, such as those found in small posterior polar cataract. In this situation, an irregularity in the posterior capsule may be preexisting or easily induced.[6] This makes presentation of vitreous a real possibility. In cases of difficult to remove posterior cortical fibers, it may be prudent to leave the cortex for later neodymium-doped yttrium-aluminum-garnet (nd:YAG) laser capsulotomy.[6]

E. Viscoelastic Removal

Following insertion of the IOL, remaining viscoelastic material must be irrigated and aspirated from the eye to prevent subsequent intraocular pressure rise.[7-9] Settings for viscoelastic removal include both high aspiration rate and vacuum to promote copious irrigation and adequate aspiration (see Table 15-1). Viscoelastic may become sequestered behind the IOL, and thus gentle rocking of the lens with the I/A tip can help free this material. Additionally, sweeping the angle with the tip aids in removing viscoelastic trapped in the anterior chamber particularly with viscodispersive and viscoadaptive agents.[10]

V. Practical Tips for Subincisional Cortex

Many cases of capsular rupture during cortex removal occur when subincisional cortex is manipulated. Given the difficult angle of approach underneath the wound, and the tendency for further compromise of adequate visualization from easily induced corneal striae, subincisional cortex poses many problems during I/A. However, by applying a systematic approach, I/A of subincisional cortex can be performed safely and efficiently.

A. Choose Proper Instrumentation

Choosing a tip angulation well-suited for subincisional cortex removal can be helpful (see Figure 15-3). Angled tips, such as the 45-degree, banana shaped, or more optimally the 90 degree tip, provide better ergonomics. Bimanual I/A systems eliminate the dilemma by allowing for entry of the aspiration port through a different incision, making access to all recesses equal (see Figure 15-1). In cases where coaxial I/A is first attempted, either automated or nonautomated bimanual I/A is an option.

B. Rotational Technique

With coaxial I/A, subincisional cortex can be stripped in an arc-like fashion to simplify removal. Cortex is first engaged with the side port facing up and toward the surgeon along one edge of the incision. Once occlusion is achieved, the I/A hand piece is rotated so that the side port swivels under the incision, until it re-emerges on the other side of the incision. The side port remains facing up and away from the posterior capsule during the entire maneuver. This technique helps strip the cortex in an arc-like fashion beneath the wound and maintains a safe aspiration port position at all times.

C. Insertion of Intraocular Lens as Tamponade

When the bulk of cortical material has been removed, the IOL can be inserted for capsular bag stability and tamponade. Then, I/A can be resumed, using the lens as a shield to posterior capsule entrapment. This technique is also helpful in cases of highly mobile posterior capsules, such as those encountered in high myopia or prior vitrectomy. The IOL can also be dragged with the I/A tip toward the capsular bag equator for added safety during aspiration. However, if a large quantity of cortical material remains, the IOL haptics can make cortical removal more difficult by trapping cortex against the capsular bag.

VI. Conclusion

Efficient I/A requires a proper understanding of the lens anatomy and facility with the instrumentation and techniques involved. A good cataract surgeon adapts the surgical technique to each individual case, modifying parameters based upon the situation at hand. There are many options and variations on I/A, a combination of which should be mastered for proficient cataract removal.

KEY POINTS

1. Choose an angled tip for easier access to subincisional cortex.
2. Consider a bimanual I/A system, especially for difficult-to-reach cortical material.
3. Avoid trauma to the capsule through diligent attention to the aspiration tip and by stripping cortical fibers toward the pupillary center.
4. Modify the I/A settings based upon the situation and particulars of each case.
5. Perform careful capsular polish with consideration to settings and specialized tips, while remembering that later nd:YAG capsulotomy is an option for resilient posterior plaques.

REFERENCES

1. Chylack LT. Surgical anatomy, biochemistry, pathogenesis, and classification of cataracts. In: Steinert RF, ed. *Cataract Surgery, 2nd Edition—Technique, Complications, and Management.* Philadelphia, PA: W.B. Saunders; 2004:9-17.
2. Fine IH. Cortical cleaving hydrodissection. *J Cat Refract Surg.* 1992;18:508-512.
3. Peng Q, Apple DJ, Visessook N, et al. Surgical prevention of posterior capsule opacification. Part 2: enhancement of cortical clean up by focusing on hydrodissection. *J Cat Refract Surg.* 2000;26:188-197.
4. Reiss G, Dulaney D, Ness J. Bimanual cortex removal. *Ophthalmic Surg.* 1994;25:659-660.
5. Fine IH, Packer M, Hoffman RS. Hydrodissection and hydrodelineation. In: Steinert RF, ed. *Cataract Surgery, 2nd Edition—Technique, Complications, and Management.* Philadelphia, PA: W.B. Saunders; 2004:147-152.
6. Fine IH, Packer M, Hoffman RS. Management of posterior polar cataract. *J Cat Refract Surg.* 2003;29:16-19.
7. Barron BA, Busin M, Page C, et al. Comparison of the effects of Viscoat and Healon on postoperative intraocular pressure. *Am J Ophthalmol.* 1985;100:377-384.
8. Pape LG. Intracapsular and extracapsular technique of lens implantation with Healon. *J Am Intraocul Implant Soc.* 1980;6:342-343.
9. Choyce DP. Healon in anterior chamber lens implantation. *J Am Intraocul Implant Soc.* 1981;7:138-139.
10. Cavallini GM, Campi L, Delvecchio G, Lazzerini A, Longanesi L. Comparison of the clinical performance of Healon 5 and Healon in phacoemulsification. *Eur J Ophthalmol.* 2002;12:205-211.

16

INTRAOCULAR LENS CALCULATIONS

Lisa Park, MD

I. INTRODUCTION

Choosing the appropriate intraocular lens (IOL) power is a major determinant of patient satisfaction with cataract surgery. The 3 main factors to consider include taking accurate measurements (biometry), selecting appropriate calculations (formulas), and assessing the patient's needs and expectations to determine the postoperative refractive target (clinical considerations).

II. BIOMETRY

At minimum, 2 measurements are required to calculate the appropriate implant power: the axial length and the corneal curvature (keratometry) of the eye. Precise measurements are critical given that an error of only 0.3 mm in axial length will result in a 1-D error in IOL power.

A. Axial Length

1. A-scan ultrasound

Axial length has traditionally been obtained utilizing A-scan ultrasound to measure the distance between the anterior surface of the cornea and the fovea. This measurement is determined by calculation; an ultrasound pulse is applied and the transit time through the eye is measured. Using estimated velocities of ultrasound waves through various media (ie, cornea, aqueous, lens, and vitreous) the distance traveled through the eye is then calculated.

1. The instrument should have an oscilloscope screen to differentiate a good measurement from a poor one. Characteristic echo peaks or spikes should be observed when the probe is aligned properly (Figure 16-1).

Henderson BA. *Essentials of Cataract Surgery, Second Edition* (pp 157-166).
© 2014 Taylor & Francis Group.

Figure 16-1. A-scan measurement of axial length. C: initial spike (probe tip and cornea). L1: anterior lens capsule. L2: posterior lens capsule. R: retina. (Reprinted with permission of Warren Hill, MD.)

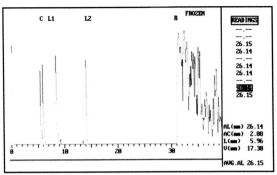

These include the following: a tall peak for the cornea, tall peaks for the anterior and posterior lens capsule, tall peak for the retina, moderate peak for the sclera, and moderate-to-low peaks for orbital fat. If these spikes are not well seen, then the probe may be misaligned.

2. The contact A-scan technique must be performed carefully, as compressing the cornea will result in a shorter-than-expected measurement. It is recommended that measurements are taken to the nearest hundredth of a millimeter, and multiple measurements should be taken and averaged. If several are taken and differ by a significant amount, they should be discarded until consistent readings can be obtained. It is also prudent to measure both eyes for comparison.

3. Measurements must be adjusted for specific clinical situations—silicone oil in the posterior chamber, aphakia, dense cataract, etc. Be sure to choose the machine settings appropriate for the eye being measured (ie, phakic, aphakic, pseudophakic). Additionally, the machine should be regularly calibrated, checking measurements against an eye of known axial length.

2. Immersion technique

1. The immersion technique of Ossoinig[1] is thought to more accurately represent the true axial length because there is no corneal compression.

2. In this technique, the patient lies in the supine position and a scleral shell is placed on the eye and filled with Goniosol. The ultrasound probe is placed in this solution and the beam is aligned with the macula by having the patient look at the probe tip fixation light.

3. Although the immersion method may be strongly advocated by some users, applanation A-scan is the more commonly used method and has provided the data for the overwhelming majority of IOL calculation research. IOL-specific A-constants and ACD-constants are based

on applanation techniques and need to be adjusted if immersion measurements are used.

3. Optical biometry: IOLMaster

In the last decade, the technique of optical coherence biometry was introduced by Haigis,[2] which utilizes light rather than ultrasound to measure the length of the eye. The first device introduced was the IOLMaster (Zeiss), based on the principle of partial coherence interferometry using a 780-nm multimode laser diode.

1. There are 2 advantages to the IOLMaster: (1) Measurements are taken without contact to the patient's eye, thus eliminating variability due to an examiner technique. (2) The distance measured lies between the anterior surface of the tear film and the retinal pigmented pigment epithelium(rather than the anterior surface of the cornea and the internal limiting membrane), which may be more physiologically accurate (refractive rather than anatomic axial length).

2. To use this instrument, the patient is asked to focus on a small red fixation light, and the examiner maneuvers the focusing spot within the measurement reticule, sampling areas until the best peak pattern is obtained. Five to 20 measurements are then obtained until the readings differ by less than 0.1 mm. Maximal axial length measured is 40 mm.

3. The primary disadvantage of this optical device is that any significant axial opacity, such as a corneal scar, dense posterior subcapsular plaque, darkly brunescent cataract, or vitreous hemorrhage, will reduce the signal-to-noise ratio (SNR) to the point that reliable measurements are not possible.

4. Optical biometry: LENSTAR

The second optical biometry device introduced was the LENSTAR (Haag-Streit). This unit utilizes optical low coherence reflectometry with a superluminescent diode laser of 820 nm.

1. Because of the spectral characteristics of this laser, a high level of resolution can be achieved and reflective structures within the cornea, anterior chamber, lens, and retina can be detected. This allows simultaneous measurements of the axial length, central corneal thickness, anterior chamber depth, and lens thickness.

2. Although both the IOLMaster and the LENSTAR measure axial length using optical biometry (maximal axial length measured is 32 mm), the LENSTAR also uses this technology to measure anterior chamber depth, while the IOLMaster uses slit lamp imagery, which is considered to be slightly less accurate.

5. Data validation

A-scans should be re-measured under the following conditions[3]:

1. Axial length is less than 22 mm or greater than 25 mm in either eye.
2. The difference between the 2 eyes is greater than 0.3 mm.
3. The measurements do not correlate with the patient's refraction (ie, hyperopes should have shorter eyes, and myopes should have longer eyes).

B. Corneal Curvature

The general principle of keratometry is the following: an illuminated object (such as a ring) is placed near the eye, and the cornea acts as a convex mirror reflecting light off of its surface, producing a virtual image. The size and position of this image are measured. Knowing the object size, the image size, and the distance between the object and the reflective surface, the radius of the reflective surface can then be calculated. It should be noted that neither manual keratometers nor automated keratometers measure the central curvature directly. Multiple intermediate areas are measured and the central corneal power is calculated.

1. Manual keratometry

The classic Bausch & Lomb keratometer is the gold standard for manual keratometry, which measures 2 reflected mires at approximately 3 to 3.2 mm. Unusual readings obtained via other methods should be checked manually.

1. The eyepiece should first be carefully focused to the examiner's eye. Failure to do so may result in errors greater than 1 D in power.
2. The keratometry measurements should be performed prior to the A-scan, as applanation may result in corneal irregularities.
3. A single reading is not satisfactory; repeat until 2 identical measurements are taken in both meridians. Measurements from both eyes should be compared and any unusual readings should be rechecked.

2. Automated keratometry

Automated keratometry is based on the same principles, utilizing optical sensors and computerized technology to measure the cornea at the flat and steep meridians. Both the IOLMaster and LENSTAR analyze a pattern of LEDs imaged on the front surface of the cornea to determine the corneal curvature.

1. The IOLMaster measures curvature based on the relative position of 6 projected light reflections at a 2.5-mm optical zone.
2. The LENSTAR makes use of 32 reference points, that are arranged on 2 concentric rings with 16 measuring points each. The outer circle is projected in a 2.3-mm diameter ring, and the inner circle is projected

in a 1.65-mm diameter ring. The small diameter can provide useful data in patients who have undergone a refractive laser procedure that has altered the central corneal curvature.

3. Topographic keratometry

Topographic analysis measures the corneal curvature over the surface at hundreds to thousands of data points. These measurements are then used to calculate a simulated keratometry value (Sim-K). This type of analysis may provide greater accuracy than keratometers in corneas with irregular astigmatism; however, the derivations vary between different topography units due to variable settings and calibrations. Therefore, care should be taken before using these interchangeably with measured keratometry readings.

4. Data validation

Manual keratometry readings should be repeated under the following conditions[3]:
1. Corneal curvature is less than 40 D or greater than 47 D.
2. The difference is greater than 1 D between 2 eyes.
3. The keratometry measurements correlate poorly with the refractive corneal cylinder.

III. FORMULAS

Lens power calculation formulas have evolved over the past 30 years, since the first theoretical formula for iris-supported lenses was published by Fyodorov and Kolonko[4] in 1967.

A. First Generation

Initial formulas were based largely on axial length, but with the availability of posterior chamber implants, consideration had to be given to the distance from the cornea to the implant (anterior chamber depth). By studying large numbers of cases, linear regression techniques were used to determine a formula for predicting emmetropic implant power. The most widely used regression formula was developed by Sanders, Retzlaff, and Kraff in 1980 and is known as the *SRK formula*.[5-7]

$$P = A - (2.5 \times AL) - (0.9 \times K)$$

where P is the lens implant power (diopters), AL is the axial length (mm), K is average keratometry (diopters), and A is the *constant* (no units), a theoretical value that relates the lens power to axial length and keratometry. It is specific to the design of the IOL and its intended position inside the eye. This number is specified by the IOL manufacturer.

B. Second Generation

The SRK formula is a linear equation derived by fitting collected data to a straight line. However, the optical system is nonlinear and begins to produce significant error with short or long eyes. To improve accuracy, the formula was modified, taking into consideration variation in axial length. This enhancement is known as the *SRK II*[8] formula in which the *A*-constant is defined at different axial lengths:

$A = A + 3$ (AL < 21 mm)
$A = A + 2$ (20 mm < AL < 21 mm)
$A = A + 1$ (21 mm < AL < 22 mm)
$A = A$ (22 mm < AL < 24.5 mm)
$A = A - 0.5$ (24.5 mm < AL)

Although the SRK II formula was an improvement, there was a push to increase accuracy and design formulas based on both empirical and theoretical data. These second-generation formulas include those pioneered by Binkhorst[9] and Hoffer,[10] which included different approaches for predicting the anterior chamber depth (*ACD constant*).

C. Third Generation

In 1988, Holladay et al[11] further refined the theoretical formulas by proposing a relationship between the steepness of the cornea and the position of the IOL. Instead of factoring in the anterior chamber depth, the formula would calculate the distance from the cornea to the iris plane and add the distance from the iris plane to the IOL. This second variable was termed the *surgeon factor*, was specific to each lens, and had the ability to be personalized and adjust for any consistent bias in the surgeon's results. Hoffer achieved the same effect via another approach in his *Hoffer Q*[12] formula. Retzlaff followed suit to take into consideration not only the position of the implant, but also incorporated a correction for the retinal thickness, thus developing the *SRK/T*[13] formula in 1990.

D. Fourth Generation

In the early 1990s, Haigis presented the notion that the individual geometry of each IOL model also should be considered in determining which formula to use. The geometry for a particular IOL model is not the same at all powers; therefore, the *Haigis*[14] formula utilizes 3 lens constants to address these issues:

a_0 constant moves the power prediction curve up or down
a_1 constant is tied to the measured anterior chamber depth
a_2 constant is tied to the measured axial length

Optimization of the Haigis formula requires collecting pre- and postoperative data from over 200 patients in order to allow surgeon-specific optimization, which is available online.

In the late 1990s, the *Holladay 2* IOL consultant software was introduced to attempt to improve upon predictability by incorporating additional optical data points. It requires 7 measurements including white-to-white corneal diameter, anterior chamber depth, lens thickness, patient's age, preoperative refraction, keratometry, and axial length. This formula may be more precise in unusual eyes such as those that have undergone refractive surgery.

One or more of the third-generation formulas (SRK/T, Holladay 1, and Hoffer Q) are generally programmed into A-scan biometers sold today. The optical biometers are now incorporating the fourth-generation formulas (Haigis and Holladay 2).

Over time, some trends have emerged regarding which formulas to use in general categories of patients:

<22 mm: Hoffer Q
22 to 23 mm: Hoffer Q or Holladay 1
24 to 26 mm: Holladay 1
>26 mm: SRK/T or Holladay 2

It is essential to use the appropriate power calculation constant (*A-constant, ACD-constant, surgeon factor*) specified by the IOL manufacturer for the specific formula, chosen IOL style, and personalized as warranted by the surgeon.

E. Intraocular Lens Calculation After Refractive Surgery

The complex scenario of a patient undergoing cataract surgery after refractive surgery is becoming increasingly common. Determining the proper IOL power in these patients is a challenge for the surgeon, and while dozens of formulas have been published to address this issue, here we will focus on the basic sources of error that can contribute to a refractive surprise.

1. Error in corneal curvature

This error is due to the fact that keratometric measurements are not taken centrally, but slightly peripherally, where the curvature may be steeper or flatter than it is in the center after a myopic or hyperopic ablation, respectively.

2. Error in corneal power

To measure true corneal power, both the anterior and posterior surfaces must be considered. Classic keratometry, however, derives the refractive power of the cornea from the anterior surface alone and assumes a fixed ratio between the anterior and posterior corneal surface. Naturally this relationship has been altered in any refractive surgery, and therefore leads to an incorrect power calculation.

3. Error from the Intraocular Lens formula

Several IOL formulas assume the effective lens position based on the corneal power, which is reasonable in normal eyes. However, after refractive surgery, the new corneal curvature does not reflect the eye's original geometry. Therefore the resulting effective lens position will be calculated incorrectly, resulting in a hyperopic error after myopic refractive surgery.

Once the source of these errors is understood, steps can be taken to minimize the possibility of a refractive surprise.

1. To address the issue of corneal curvature: With the increased optical zones of refractive laser treatment, this error is becoming less of an issue. Measurements from the internal ring of the LENSTAR may contribute to more accurate data.

2. To address the issue of corneal power: Classically, this can be achieved using the refractive history method. Recent advancements in instrumentation have allowed direct measurements of both the anterior and posterior corneal surfaces that can overcome this error.

3. To address the issue of the IOL formula: A formula should be selected that does not use keratometric readings to predict the effective lens position, such as the Haigis formula.

The IOLMaster and the LENSTAR include software to address the postrefractive patient, and there are a number of free online IOL calculators that can be used, including on the ASCRS Web site: http://www.ascrs.org/.

IV. CLINICAL CONSIDERATIONS

Although emmetropia is often desirable, it may not always be the ideal postoperative refraction for all patients undergoing cataract extraction with IOL implantation. A thoughtful decision-making process should involve discussion with the patient, with adequate time to confirm the desired target refraction. A number of factors should be considered.

A. Visual Acuity and Refraction of the Other Eye

Consideration must be given to the refraction of the fellow eye particularly when surgery is being performed on only one eye, to avoid significant postoperative anisometropia (usually no more than 2 to 3 D difference).

B. The Refraction the Patient Has Been Accustomed to for Most of His or Her Life

It might be anticipated that a patient who is +6.00 or −6.00 would appreciate being plano OU after surgery. However, there are many patients who would not want to be changed from −2.50 to plano OU, necessitating reading glasses when they never needed them before.

C. The Lifestyle and Desires of the Patient, Including Occupational and Recreational Needs

Attention must be given to the patient's most frequent vision needs. For example, an attorney who reads many hours a day may prefer a myopic target refraction. Certain patients may also prefer monovision or blended vision, with a slightly higher power IOL in the nondominant eye to eliminate the need to wear glasses for most daily activities.

D. Availability of Premium Intraocular Lenses

There are now a number of IOLs that can address issues of presbyopia and astigmatism. These require an in-depth evaluation and counseling to determine the ideal candidate for these specialized implants.

KEY POINTS

1. Choosing the correct IOL power requires accurate biometry. The method chosen to obtain these measurements may not be as critical as careful technique. Small errors in axial length and keratometry can result in significant IOL power errors.

2. Third- or fourth-generation formulas should be used and data collected to optimize surgeon-specific outcomes.

3. Careful consideration of a patient's specific vision needs and expectations is a critical component of IOL power selection.

4. Incorrect IOL implantation does occur; "refractive surprise" is a complication that can occur with even the most careful planning. Once an IOL power has been chosen, this selection should be verified for each patient in the operating room and the packaging inspected prior to implantation.

REFERENCES

1. Ossoinig KC. Standardized echography: basic principles, clinical applications, and results. *Int Ophthalmol Clin.* 1979;19:127.
2. Haigis W. Optical coherence biometry. *Dev Ophthalmol.* 2002;34:119-130.
3. Holladay JT, Prager TC, Ruiz RS, Lewis JW, Rosenthal H. Improving the predictability of intraocular lens power calculations. *Arch Ophthalmol.* 1986;104:539-541.
4. Fyodorov SN, Kolonko AI. Estimation of optical power of the intraocular lens. *Vestnik Oftalmologic (Moscow).* 1967;4:27.
5. Retzlaff J. A new intraocular lens calculation formula. *J Am Intraocul Implant Soc.* 1980;6:148-152.
6. Sanders DR, Kraff MC. Improvement of intraocular lens calculation using empirical data. *J Am Intraocul Implant Soc.* 1980;6:263-267.

7. Retzlaff J. Posterior chamber implant power calculation: regressive formulas. *J Am Intraocul Implant Soc.* 1980;6:268-270.

8. Sanders DR, Retzlaff J, Kraff MC. Comparison of the SRK II formula and the other second generation formulas. *J Cataract Refract Surg.* 1988;14:136-141.

9. Binkhorst RD. *Intraocular Lens Calculations Manual: A Guide to the Author's TI 58/59 IOL Power Module.* 2nd ed. New York: RD Binkhorst, 1981.

10. Binkhorst RD. Biometric A-scan ultrasonography and intraocular lens power calculation. In: Emery JE, ed. *Current Concepts in Cataract Surgery: Selected Proceedings of the Fifth Biennial Cataract Surgical Congress.* St. Louis: Mosby; 1987:175-182.

11. Holladay JT, Prager TC, Chandler TY, et al. A three-part system for refining intraocular lens power calculations. *J Cataract Refract Surg.* 1988;14:17-24.

12. Hoffer KJ. The Hoffer Q formula: a comparison of theoretic and regression formulas. *J Cataract Refract Surg.* 1993;19:700-712.

13. Retzlaff JA, Sanders DR, Kraff MC. Development of the SRK/T intraocular lens implant power calculation formula. *J Cataract Refract Surg.* 1990;16:333-340.

14. Haigis W: Einfluß der Optikform auf die individuelle Anpassung von Linsenkonstanten zur IOL-Berechnung. In: 9. Kongreß d. Deutschen Ges. f. Intraokularlinsen Implant., Kiel 1995 , hrsg.v. R Rochels, GIW Duncker, Ch Hartmann, Springer Heidelberg, 183-189, 1996.

17

Intraocular Lens Design, Material, and Delivery

Thomas A. Oetting, MS, MD; Hilary Beaver, MD;
and A. Tim Johnson, PhD, MD

I. Intraocular Lens Design

The importance of the contribution made by Dr. Harold Ridley cannot be overstated. He was the first surgeon to implant an artificial intraocular lens (IOLs) after he noticed that injured British pilots tolerated retained plastic intraocular fragments from their airplane canopies. Dr. Ridley postulated that an IOL could be developed using a similar inert material. Dr. Ridley's persistence despite significant problems with his initial IOL design led to our modern IOLs.

A. Early Lens Development

1. Harold Ridley IOL

1. History
   - First implanted November 29, 1949
   - Very controversial with established ophthalmology
   - 1981 IOL approved by the US FDA
   - 2000 Ridley knighted by Queen Elizabeth II
2. Design: polymethylmethacrylate (PMMA) disc
3. Advantages: innovative approach to aphakia
4. Disadvantages
   - Dense capsular fibrosis
   - Excess weight and poor capsular fixation allowed dislocation into the vitreous cavity, anterior chamber collapse, glaucoma, uveitis, and iris atrophy

Henderson BA. *Essentials of Cataract Surgery, Second Edition* (pp 167-182).
© 2014 Taylor & Francis Group.

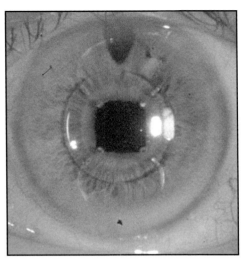

Figure 17-1. Binkhorst-style IOL with haptics straddling the pupil margin to provide fixation.

2. Anterior chamber lens (AC IOL)

1. Design: central optic, multiple haptics for angle fixation
2. Advantages:
   - Stable fixation in angle preventing dislocation
   - Easy to insert
3. Disadvantages:
   - Rigid haptic structure damaged tissue adjoining IOL
   - Size: undersized IOLs rotated causing corneal endothelial touch and pseudophakic bullous keratopathy; oversized IOLs caused chronic pain and inflammation
   - Vaulting: excessive vaulting damaged endothelium; inadequate vaulting caused iris damage and pupillary block glaucoma
   - Finish: initial poor quality IOL finish caused uveitis, hyphema, and glaucoma (UHG) syndrome

3. Iris-supported IOL

1. Design: iris fixation with sutures, metal clips, or haptics that straddled the iris through the pupil (Figure 17-1)
2. Advantages: avoids anterior chamber angle contact
3. Disadvantages:
   - Corneal decompensation
   - Cystoid macular edema
   - Dislocation common

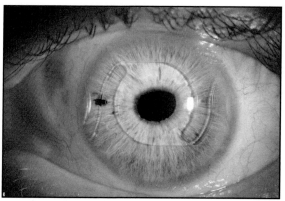

Figure 17-2. Modern AC IOL.

- Pupillary block
- Difficult to place

B. Diverging Surgical Techniques

Diverging surgical techniques (intracapsular cataract extraction [ICCE] versus extracapsular cataract extraction [ECCE]) led to 2 IOL approaches: anterior chamber (ICCE) and posterior chamber (ECCE).

1. Intracapsular cataract extraction

ICCE led to improved AC IOL.
1. AC IOL design
   - Improved polish, fixation, and vault
   - Improvements culminated with the modern Kelman AC IOL: one-piece PMMA lens with 2- or 3-point fixation via flexible haptics and small footplates resting on the scleral spur (Figure 17-2)
2. Advantages:
   - Haptic flexibility decreased ocular pain and corneal decompensation
   - Multiple haptic diameters available improved sizing

2. Extracapsular cataract extraction

ECCE led to improved PC IOL.
1. Posterior chamber IOL design
   - IOL fixed in the posterior chamber
   - Small optic and compressible haptics compatible with both capsular bag and sulcus, with or without iris sutures
   - Posterior vaulting avoids iris contact, inflammation, and pupil capture

2. Advantages:
   - Capsular bag yields best optical performance
   - Least collateral tissue damage
3. Disadvantages:
   - Capsular fixation requires intact posterior capsule
   - Sulcus fixation places IOL adjacent to iris tissue

C. Modern IOL Design

1. One-piece versus three-piece design
1. One-piece design with PMMA, acrylic, or silicone material
2. Three-piece design with PMMA, silicon, or acrylic optic, flexible PMMA polymer or polypropylene haptics

2. Haptic shape
The haptic shape is J- or C-loop configuration.

3. Fixation
1. Capsular bag: best location for all posterior chamber IOLs
2. Sulcus:
   - Large 1-piece PMMA, 3-piece silicone foldable, or 3-piece acrylic foldable IOL
   - Cannot use plate haptic silicon or one-piece acrylic in sulcus
3. No capsular support
   - Trans-scleral sutured sulcus lenses (haptic eyelets available on some PMMA IOL)
   - Iris fixated: McCannel suture versus iris claw lens
   - Anterior chamber lens

D. Foldable IOL Designs

1. Plate haptic silicone IOL (original foldable IOL)
1. Design: one-piece, silicone, foldable, and plate-haptic lens (Table 17-1 and Figure 17-3)
2. Advantages:
   - Smallest incisions with simple lens inserter
   - IOL flexes with capsular contraction, may decrease posterior capsular opacification (PCO)

TABLE 17-1. INTRAOCULAR LENS DESIGN CONSIDERATIONS		
Foldable Lens Design	Advantages	Disadvantages
Single piece: Foldable	Smaller incision, easy to inject	Sulcus incompatible
3 piece: Foldable	Sulcus compatible	Larger incision, tricky to inject
Square edge	Less PCO	Dysphotopsia
Round edge	Less dysphotopsia	More PCO

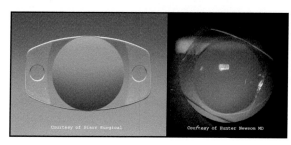

Figure 17-3. Plate-haptic IOL shown inserted in eye on right. (Reprinted with permission of STAAR Surgical and Hunter Newsom, MD.)

3. Disadvantages:
  ¤ Plate haptic defies tight capsular fixation: lens can rotate in capsular bag and can dislocate following posterior capsulotomy despite modern enlarged fixation hole
  ¤ Short haptic diameter does not allow sulcus fixation
  ¤ Requires intact anterior capsulorrhexis

2. Three-piece foldable IOL

Three-piece foldable IOL of silicone (Figure 17-4) or acrylic (see "Material" section on p. 173).
  1. Advantages:
    ¤ Excellent capsular fixation
    ¤ Haptics (often sturdy PMMA) allow sulcus fixation
    ¤ Compatible with iris and trans-scleral fixation
  2. Disadvantages:
    ¤ Require larger incision than plate haptic IOLs
    ¤ Haptic fragility with insertion
    ¤ Insertion systems more complicated

Figure 17-4. Three-piece, silicon IOL. (Reprinted with permission of STAAR Surgical.)

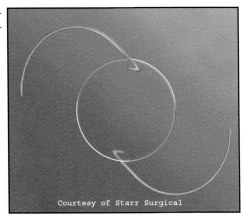

Courtesy of Starr Surgical

Figure 17-5. Single-piece acrylic IOL stable in bag with anterior capsular tear.

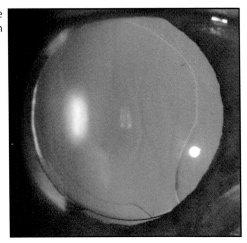

3. Single-piece acrylic IOL

1. Advantages:
   ▫ Small incision size
   ▫ Easy insertion as haptics are resistant to plunger damage
   ▫ Stable centration even with anterior capsular tear (Figure 17-5)
2. Disadvantages: cannot place thick square haptics in the sulcus

E. Optic Design Advances

1. Square optic edge on several silicone and acrylic IOLs

1. Advantages: sharp barrier to lens epithelial cell migration behind IOL decreases PCO (Figure 17-6)

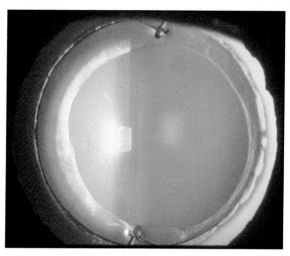

Figure 17-6. Three-piece acrylic IOL with capsular opacity only at margin blocked by square edge of optic.

2. Disadvantages:
   - Dysphotopsia, a positive and negative peripheral visual phenomena, more frequent and bothersome with smaller optic size IOLs and acrylic IOLs that can lead to IOL explantation (different IOL manufacturers have decreased dysphotopsia by enlarging the optic diameter, clouding the optic edge, and rounding the anterior optic edge)
   - Thick, sharp-edged haptics of one-piece acrylic IOL design cause iris chafe, irritation with sulcus fixation

2. Anterior or posterior IOL optic surface modified to counteract the spherical aberration of the cornea

1. Advantages: improved contrast sensitivity and mesopic acuity
2. Disadvantages: increased susceptibility to higher-order aberrations with lens tilt or decentration
3. Multifocal optic designs

They are covered in Chapter 29.

II. INTRAOCULAR LENS MATERIAL

A successful IOL must maintain optical clarity long after implantation within the eye. The evolution of the modern IOL began in 1949 with Dr. Ridley's implantation of IOLs made of PMMA. His persistence with this material eventually demonstrated the high degree of biocompatibility of PMMA within the human eye. This polymer needs to be free of pigments, plasticizers, and other additives to be tolerated within the human eye. Lens styles today continue to rely on PMMA, including anterior chamber, iris fixated, and

TABLE 17-2. INTRAOCULAR LENS MATERIAL CONSIDERATIONS		
Lens Material	Advantages	Disadvantages
PMMA	Time tested, least expensive, little inflammation	Wound size ≥ optic diameter
Acrylic	Wound <3.0 mm, least inflammation	Cost, dysphotopsia
Silicone	Inexpensive, wound <3.0 mm	More inflammation, silicone oil (for RD repair) can adhere to silicone IOL

posterior chamber designs. The most common IOLs used today, however, have optics made from foldable material to allow for a smaller incision (Table 17-2).

A. Optic Materials

1. PMMA
2. Foldable material: silicone, hydrophilic and hydrophobic acrylic

B. Haptic Materials

1. Nylon: degraded and was abandoned by most manufacturers in 1979
2. Polyamide
3. Polypropylene: found to increase bacterial adhesion and has been associated with an increased risk of endophthalmitis
4. PMMA: most common

C. Chromatophores

1. Included in optic polymer, absorb ultraviolet radiation. Reduced transmission of ultraviolet light to the retina in theory lowers the incidence of cystoid macular edema and age-related macular degeneration
2. Recent acrylic chromatophores remove additional blue light from the transmission spectrum, in theory protecting retinal cells from near ultraviolet blue light toxicity

D. Foldable Optic Materials

IOLs that could be folded into a small profile and implanted through small incisions near the size of the phacoemulsification needle revolutionized cataract surgery.

1. Silicone

Silicone is manufactured from polymers of highly cross-linked siloxanes, frequently with benztriazole (an UV absorbing chromophore). Early silicone materials had impurities that led to IOL discoloration. These impurities are now filtered out, resulting in siloxanes that remain clear. Silicone oil used in some complex retinal surgeries can irreversibly bind to the silicone IOL. As such, many surgeons do not use silicone IOLs in cases such as severe diabetic retinopathy where silicone oil may be required in the future.

2. Hydrogel

Hydrogen is a hydrophilic acrylic material, is a polymer of hydroxy-ethylmethacrylate (HEMA), alone or in combination with another acrylic monomer such as methylmethacrylate (MMA), which is flexible at body temperature, but rigid below 10°C.

1. Higher water content than other IOL materials
2. Calcification of the optic surface has been reported. Various surgical- and patient-related factors have been proposed in the etiology of the calcification, but the exact mechanism is not clear

3. Hydrophobic acrylic

Not a single molecule but a blend of different polymers. For example, copolymers of phenylethyl acrylate and phenylethyl methacrylate are used in the Alcon AcrySof, and ethylacrylate, ethylmethacrylate, and trifluorethyl-methacrlate are used for the Advanced Medical Optics (AMO) Sensar.

1. High index of refraction, allowing a thinner IOL to fold into a small profile to pass through a smaller incision
2. Glistenings are microscopic pockets of water within the matrix of the lens polymer. Although seen most frequently in hydrophobic acrylic lenses, they are seen in all lens materials. In rare instances, glistenings are severe enough to affect contrast sensitivity and visual acuity.

4. Collamer

Collamer is a collagen polymer that is very thin and translucent.

E. Biocompatibility

1. IOL biocompatibility is based on the material and on the IOL design
2. The relative adhesion of macrophages to various lens materials (in decreasing order of number of cells):
   ¤ Hydrogel: this material can allow lens epithelial cells to migrate from the edge of the anterior capsule onto the anterior optic surface, which may compromise visual acuity
   ¤ PMMA
   ¤ Hydrophobic acrylic

◻ Silicone: relatively hydrophobic, which decreases cell adhesion. The reduced biocompatibility of silicone induces a greater cellular reaction along the anterior capsular leaflet.

Studies of anterior chamber inflammatory response, including measurement of aqueous flare and deposition of cells on the anterior optic, showed no consistent differences among different lens materials.

F. Posterior Capsular Opacity and YAG Capsulotomy Rates

1. Highest for hydrogel
2. Intermediate for PMMA and silicone
3. Lowest for hydrophobic acrylic

G. Anterior Capsular Contraction

1. Greatest with hydrogel and silicone
2. Lower with PMMA and hydrophobic acrylic

III. IOL PLACEMENT

A. Fill Bag With Ophthalmic Viscosurgical Device

- Form capsular bag not sulcus
- Use cohesive ophthalmic viscosurgical device (OVD) in bag
- Consider dispersive OVD at wound to seal
- Place OVD ahead of the cannula—as cannula can pierce the posterior capsule (Table 17-3)

B. Wound May Need to Be Extended (From Size for Phaco Needle)

- PMMA (does not fold) extend to optic size (typically 6 mm)
- Most injected IOLs do not need wound extension
- Bigger, appropriately sized wound seals better than stretched small wound

C. Lens Is Placed Into Capsular Bag

1. PMMA IOL

◻ Grasp IOL and trailing haptic with forceps (eg, Kelman-McPherson)
◻ Place leading haptic into bag, optic into anterior chamber, and release forceps
◻ Place trailing haptic into bag with hook or forceps

Table 17-3. Intraocular Lens Placement Complications

Complication	What to Do About It
Placed IOL upside down	Can leave as is —accept myopic shift, or take one haptic out of the wound with a Sinskey hook Fill with OVD above and below the IOL One hook above and one below and then flip the IOL
Inadvertent sulcus placement	Fill with OVD Rotate into capsular bag with hook Do not leave single piece acrylic in sulcus
IOL does not center	Usually one haptic in sulcus, one in bag Dial both into bag or both into sulcus Possible zonular dialysis: If nearly centered, leave it alone Rotate IOL carefully for best centration with 3-piece; often haptics best at weak area Check wound for vitreous Consider placement of capsular tension ring (CTR) Place miochol to help check for vitreous haptic damage (especially with 3-piece IOL); may have to replace IOL
Tear in Descemet's membrane	Use care to not extend the tear Place an air bubble at the end of case, postoperative Position wound up, bubble seals Descemet's membrane
Marred IOL	If not central, forget about it If central, replace the IOL
Lens material behind IOL	Rotate haptic 90 degrees from the wound Toe down with I/A and get under the IOL Aspirate with the aspiration tip visible at all times

2. Folded IOL (rarely used now as injectors are more common)

- Folded and placed in special forceps
- Incision size grows a bit with increased power of IOL—3.5 mm range

- Moustache-style fold: wider incision but haptics flow into bag
- Axial-style fold: smaller incision but haptics need guidance

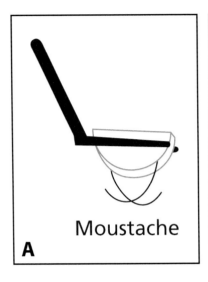

A Moustache

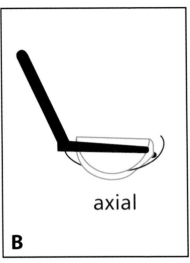

B axial

3. Injected IOL
- Many different systems
- Single-piece acrylic and plate haptic IOL most simple
- Three-piece IOL requires some haptic care and manipulation

4. Be careful of Descemet's membrane with IOL insertion (especially with injectors)

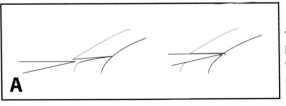

A

Toe up on injector can tear Descemet's membrane

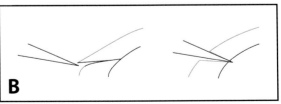

B

Toe down slips under Descemet's membrane

D. Is the IOL Right Side Up?

1. Correct side up looks like 7 O Leven

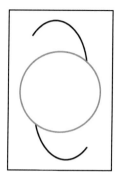

Top haptic looks like a 7

Optic looks like an O

bottom haptic looks like an L

2. IOL is designed for the right-handed surgeon to easily rotate

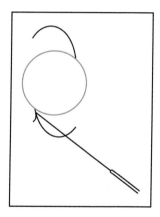

3. When upside down the IOL looks like an S so Stop

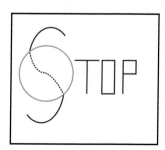

4. Upside down 3-piece IOL with angulated haptics creates myopic shift as optic is more anterior than expected (shifts effective lens position)

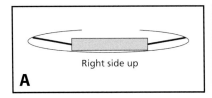

Right side up

A

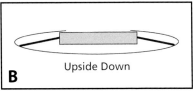

Upside Down

B

E. Make Sure That Both Haptics Are in the Bag

1. May need to add OVD: often some is lost during insertion of IOL
2. Most common cause of decentration: one haptic in bag; one in sulcus
3. Bag has less space than sulcus: ½ in IOL shifts toward sulcus haptic

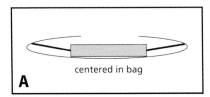

centered in bag

A

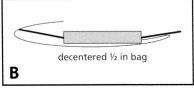

decentered ½ in bag

B

F. Rotate IOL So That Haptics Are 90 Degrees From the Wound

- Set yourself up for the next step: irrigation and aspiration I/A
- Allows I/A tip to get under IOL to remove OVD under IOL
- Frees most common site of residual cortical material from haptic

G. Special IOL Placement Conditions

1. Anterior capsular tear

- ¤ Consider using a single piece acrylic in the bag—the flexible haptics create little tension on the bag, limiting the risk of the tear extending posterior
- ¤ Could also use a 3-piece IOL with both haptics in the sulcus

2. Zonular dialysis

- ¤ Capsular tension ring with any IOL
- ¤ 3-piece IOL with PMMA haptic oriented toward weak area of zonules

3. Posterior capsular tear

◻ Dispersive OVD in the postcapsular hole: gently place IOL into bag

◻ Place 3 piece in sulcus ± capture of optic by centered anterior continuous curvilinear capsulorrhexis (CCC)

4. No capsular support

◻ AC IOL: 3 sizes depending on white-to-white size

◻ Iris-sutured PC IOL

◻ Scleral sutured PC IOL

◻ Iris clip IOL (Artisan—not approved for aphakia by FDA yet)

◻ Glue haptics of 3-piece IOL into a scleral pocket (Agarwal technique)

KEY POINTS

1. IOL designs have evolved with regard to safety, stability, and versatility.
2. Advances in design, including foldable lenses, square edges, and aspheric lenses, have advantages and disadvantages.
3. IOL materials include PMMA, acrylic, and silicone.
4. Successful IOL delivery requires adequate capsular bag inflation, possible wound enlargement, and proper orientation.
5. Misplaced haptics can result in IOL decentration.

BIBLIOGRAPHY

Agarwal A, Kumar DA, Jacob S, Baid C, Agarwal A, Srinivasan S. Fibrin glue assisted sutureless posterior chamber intraocular lens implantation in eyes with deficient posterior capsules. *J Cataract Refract Surg.* 2008;34(9):1433-1438.

Chang DF, Masket S, Miller KM, et al. Complications of sulcus placement of single-piece acrylic intraocular lenses: recommendations for backup IOL implantation following posterior capsule rupture. *J Cataract Refract Surg.* 2009;35(8):1445-1458.

Chehade M, Elder MJ. Intraocular lens materials and styles: a review. *Aust N Z J Ophthalmol.* 1997;25(4):255-263.

Davison JA. Positive and negative dysphotopsia in patients with acrylic intraocular lenses. *J Cataract Refract Surg.* 2000;26:1346-1355

Doan KT, Olson RJ, Mamalis N. Survey of intraocular lens material and design. *Curr Opin Ophthalmol.* 2002;13(1):24-29.

Harstall C, Schneider WL. Intraocular lenses for uncomplicated senile cataract. *Intraocular lenses for Uncomplicated Senile Cataract: A Health Technology Report, Alberta Heritage Foundation for Medical Research.* June 1999. Available at: http://www.ahfmr.ab.ca/hta/hta-publications/reports/intraocular99. Accessed 25.03.06.

Hayashi K, Hayashi H, Nakao F, Hayashi F. Comparison of decentration and tilt between one piece and three piece polymethyl methacrylate intraocular lenses. *Br J Ophthalmol.* 1998;82(4):419-422.

LeBoyer RM, Werner L, Snyder ME, Mamalis N, Riemann CD, Augsberger JJ. Acute haptic-induced ciliary sulcus irritation associated with single-piece AcrySof intraocular lenses. *J Cataract Refract Surg.* 2005;31(7):1421-1427.

Oetting TA, Beaver HA. Protecting the haptic when a Monarch injector is used. *J Cataract Refract Surg.* 2005;31:258-259.

Oetting TA. *Cataract Surgery for Greenhorns.* MedRounds Publishing; 2005. Available at http://www.medrounds.org/cataract-surgery-greenhorns.

Paleokastritis GP, Glazer LC, Papadopoulos GP, Azar DT, Adamis AP. History of cataract surgery and intraocular lenses. In: Azar DT, Stark WJ, Azar NF, Pineda R, Yoo S, eds. *Intraocular Lenses in Cataract and Refractive Surgery.* Philadelphia, PA: W.B. Saunders Company; 2001:3-27.

Pandey SK, Apple DJ, Werner L, Maloof AJ, Milverton EJ. Posterior capsule opacification: a review of the aetiopathogenesis, experimental and clinical studies and factors for prevention. *Indian J Ophthalmol.* 2004; 52:99-112.

Patel CK, Ormonde S, Rosen PH, Bron AJ. Postoperative intraocular lens rotation: a randomized comparison of plate and loop haptic implants, *Ophthalmology.* 1999;106(11):2190-2195; discussion 2196.

Peterson AM, Bluth LL, Campion M. Delayed posterior dislocation of silicone plate-haptic lenses after neodymium:yag capsulotomy. *J Cataract Refract Surg.* 2000;26(12):1827-1829.

Raskin EM, Speaker MG, McCormick SA, Wong D, Menikoff JA, Pelton-Henrion K. Influence of haptic materials on the adherence of staphylococci to intraocular lenses. *Arch Ophthalmol.* 1993;111(2):250-253.

Schmidbauer JM, Vargas LG, Peng, Q, et al. Posterior capsule opacification. *Int Ophthalmol Clin.* 41(3):109-131.

Vargas LG, Peng Q, Apple DJ, et al. Evaluation of 3 modern single-piece foldable intraocular lenses: clinicopathological study of posterior capsule opacification in a rabbit model. *J Cataract Refract Surg.* 2002;28(7):1241-1250.

Werner L, Pandey SK, Escobar-Gomez M, Visessook N, Peng Q, Apple DJ. Anterior capsule opacification: a histopathological study comparing different IOL styles. *Ophthalmology.* 2000;107(3):463-471.

Wolken MA, Oetting TA. Linear posterior capsule opacification with the AcrySof intraocular lens. *J Cataract Refract Surg.* 2001;27:1889-1891.

Drawings and tables reprinted with permission from Oetting TA. *Cataract Surgery for Greenhorns.* MedRounds Publishing; 2005 (available at http://www.medrounds.org/cataract-surgery-greenhorns).

18

SUTURING IN CATARACT SURGERY

Chi-Wah (Rudy) Yung, MD, FACS; Clark Springs, MD;
and Dongmei Chen, MD, PhD

I. INTRODUCTION

With advancements in phacoemulsification, wound closure with sutures in cataract surgery has become less common. Small incisions ranging from 2 to 4 mm, together with proper wound construction, have made cataract incision wounds self-sealing. There remain a few circumstances, however, that require placement of sutures in order to ensure wound security. The primary reasons for suturing in cataract surgery are to minimize wound leak and to decrease the risk of endophthalmitis.

Indications for suturing after cataract surgery:

1. Pediatric cataract surgery

2. Combined cataract surgery with other intraocular surgery, for example glaucoma surgery (including trabeculectomy or drainage device), cornea transplant surgery such as descemet's stripping endothelial keratoplasty (DSEK), and pars plana vitrectomy.

3. Compromised phacoemulsification wound: These include wound gaping as a result of a poorly constructed wound; thermal wound burns; and wound enlargement after conversion from phacoemulsification to extracapsular cataract extraction.

II. CHARACTERISTICS OF A NEEDLE

An ideal needle should be sharp with the smallest possible wire size. It should be strong enough to resist bending, deformation, or breaking and be free of mechanical defects.[1]

Henderson BA. *Essentials of Cataract Surgery, Second Edition* (pp 183-192).
© 2014 Taylor & Francis Group.

Figure 18-1. Reverse cutting.

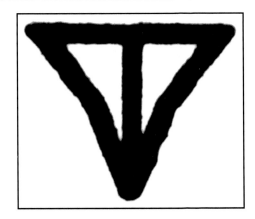

Figure 18-2. Conventional spatula needle.

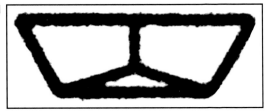

A. Point Cutting Edge

1. Cutting

The cutting edge has a triangular configuration at the tip with 2 sharpened edges. The conventional cutting needle has a third cutting edge on its concave surface. A reverse cutting needle has this third cutting edge on its convex surface (Figure 18-1). Cutting needles can cut through tissue more easier than taper-point needles but will leave larger tracks.

2. Spatula

The spatula edge is best for lamella work. It forms a slit-like track (Figures 18-2 and 18-3).

3. Round (taper-point)

Known as a cardiovascular needle, the round or taper-point edge is best for watertight closure. It penetrates tissue by blunt dissection and requires force for passage.[2] One modification of a taper-point needle is a tapercut needle, which has a short reverse cutting surface at the tip and a taper-point body (Figure 18-4).[3]

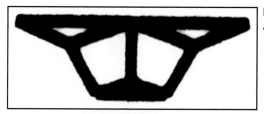

Figure 18-3. Reduced edge-angled spatula needle.

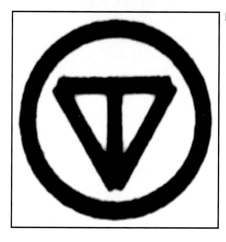

Figure 18-4. Tapercut.

B. Curvature

Needle curvature and length of needle are defined in terms of circle arc and circle degrees. Half-circle needles are good for deep and short bites, while one-quarter and three-eighths needles are good for shallower and larger bites. The less curved, lower arc needles are better for more shallow tissue penetration (Figure 18-5).[4]

C. Chord Length and Radius

Chord length is the distance measured in a straight line between the tip and swage of the needle.

III. CHARACTERISTICS OF A SUTURE

Suture materials can be categorized into 2 main groups: absorbable and nonabsorbable. A suture is said to be absorbable if it loses most of its tensile strength within 2 months. Sutures can be further classified according to other properties: configuration (monofilament or multifilament), tensile strength, elasticity and plasticity, inherent memory of suture material, and knot strength.

Figure 18-5. Needle circle and degrees.

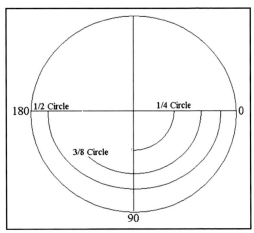

An ideal suture should be strong, easily manipulated, and able to form knots that tie easily and with minimal bulk and slippage. It should also provoke minimal tissue reaction.

Sutures commonly used in cataract surgery include Nylon or Vicryl for wound closure and Prolene or Gore-Tex for sutured intraocular lens (IOL) implant. The following is a brief review of various types of sutures that are used in ophthalmic surgery.

A. Gut

Gut is a classic absorbable suture. It retains its original tensile strength for only 4 to 5 days. When treated with chromic acid (chromic gut), tensile strength lasts from 14 to 21 days. It is commonly used for skin closure in eyelid surgery. It has limited use in ophthalmic surgery due to its stiffness and inflammatory response.

B. Polyglycolic Acid

Polyglycolic acid (Dexon) is stiff and generally braided for use. It retains approximately 20% of its strength at 14 days and about 5% at 1 month. It can be used for skin closure. It induces less inflammation than gut suture.[5,6]

C. Polyglactic Acid

Polyglactic acid (Vicryl) has properties similar to polyglycolic acid but has slightly less overall tensile strength. Tissue inflammatory response is similar to polyglycolic acid.[7] Vicryl suture has extensive use in ophthalmic surgery for soft tissue approximation. It is absorbed in 6 to 8 weeks. Most pediatric ophthalmologists prefer one simple stitch with 8-0 or 9-0 Vicryl suture for wound closure in pediatric cataract surgery.

D. Polydioxanone

Polydioxanone (PDS) is a monofilament polyester. It retains 75% of original tensile strength at 14 days and 40% at 6 weeks. It is stiffer than other polyesters and therefore more difficult to manipulate. One advantage of this suture material is that it induces minimal tissue reaction.[8]

E. Polytrimethylene Carbonate

Polytrimethylene carbonate (Maxon) is a monofilament suture. Tensile strength is better than PDS. It retains 80% strength at 14 days and 30% at 6 weeks. It is easier to manipulate than PDS.[9]

F. Nylon

Nylon is a polyamide monofilament suture. Although it is classified as nonabsorbable, it retains only 70% of its initial tensile strength at 2 years. It is degraded by hydrolysis at a rate of 15% to 20% per year.[10,11] It has inherent memory that makes knotting more difficult and additional throws are needed to attain knot security. Tissue inflammation typically is minimal but an exposed suture can induce a reaction such as giant papillary conjunctivitis. Nylon is frequently used in ocular surgery for wound closure. It is, however, not an ideal suture to use for suture iris fixation implant or sclera fixation implant because of the continued degradation over time.

G. Polypropylene

Polypropylene (Prolene) is inert and smooth. It has low tissue adherence. Tensile strength is comparable to nylon but has more slippage of knotting than nylon.[12] Additional throws are required for knot security. It is classified as nonabsorbable but slow degradation does occur.[13] It is a better suture than nylon for intraocular use, such as fixating an implant to the iris or sclera.

H. Braided Polyester

Braided polyester (Mersilene, Dacron) is a multifilament suture. Its tensile strength is comparable to monofilament polyesters but with improved handling due to the multifilament configuration. Tissue reaction to the suture material is minimal.[14] It is used in surgery such as frontalis suspension.

I. Polybutester

Polybutester (Norafil) is an elastic monofilament suture. It has better elasticity than nylon or polypropylene. This allows a stretching response to tissue edema and is therefore better able to maintain wound closure during healing. It has minimal degradation, which is a distinct advantage over nylon.[15]

J. Surgical Silk

Surgical silk is processed protein treated with silicone or wax to enhance handling. It is slowly hydrolyzed over time with complete degradation in 2 years. It has relatively low tensile strength and little memory.[16] It may elicit a significant inflammatory response.[17]

K. Gore-Tex

Gore-Tex is a unique, microporous, nonabsorbable monofilament made of expanded polytetrafluoroethylene (ePTFE). This unique material offers the benefits of both monofilament and multifilament sutures with the excellent material properties of PTFE: soft and supple for excellent handling and minimizing the irritation caused by knots, no out of package memory. Given these advantages, it is gaining more interest as the suture of choice in sutured IOL implant.

IV. SUTURING TECHNIQUE

For most circumstances in cataract surgery, simple interrupted radial sutures are sufficient and appropriate. The goal of suturing is to adequately oppose tissue so as to ensure watertight closure, while minimizing induced astigmatism.

There are rare situations, beyond the scope of this text, where alternative suturing techniques may be preferable to simple interrupted closure. These include running sutures or mattress sutures, where several passes are made prior to securing the suture with a knot. The potential benefit of a running suture is that less astigmatism may be induced since suture tension is equally distributed over the length of the wound, as in a larger extracapsular cataract wound. Mattress sutures or figure-of-eight sutures are useful when there is wound gape or tissue maceration, as in thermal wound burns or late wound dehiscence.

Effective suturing incorporates 3 essential maneuvers: grasping tissue, placing the suture and securing the suture.

A. Grasping Tissue

1. Cornea/sclera

1. Fine-toothed forceps, such as 0.12 forceps or Colibri-style forceps, are used on rigid tissue, such as cornea and sclera.
2. Grasp tissue only with the tips of the forceps. Behind the tips of most toothed forceps are tying platforms, which are ineffective for stabilizing tissue.

3. Attempt to minimize tissue distortion when holding tissue. Otherwise, the wound is opened during closure, allowing fluid to escape and leading to anterior chamber shallowing.

2. Conjunctiva

Smooth or ridged platform forceps are used to grasp pliable tissue such as conjunctiva. Toothed forceps will unnecessarily damage conjunctiva.

B. Placing the Suture

1. Grasping the needle

1. Fine-toothed needle holders are generally used in cataract wound closure. Whether they are locking or nonlocking is a matter of surgeon preference.

2. Grasp needle one-half to two-thirds from needle tip on the flat platform of the needle. If the suture is grasped too posteriorly on the round swage of the needle (the connection of the needle to the suture), the suture will twist as it is passed through the tissue.

3. When the suture is properly seated in the needle holder, a 90-degree angle exists between the needle and the needle holder. This ensures that the vector forces of passing the suture will be properly transmitted and prevent needle twisting.

4. Do not use anything other than needle drivers to handle needles. Forceps are ineffective tools to retrieve needles, and damage will result to the forceps.

2. Needle pass

1. Cornea/sclera

   ¤ The tissue is fixated with forceps directly at the position where the needle is to be placed.

   ¤ The tip of needle enters and exits tissue at a 90-degree angle, underneath the tips of stabilizing forceps.

   ¤ The suture is placed perpendicular to the wound edge and radially.

   ¤ The suture depth is 90%. Shallow bites can cause posterior wound gape, cheese-wiring, and induced astigmatism. Full thickness bites could provide pathogens access to the anterior chamber. The suture must be equal depth on proximal and distal aspects of the wound. Unequal depth bites will result in tissue override.

   ¤ The surgeon rotates the needle with his or her fingers on the needle holder to coincide with the needle arc.

      ◻ Adequate and approximately equal length bites of tissue are engaged on proximal and distal aspects of the wound (approximately 1 to 2 mm). Too short of a bite can lead to cheese-wiring and difficulty in rotating the suture to bury the knot. Too long of a bite results in excess tissue compression.

2. Conjunctiva

      ◻ The goal is to cover cataract incision and restore anatomy.

      ◻ Use full thickness bites.

      ◻ Suture approximate edge-to-edge. The conjunctiva has a tendency to curl, which can lead to inclusion cysts.

C. Securing the Suture

1. The globe is pressurized to physiological tension.

2. Smooth, nonserrated forceps or tying platforms are used to handle suture material.

      ◻ Use tying forceps.

      ◻ Alternatively, needle driver and tying platforms of 0.12 or Colibri-style forceps may be used.

3. Knot formation

      ◻ Surgeon's knot: Three loops to set tension, followed by 2 opposing securing throws (3-1-1, each in opposite direction). Useful for wounds under tension, but the knot is bulky and can be difficult to bury.

      ◻ Slip knot: Two throws in the same direction to set tension, followed by one throw in the opposite direction to secure knot (1 to 1 in the same direction, 1 in the opposite direction).

4. Suture tension: The goal is to approximate wound edges but not to over tighten, which can result in induced astigmatism and wound gape, if severe.

5. Suture burial of corneal/scleral sutures

The suture is buried with suture tips facing the direction of expected removal. If the tips are in the opposite direction of suture removal, wound dehiscence can occur during suture removal.

Appropriate knot placement is on either side of the wound but not in the wound, which could cause wound leakage.

D. Suture Removal

Since 10-0 nylon suture used for wound closure is usually well tolerated, it can be left in place for a long time. However, there are rare case reports of cataract suture-related cornea ulcer. It is better to remove these sutures once the wound is healed, for phacoemulsification, usually between 1 and 3 weeks postoperatively. For large incision ECCE, start suture removal at 6 to 8 weeks if needed to correct astigmatism.

KEY POINTS

1. There are 3 main cutting edges of a needle: cutting, spatula, and round. Each is designed for a specific purpose.

2. Nylon, a monofilament suture, though classified as nonabsorbable, does degrade over time and retains only 70% of its initial strength at the end of 2 years.

3. Polypropylene (Prolene) degrades much more slowly than nylon and is more suitable for intraocular use such as fixating a lens implant to an iris.

4. Simple, interrupted radial sutures are appropriate for uncomplicated, small incision cataract wound closure.

5. The goal of suturing in cataract surgery is to oppose tissue to ensure watertight closure while minimizing induced astigmatism.

REFERENCES

1. Polack FM, Sanchez J, Eve FR. Microsurgical sutures: I. evaluation of various types of needles and sutures per anterior segment surgery. *Can J Ophthalmol.* 1974;942-947.
2. Hoard MA, Bellian KT, Powell DM, Edlich RF. Biomechanical performance of taper-cut needles for oral surgery. *J Oral Maxillofac Surg.* 1991;49:1198-1203.
3. McClelland WA, Towler MA, Kaulbach HC, et al. Biomechanical performance of cardiovascular needles. *Am Surg.* 1990;56(10):632-638.
4. Frank M. Pollack, Pedersen NC, & Morris B, eds Microsurgical instrumentation and sutures. In: *Coneal Transplantation.* New York: Grune & Stratton; 1977:114-121.
5. Morgan MN. New synthetic absorbable suture material. *Br J Med.* 1969;2:308-313.
6. Herman JB, Kelly RJ, Higgins GA. Polyglycolic acid sutures. *Arch Surg.* 1970;100:486-490.
7. Blomstedt B, Jacobson S. Experiences with polyglactin 910 in general surgery. *Acta Chir Scand.* 1977;143:259-263.
8. Ray JA, Doddi N, Regula D, Williams JA, Melvegar A. Polydioxanone (PDS), a novel monofilament synthetic absorbable suture. *Surg Gynecol Obstet.* 1981;153:497-503.
9. Moy RL, Kaufman AJ. Clinical comparison of polyglactic acid (Vicryl) and polytrimethylene (Maxon) suture material. *J Dermatol Surg Oncol.* 1991;17:667-669.
10. Postlethwaite RW. Long term comparison study of nonabsorbable sutures. *Ann Surg.* 1970;271:892-898.
11. Ethicon, Inc. *Wound Closure Manual.* Somerville, NJ: Author; 1985:1-101.
12. Bennett R. Selection of wound closure materials. *J Am Acad Dermatol.* 1988;18;619-637.
13. Jongebloed WL, Worst JGF. Degradation of polypropylene in the human eye: a SEM study. *Doc Ophthalmol.* 1986;64:143-152.
14. Macht SD, Krizek TJ. Sutures and suturing: current concepts. *J Oral Maxillofacial Surg.* 1978;36:710-712.

15. McClellan KA, Billson FA. Long-term comparison of Novafil and nylon in corneoscleral sections. *Ophthalmol Surg.* 1991;22(2):74-77.
16. Herman JB. Tensile strength and knot security of surgical suture materials. *Am Surg.* 1971;37:209-217.
17. Soong HK, Kenyon KR. Adverse reaction to virgin silk sutures. *Ophthalmology.* 1984;91:479.

19

SUTURED INTRAOCULAR LENSES

Bryan D. Edgington, MD; Sankaranarayana Mahesh, MD;
and Michael H. Goldstein, MD, MBA

I. INTRODUCTION

Sutured intraocular lenses (IOLs) are indicated for the correction of aphakia in eyes without adequate capsular support for placement of a posterior chamber lens in the capsular bag or sulcus. It is also possible to place an anterior chamber IOL in many of the clinical situations in which a sutured IOL is used. There is currently insufficient evidence to demonstrate the superiority of any single lens type or fixation site. The decision regarding which type of fixation to use rests largely on the clinical examination and prior surgical experience of the primary surgeon.

The 2 main locations to suture a posterior chamber IOL are the iris and the sclera. There are multiple techniques and variations for securing an IOL in either location. There are advantages and disadvantages to suturing a posterior chamber IOL in either location, and these will be discussed in the body of each section. Potential complications from placement of sutured posterior chamber IOLs include hyphema, corneal edema or graft failure, glaucoma, cystoid macular edema (CME), lens tilt or dislocation, vitreous hemorrhage, retinal detachment, and endophthalmitis.[1-3]

II. IRIS-SUTURED POSTERIOR CHAMBER INTRAOCULAR LENS

A. Indications

This lens is useful for eyes without capsular support and with normal iris integrity and anterior chamber structures, for securing dislocated posterior chamber IOLs (eg, with zonular dehiscence secondary to pseudoexfoliation),

Henderson BA. *Essentials of Cataract Surgery, Second Edition (pp 193-206)*.
© 2014 Taylor & Francis Group.

and for secondary implantation at the time of penetrating keratoplasty. It is not useful for eyes with significant disruption of the anterior chamber or iris from congenital defects or trauma. It can be performed in patients with a functioning filtering bleb. (Note: The same suture techniques can be used for reconstruction of iris defects after complicated surgery or trauma.)

B. Advantages

Posterior chamber location theoretically decreases the risks of corneal decompensation and bullous keratopathy. They may be performed through a smaller incision using a foldable IOL. There is better visualization of suture passes than with scleral-fixated posterior chamber IOL.

C. Disadvantages

Placement of these lenses is technically more challenging than placement of an open-loop anterior chamber IOL. Iris chafing can result in chronic inflammation and increased risk of CME when compared with either open-loop anterior chamber IOLs or scleral-fixated posterior chamber IOL.[1]

D. Results

- Primary—complicated cataract extraction: Little data available.
- Secondary—uncomplicated/complicated cataract extraction: 95% with best-corrected visual acuity (BCVA) within 1 line of preoperative BCVA.[1]
- Secondary—penetrating keratoplasty: No increased rate of glaucoma. CME rates were variable depending upon the source. Some studies reported a lower rate of CME with iris-fixated posterior chamber IOLs while others reported that CME was a significant cause of a poor visual outcome in these patients.[1]

E. Lens Selection

The lens design used most frequently is a 3-piece foldable acrylic lens with round haptics (eg, Alcon MA60AC). The lens is usually folded along the 3:00 to 9:00 meridian using a "moustache technique" to facilitate placement of the haptics posterior to the iris (Figure 19-1). The use of single-piece acrylic lenses has been reported as well. However, the soft haptics and square edges make these lenses less desirable (eg, Alcon SA60AT, SN60AT). Silicone lenses are not recommended because they tend to be more slippery and difficult to control during fixation.

F. Suture Selection

Polypropylene (Prolene; Ethicon) is the preferred suture material because the suture will need to maintain its strength and integrity for a long duration.

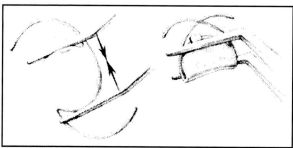

Figure 19-1. Folding technique for IOL. (Reprinted with permission from Stutzman RD, Stark WJ. Surgical technique for suture fixation of an acrylic intraocular lens in the absence of capsular support *J Cataract Refract Surg.* 2003;29(9):1658-1662.)

Single-armed 10-0 and 9-0 are both acceptable. Both Vicryl (Ethicon) and nylon degrade too rapidly for long-term secure fixation. Silk causes excessive inflammation. The procedure requires a long suture needle with minimal curvature (eg, Ethicon's CIF-4, Alcon's PC-7).

G. Techniques

1. Modified McCannel suture

- A standard 3.2-mm scleral or clear corneal incision is made with a paracentesis opposite the corneal wound.
- A miotic agent is used to constrict the pupil (pilocarpine preoperative or acetylcholine or carbachol intraoperative).
- Viscoelastic is injected into the anterior chamber to maintain the anterior chamber space.
- The IOL is folded along the 3:00 to 9:00 meridian so that the haptics can both be inserted through the constricted pupil (as described previously).
- The lens is inserted through the corneal incision and a second instrument is inserted through the paracentesis.
- The haptics are directed through the pupil, and the lens is allowed to slowly unfold. The second instrument is inserted behind the optic to ensure the IOL does not fall into the vitreous.
- The optic is captured on the pupil margin to maintain the lens position during suturing (Figure 19-2).
- A 10-0 polypropylene suture is passed through the clear cornea and iris, under the peripheral aspect of the haptic, then out through the iris and clear cornea (Figure 19-3).

Figure 19-2. IOL, optic captured over the iris. (Reprinted with permission from Stutzman RD, Stark WJ. Surgical technique for suture fixation of an acrylic intraocular lens in the absence of capsular support *J Cataract Refract Surg.* 2003;29(9):1658-1662.)

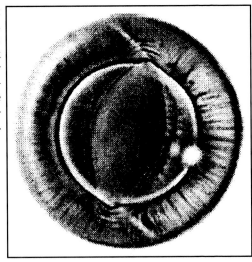

Figure 19-3. Passing 10-0 Prolene suture under the haptic and capturing the iris. (Reprinted with permission from Stutzman RD, Stark WJ. Surgical technique for suture fixation of an acrylic intraocular lens in the absence of capsular support *J Cataract Refract Surg.* 2003;29(9):1658-1662.)

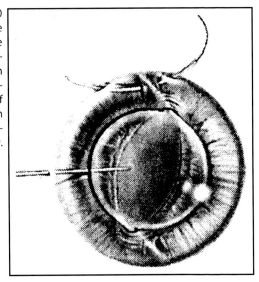

- A paracentesis is created over the haptic and the suture ends are pulled out and then tied (Figure 19-4). This is repeated for the second haptic.
- The optic is then prolapsed posteriorly and the iris is gently manipulated to minimize ovalization of the pupil. The anterior chamber is inspected for vitreous and a limited vitrectomy is performed as necessary.

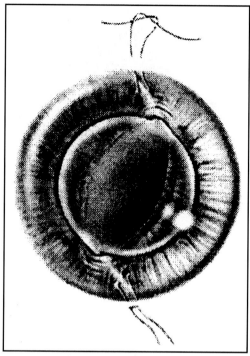

Figure 19-4. Tying the suture outside of the paracentesis. (Reprinted with permission from Stutzman RD, Stark WJ. Surgical technique for suture fixation of an acrylic intraocular lens in the absence of capsular support *J Cataract Refract Surg.* 2003;29(9):1658-1662.)

- The anterior chamber is irrigated and any residual viscoelastic material is aspirated.[4,5]

2. Siepser slip-knot technique

The initial steps are similar to those described for the modified McCannel suture.

- The optic is captured on the pupil margin to maintain the lens position during suturing. An additional paracentesis is made slightly oblique to the meridian of the haptic.
- The needle is passed through the paracentesis, through the iris perpendicular to the haptic, under the haptic, and out through the iris and clear cornea.
- An iris hook is then used to retrieve the distal end of the suture and create a loop in the paracentesis (Figure 19-5).
- The proximal suture end is passed through the loop in 2 throws. The proximal and distal ends of the suture are pulled, and the knot slides into place over the haptic with minimal iris manipulation and trauma (Figure 19-6).

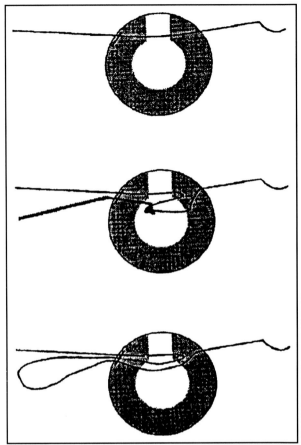

Figure 19-5. Creation of the loop. (Reprinted with permission from Osher RH, Snyder ME, Cionni RJ. Modification of the Siepser slip knot technique. *J Cataract Refract Surg.* 2005;31(6):1098-1100.)

- The maneuver is repeated for additional passes.
- Long Vannas or angled Gills scissors are used to trim the suture ends. This is repeated for the second haptic.
- The optic is then prolapsed posteriorly and the iris is gently manipulated to minimize ovalization of the pupil. The anterior chamber is inspected for vitreous and a limited vitrectomy is performed as necessary.
- The anterior chamber is irrigated and any residual viscoelastic material is aspirated. (Note: Due to the minimal traction on the iris,

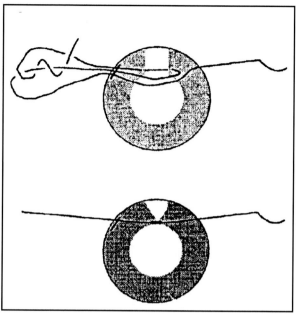

Figure 19-6. Tying the knot. (Reprinted with permission from Osher RH, Snyder ME, Cionni RJ. Modification of the Siepser slip-knot technique. *J Cataract Refract Surg.* 2005;31(6):1098-1100.)

this technique is especially useful in iris reconstruction where atrophy of the iris stroma can make the tissue friable.)[6,7]

III. SCLERAL-SUTURED POSTERIOR CHAMBER INTRAOCULAR LENS

A. Indications

These lenses are useful for eyes without capsular support, with significant disruption of the anterior chamber or iris from congenital defects or trauma, where silicone oil is placed posteriorly to help prevent the oil from entering the anterior chamber (in eyes that lack capsular support), and for secondary implantation at the time of penetrating keratoplasty (in eyes that lack capsular support).

B. Advantages

The location of the posterior chamber theoretically decreases the risks of corneal decompensation, bullous keratopathy, and glaucoma. Lack of iris manipulation theoretically reduces the risks of prostaglandin release and CME.

C. Disadvantages

Scleral-sutured posterior chamber IOLs are significantly more challenging technically than placement of an open-loop anterior chamber IOL. They require larger incisions than iris-fixated posterior chamber IOLs and have higher rates of lens tilt and lens dislocation than with open-loop anterior chamber IOL or with iris-fixated posterior chamber IOL (variable rates reported in different studies[1,3]) and higher rates of vitreous hemorrhage, hyphema, and retinal detachment related to placement of the scleral fixation sutures.[1] Erosion of the fixation suture through the conjunctiva may lead to endophthalmitis. Breakage of the suture can lead to lens dislocation.

D. Results

- Primary—complicated cataract extraction: BCVA >20/40 in 80%. Retinal detachment in 4.6%. Lens tilt and dislocation in 7.8%. Studies report low rates of corneal edema, glaucoma escalation, and CME.[1]
- Secondary—uncomplicated/complicated cataract extraction: BCVA within 1 line of preoperative BCVA in 95%. BCVA >20/40 in 90% if no predisposing risk factors were present. Retinal detachment in 3.5% to 6%, 2.6% to 12% lens tilt/dislocation, and 0.9% endophthalmitis.[1]
- Secondary—penetrating keratoplasty: Visual outcomes consistent with guarded prognosis. Studies report lower rate of retinal detachment, lens tilt or dislocation, and endophthalmitis when compared with scleral-sutured posterior chamber IOLs using a closed system. This may be due to improved access to sulcus using the open-sky technique.[1,2]

E. Lens Selection

The lens utilized most frequently is a single-piece acrylic IOL with eyelets located at the apex of the haptic (eg, Alcon CZ70BD, Bausch & Lomb 6190B, Storz P366UV [Bausch & Lomb]) (Figure 19-7). These haptics are rigid and easily broken, so care must be taken to ensure that the incision is large enough to facilitate easy placement within the eye without excessive pressure or force.

F. Suture Selection

As is the case with iris fixation, the sutures need to maintain strength and integrity over time. Two double-armed 10-0 or 9-0 polypropylene (Prolene)

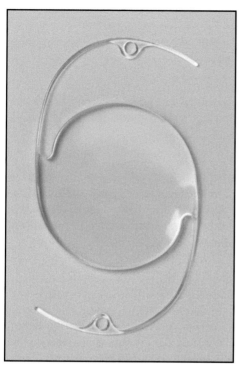

Figure 19-7. Single-piece IOL with eyelets. (Reprinted with permission from Alcon Laboratories.)

sutures on a long, tapered minimally curved needle are preferable for most techniques (eg, Ethicon CIF-4, Alcon PC-7).

G. Techniques

1. Pupil

The pupil should be maximally dilated to facilitate placement of both the scleral passes and the rigid lens. Dilation can be facilitated both pharmacologically and with manual iris retraction using multiple flexible iris hooks.

2. Flap creation

Not all techniques described in the literature utilize scleral flaps. Triangular 50% thickness limbal-based scleral flaps are created exactly 180 degrees apart. The advantage of scleral flaps is to reduce the chance of erosion of the suture through the conjunctiva. Exposure through the conjunctiva can increase the risk of endophthalmitis and broken suture with resulting lens dislocation. Alternatively, circumferential 60% thickness scleral incisions can be created 1 to 1.5 mm posterior to the limbus. Scleral incisions provide a groove where the suture can recess below the ocular surface, again minimizing erosion of the suture through the conjunctiva.

3. Vitrectomy

If the eye has not already undergone a vitrectomy, an anterior vitrectomy or standard 3-port vitrectomy is required.

4. Incision

A scleral tunnel or partial-thickness beveled limbal incision is created for the posterior chamber IOL insertion. The incision must be of sufficient length to allow placement of a rigid lens.

5. Scleral passes

The 2 main techniques for placing the scleral passes are ab interno and ab externo. Multiple variations and combinations of ab interno and ab externo procedures are described in the literature. With either technique, after placement of the scleral passes, all 4 suture needles are external to the eye and suture loops are present within the anterior chamber.

a. Ab interno

Once the scleral incision is created, the first needle is passed into the anterior chamber and directed toward the scleral flap or groove. The sclera is observed as the needle is carefully passed 1.0 to 1.5 mm posterior to the limbus. The procedure is repeated for the second arm of the same suture, ensuring the exit points are separated by approximately 3.0 mm. It is possible to provide better tangential support and minimize lens tilt by separating the suture passes, one of the significant possible complications of a scleral-sutured IOL. The procedure is repeated with the second double-armed suture directed to the second scleral flap or groove. Most procedures are performed without direct visualization of the suture site. Endoscopic visualization of the suture pass has been described.[8]

b. Ab externo

The placement of the scleral passes can be aided by passing a 25- or 27-gauge hollow bore needle ab externo 1.0 to 1.5 mm posterior to the limbus. The suture needle is then directed into the bore of the needle, which is then carefully withdrawn, pulling the suture through at a precise location (Figure 19-8). This is repeated for both arms of both sutures.[9,10]

c. Hoffman pocket

In this modification of transscleral fixation of IOLs, a scleral pocket created through a peripheral clear corneal incision obviates the need for conjunctival dissection or burying the knot. Though it can be more useful for dislocated IOL bag complex, it can be also used for any IOL that requires trans-scleral fixation. For secondary IOL implantation, an additional step involves insertion of the IOL through a standard corneoscleral incision. Clear corneal incisions up to a

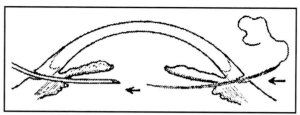

Figure 19-8. Variation of an ab externo technique. (Reprinted with permission from Lin C-P, Tseng H-Y. Suture fixation technique for posterior chamber intraocular lenses. *J Cataract Refract Surg.* 2004;30(7):1401-1404.)

depth of 400 μm, 180 degrees apart are made with #64 blade anterior to the conjunctival insertion of limbus.[11] Scleral pockets are fashioned by posterior dissection (~3 mm) using a crescent knife or diamond blade helps in burying the fixation sutures.[11] A 1-mm paracentesis is placed adjacent to the corneal incisions that aids in the placement of the polyproplene fixation suture used in fixation of the IOL. A 27-G needle passed through the conjunctiva and scleral pocket 1 mm posterior to the limbus directed behind the iris and in front of the capsular bag.[11] A double-armed 10-0 or 9-0 polyproplene on a straight needle (STC-6 Ethicon) inserted through the opposite paracentesis is guided to the 27-gauge needle and retrieved externally. The second arm of the double-armed needle is similarly passed through the paracentesis, behind the capsular bag and retrieved 1 mm adjacent to the previous suture.[11] The needles are removed and suture ends retrieved through the corneal incisions for tying. The same technique is performed for fixing the opposite haptic 180 degrees apart. The advantages of this technique include that there is no need for conjunctival dissection, cauterization, or sutured wound closure and it can be performed with topical anesthesia. The wounds cause less astigmatism due to shorter arc length compared to traditional limbal relaxing incisions.

d. Sutureless intrascleral haptic fixation

Another method that has evolved in recent years is the transscleral fixation of haptics in scleral pocket with or without sutures. The basic technique involves creating two 2- to 3-mm lamellar scleral flaps 180 degrees apart. In addition, sclerotomies are fashioned underneath the flaps, 1.5 mm from the limbus for trapping the IOL haptics. A 3-piece IOL can be inserted through a corneoscleral incision. With a help of 26-gauge needle, the leading and trailing haptics are externalized through the sclerotomies and fixed to the scleral pockets. The flaps can be sutured or held down with fibrin glue. The

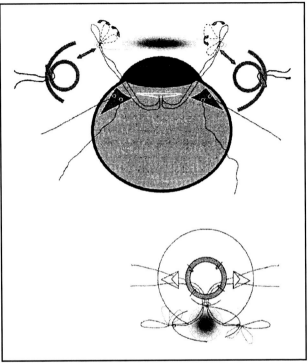

Figure 19-9. Hitch technique for securing the lens. (Reprinted with permission from Grigorian R, Chang J, Zarbin M, Del Priore L. A new technique for suture fixation of posterior chamber intraocular lenses that eliminates intraocular knots. *Ophthalmology.* 2003;110(7):1349-1356.)

advantage of this technique in theory at least is no risk of late suture breakage and less pseudophacodonesis as the haptics are tucked into scleral tunnels parallel to the limbus, affording more stability. Long-term studies are warranted on the decentration and subluxation rates with this newer technique.[12]

6. IOL

Once the sutures are in place, they can be attached to the IOL. This can be accomplished by cutting the loops and tying each end to the eyelet of the haptic. Care must be taken to ensure that the knots are secure. Alternatively, a hitch can be created by passing the loop through the eyelet and then wrapping it around the haptic (Figure 19-9). This has the advantage of securing the lens without creating an intraocular knot.[13] The lens is then carefully inserted into the sulcus and the external sutures are carefully tied. The suture ends can be cut slightly long so that they lie flat either underneath the partial thickness scleral flap or within the scleral groove. It is not always necessary to suture scleral flaps closed, but it is easily accomplished using one or two 10-0 nylon sutures. The conjunctiva should be sutured in place over the scleral flaps using 8-0 Vicryl suture.

IV. CONCLUSION

Iris-sutured and scleral-sutured posterior chamber lenses can both be used for patients with poor capsular support or aphakia. They are both technically more difficult than placing an open-loop anterior chamber IOL. All 3 techniques may have similar rates of success, and there is no clear consensus as to which technique is superior. The decision as to which technique to use should be tailored to meet the individual needs of each patient.

KEY POINTS

1. Sutured IOLs are a useful technique for patients with poor capsular support or aphakia.

2. The placement of sutured IOLs is technically more challenging than the placement of an open-loop anterior chamber IOL.

3. Visual outcomes, glaucoma, CME, and endothelial cell loss rates appear to be similar for open-loop anterior chamber IOLs, iris-fixated posterior chamber IOLs, and scleral-fixated posterior chamber IOLs (studies report variable rates). Lens dislocation rates are higher for sutured lenses than for open-loop anterior chamber IOLs.

4. McCannel suture techniques and Siepser slip-knot techniques are useful both for securing iris-fixated posterior chamber IOLs and for repairing iris defects.

5. Scleral-sutured posterior chamber IOLs can be placed using ab interno or ab externo techniques.

REFERENCES

1. Wagoner MD, Cox TA, Ariyasu RG, Jacobs DS, Karp CL. Intraocular lens implantation in the absence of capsular support: a report by the American Academy of Ophthalmology. *Ophthalmology*. 2003;110:840-859.

2. Schein OD, Kenyon KR, Steinert RF, et al. A randomized trial of intraocular lens fixation techniques with penetrating keratoplasty. *Ophthalmology*. 1993;100:1437-1443.

3. Hayashi K, Hayashi H, Nakao F, Hayashi F. Intraocular lens tilt and decentration, anterior chamber depth, and refractive error after trans-scleral suture fixation surgery. *Ophthalmology*. 1999;106:878-882.

4. Stutzman RD, Stark WJ. Surgical technique for suture fixation of an acrylic intraocular lens in the absence of capsular support. *J Cataract Refract Surg*. 2003;29:1658-1662.

5. Condon GP. Iris-sutured PCIOLs: a modified McCannel slip-knot suture makes the iris fixation of a multipiece AcrySof lens possible without capsular support. *Cataract Refract Surg Today*. 2004;May:1-4.

6. Chang DF. Siepser slip-knot for McCannel iris-suture fixation of subluxated intraocular lenses. *J Cataract Refract Surg*. 2004;30:1170-1176.

7. Osher RH, Snyder ME, Cionni RJ. Modification of the Siepser slip-knot technique. *J Cataract Refract Surg*. 2005;31:1098-1100.

8. Sasahara M, Kiryu J, Yoshimura N. Endoscope-assisted transscleral suture fixation to reduce the incidence of intraocular lens dislocation. *J Cataract Refract Surg*. 2005;31:1777-1780.

9. Lewis JS. Ab externo sulcus fixation. *Ophthalmic Surg*. 1991;22:692-695.

10. Lin CP, Tseng HY. Suture fixation technique for posterior chamber intraocular lenses. *J Cataract Refract Surg*. 2004;30:1401-1404.

11. Hoffman RS, Fine IH, Packer M. Scleral fixation without conjunctival dissection. *J Cataract Refract Surg*. 2006;32(11):1907-1912.

12. Agarwal A, Kumar DA, Jacob S, Baid C, Agarwal A, Srinivasan S. Fibrin glue-assisted sutureless posterior chamber intraocular lens implantation in eyes with deficient posterior capsules. *J Cataract Refract Surg*. 2008;34(9):1433-1438.

13. Grigorian R, Chang J, Zarbin M, Del Priore L. A new technique for suture fixation of posterior chamber intraocular lenses that eliminates intraocular knots. *Ophthalmology*. 2003;110:1349-1356.

PERIOPERATIVE AND POSTOPERATIVE MEDICATIONS

John J. DeStafeno, MD and Terry Kim, MD

I. INTRODUCTION

The use of medications in the peri- and postoperative period of cataract surgery can affect the desired surgeon experience and patient outcome. Commonly used medications include anesthetics, antibiotics, anti-inflammatories, and pharmacologic dilating and miotic agents. We will review the indications, benefits, risks, and evidence for the use of these various agents in cataract surgery.

II. PERIOPERATIVE MEDICATIONS

A. Intracameral Lidocaine 1%

Topical anesthesia is a routinely used and effective method of pain control prior to cataract surgery today. Corneal and conjunctival sensation are greatly diminished with the use of these topical medications (refer to Chapter 4). However, insufficient iris and ciliary body anesthesia is often encountered with topical anesthesia alone.

Gills et al[1] introduced the concept of using unpreserved lidocaine 1% intracamerally in addition to topical anesthesia for cataract surgery in 1995. The safety and efficacy of intracameral lidocaine has been studied and found to be well tolerated and effective for pain control. Kim et al[2] found that transient and reversible endothelial swelling occurred after unpreserved intracameral lidocaine. Others have agreed that there is no toxicity to the endothelial cells with use of unpreserved lidocaine. Martin et al[3] studied aqueous cell/flare and demonstrated no increase in patients receiving intracameral lidocaine. Increased pain control has been demonstrated with unpreserved

Henderson BA. *Essentials of Cataract Surgery, Second Edition (pp 207-217).* © 2014 Taylor & Francis Group.

lidocaine and topical anesthesia versus topical anesthesia alone.[4-6] This can become especially useful in patients in whom iris or extensive IOL manipulation is expected. An additional benefit has been the finding that intraoperative dilation can be enhanced with intracameral lidocaine 1%.[7,8]

1. Techniques for unpreserved intracameral lidocaine 1% administration

1. Sterile skin preparation with povidone-iodine 5%
2. Speculum placement
3. A paracentesis is created and 0.3 to 0.5 mL of unpreserved lidocaine 1% is slowly injected into the anterior chamber. Alert the patient that he or she may feel a slight burning sensation during injection
4. Wait 10 to 20 seconds
5. Inject viscoelastic and proceed with cataract surgery

B. Intracameral Mydriatics

Pupillary constriction during cataract surgery is a major cause of complications including iris damage, incomplete cortex removal, posterior capsule rupture, and vitreous loss. Intracameral agents have been shown to be a safe and effective alternative to conventional topical mydriatics.[7-11] These agents can be injected during the perioperative period to induce or maintain dilation. In addition, mydriatic agents (ie, epinephrine 1:100,000) can be instilled in the irrigation bottle to decrease pupillary miosis during cataract surgery. A decreased risk of cardiovascular events and increased operating room efficiency are distinct advantages to intracameral therapy.

C. Examples of Intracameral Agents

- *Epinephrine 1:100,000 in irrigation bottle*
- *Adrenaline 1:1,000,000 in irrigation bottle*
- *Nonpreserved 1% lidocaine*
- *Epi-Shugarcaine*

Intraoperative floppy iris syndrome (IFIS) has become increasingly common due to widespread use of tamsulosin (Flomax) for treatment of benign prostatic hypertrophy. The introduction of Shugarcaine, a buffered lidocaine mixture, by the late Joel Shugar and the subsequent evolution into epi-Shugarcaine has helped to minimize intraoperative miosis and iris flaccidity from IFIS.

1. Techniques for epi-Shugarcaine administration

1. Mix 1 cc of nonpreserved 4% lidocaine with 3 cc of BSS Plus
2. Discard 1 cc of above mixture

3. Add 1 cc of nonpreserved epinephrine 1:1000 to lidocaine/BSS Plus mixture

4. Inject into anterior chamber ± underneath iris

Lundberg et al[11] reported no increase in endothelial cell loss, postoperative inflammation, corneal swelling, or surgical complications when compared to topical agents. Caution must be taken to ensure the proper use of nonpreserved medications and accurate concentrations when using intracameral medications.

D. Intracameral Miotics

Intracameral miotics have historically been used to prevent postoperative pressure spikes after cataract extraction and prevent optic nerve damage with resultant visual field loss. Acetylcholine 1% (Miochol) and carbachol 0.01% (Miostat) are commonly used agents. Both agents have clearly been shown to decrease early postoperative intraocular pressure after cataract surgery, although carbachol may have a greater duration of effect.[12] In addition, Solomon et al suggested carbachol use may improve visual function (acuity, glare) in the first postoperative week.[13]

E. Intracameral Antibiotics

The use of intracameral antibiotics in the infusion bottle or injected into the eye as a prophylactic agent against endophthalmitis remains an area of controversy today. Conflicting evidence regarding the effectiveness exists. Mendivil Soto and Mendivil[14] found a reduction in positive intraocular cultures and a decreased incidence of endophthalmitis after vancomycin was used in the irrigating fluid. Gills also noted decreased rates using intraocular filtration and adding gentamicin and vancomycin to the irrigating fluid.[6]

The European Society of Cataract and Refractive Surgeons conducted a multinational study of over 16,000 patients to evaluate the effectiveness of intracameral cefuroxime in reducing endophthalmitis. Preliminary results suggest a nearly 5-fold decrease in endophthalmitis in patients receiving intracameral cefuroxime. In addition, clear corneal incisions and use of silicone intraocular lenses were associated with an increased risk of endophthalmitis.[15]

The CDC issued a statement advising against the routine use of vancomycin as prophylaxis in all surgical procedures due to increasing concerns over resistance. In addition, bactericidal effects and drug stability in the anterior chamber suggest that the exposure of organisms to intracameral medications may be too brief to be effective.[16] Excellent arguments can be made for and against the effectiveness of these agents and the decision will be based on surgeon preference. Attention to spectrum of activity and potential for toxic and/or allergic reactions should be noted.

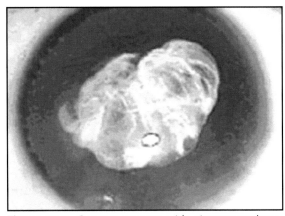

Figure 20-1. Cataract surgery with vitreous prolapse. Vitreous "stained" with triamcinolone (Kenalog) can clearly be visualized in the anterior chamber.

F. Intracameral Triamcinolone Acetonide (Kenalog)

Vitreous prolapse during cataract surgery is a well-known complication when the posterior capsular bag is compromised. Anterior vitrectomy is performed to remove all vitreous from the anterior chamber to reduce vitreous traction, pupillary irregularities, and incarceration to the wound. The optical clarity of the vitreous often makes its presence in the anterior chamber difficult to detect. Subtle clues such as peaked pupils and irregular currents around vitreous after injection of miotic agents can be used to identify remaining vitreous.

Triamcinolone acetonide (Kenalog) has been used in pars plana vitrectomies to increase visibility of the hyaloid.[17] It has been shown to be nontoxic to the eye.[18] In 2003, Burk et al[19] described the use of Kenalog to "stain" vitreous that has prolapsed into the anterior chamber. The Kenalog particles adhere to the vitreous and aid in visualization and subsequent removal (Figure 20-1). Although Kenalog is safe for intraocular use, some surgeons believe that the preservative should be removed prior to use in the anterior chamber while others will simply dilute the preparation with BSS. In 2007 Triescence (Alcon), a nonpreserved triamcinolone acetonide, was released and allows for direct injection without the need to remove preservatives. The method of use is based on surgeon preference.

1. Technique for Kenalog administration

a. Preservative removal

1. Using a tuberculin syringe, draw off 0.2 mL of well-shaken 40 mg/mL bottle

   2. Remove the needle and replace with a 5-μm syringe filter
   3. Depress the syringe to capture the Kenalog particles in the filter
   4. Remove the filter and transfer to a 5-mL syringe of BSS
   5. Depress the syringe to fully wash the Kenalog particles
   6. Transfer the filter to an empty 5-mL syringe and draw sterile BSS through the filter to resuspend the cleaned, preservative-free particles

b. Administration and removal

   1. Approximately 1 to 2 mL of the "washed" Kenalog in a syringe with a blunt cannula can be injected into the AC
   2. Perform anterior vitrectomy
   3. Ensure complete removal of vitreous and Kenalog suspension. Incomplete Kenalog removal can lead to elevated intraocular pressure[20]

G. Subconjunctival Medications

1. Antibiotics

The administration of subconjunctival antibiotics was one of the earliest prophylactic techniques for endophthalmitis after cataract surgery.[21] Again, evidence in the literature argues for and against their efficacy in preventing endophthalmitis.[22,23] Ciulla et al[24] conducted an extensive review of the literature and found a slight decrease in endophthalmitis that did not reach statistical significance in the majority of studies. It was concluded that subconjunctival antibiotics may be relevant but could not be definitely related to clinical outcome. Caution should be taken when administering subconjunctival medications. Common side effects include hyperemia, burning upon injection, allergic reactions, and ocular toxicity, especially secondary to gentamicin.

2. Corticosteroids

Local administration of corticosteroids to control intraocular inflammation after cataract surgery is preferred as systemic absorption can be reduced with less risk of side effects. Corticosteroids act as both cyclooxygenase and lipoxygenase inhibitors, thus reducing mediators of inflammation such as prostaglandins and leukotrienes.

Several studies support the belief that a subconjunctival route of administration will reduce inflammation.[25,26] Corbett et al[26] reported a significant decrease in postoperative inflammation after subconjunctival betamethasone injection. Aqueous and vitreal levels of dexamethasone were found to be increased after subconjunctival use when compared to peribulbar administration.[27] Other investigators have argued that subconjunctival steroids do not aid in recovery of the blood-aqueous barrier.[28] In addition, one report found no decrease in postoperative inflammation when studying diabetic patients.[29]

III. Postoperative Medications

A. Topical Corticosteroids

The anti-inflammatory effects of topical corticosteroids in ophthalmic surgery are well known. It works by blocking phospholipase A2. Benefits include decreased intraocular inflammation and treatment and prevention of cystoid macular edema (CME). Corticosteroids are often employed 2 to 6 weeks postsurgery in uncomplicated cataract surgeries. Although very effective, corticosteroids can induce elevated intraocular pressure, impaired wound healing, and bacterial and viral infections.

Several topical preparations are available. Prednisolone 1% was compared to rimexolone 1% and loteprednol etabonate 0.5% to determine efficacy in controlling inflammation and side effect profile.[30,31] Prednisolone more effectively controlled inflammation but may raise intraocular pressure when compared to the other agents. Recently, difluprednate (Durezol; Alcon) has been shown to be effective in controlling postoperative pain and inflammation after cataract surgery.[32] There has been little head-head comparison between difluprednate and other available corticosteroids for use after cataract surgery.

B. Nonsteroidal Anti-Inflammatories

The role of topical nonsteroidal anti-inflammatory drugs (NSAIDs) in ophthalmology has largely increased since their introduction and can play an important pre-, peri-, and postoperative role (please refer to earlier Chapter 3 for preoperative use). They are commonly used today to reduce intraoperative miosis, decrease discomfort after refractive surgery, control postoperative inflammation, and prevent and treat CME after intraocular surgery.

NSAIDs' primary mechanism of action is to act as a cyclooxygenase inhibitor thus reducing the formation of prostaglandins (Figure 20-2).[33] Prostaglandins are responsible for miosis, increased pain and allergic response, and increased permeability of the blood-ocular barrier and can serve to activate arms of the inflammatory response.[34] In addition, some NSAIDs may have an indirect role in leukotreine inhibition.[35]

Many of the studies regarding NSAIDs effects on postoperative inflammation include use with topical corticosteroids. Studies suggest these 2 medications act in synergy to decrease inflammation and reduce the incidence of CME (Figure 20-3).[36] Additional, randomized studies have confirmed a definite anti-inflammatory effect of NSAIDs and a greater ability to reestablish the blood-aqueous barrier when compared to steroids. Several topical formulations are available today, each with specific dosing and activity (Table 20-1).

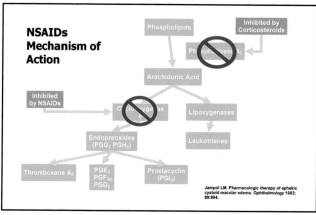

Figure 20-2. Mechanism of inhibition of corticosteroids and NSAIDs. The primary mechanisms of action of corticosteroids (inhibition of phospholipase A2) and NSAIDs (cyclooxygenase) with resultant inhibition of leukotrienes (corticosteroids only) and prostaglandins is depicted. (Reprinted with permission from Jampol LM. Pharmacologic therapy of aphakic cystoid macular edema. *Ophthalmology.* 1982;89:894.)

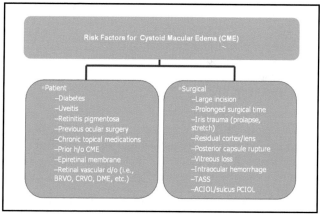

Figure 20-3. Patient and surgical risk factors increasing the risk of developing CME.

Topical NSAIDs are generally well tolerated. There have been reports of corneal melting with prolonged NSAID use, especially with earlier generic formulations and patients with ocular surface disease.[37] Although the incidence is rare, physicians should be aware of this complication and monitor patients for any signs of corneal toxicity (Table 20-2).

TABLE 20-1. TOPICAL NONSTEROIDAL ANTI-INFLAMMATORY MEDICATIONS

FDA-Approved NSAIDs	Postoperative Dosing
Diclofenac (Voltaren)	QID
Ketorolac (Acular)	QID
Ketorolac (Acuvail)	BID
Nepafenac 0.1% (Nevanac)	TID
Bromfenac 0.09% (Bromday)	BID
Bromfenac 0.07% (Prolensa)	QD
Nepafanac 0.3% (Ilevro)	QD

QID: Four times per day, TID: Three times per day, BID: Two times per day, QD: One time per day

TABLE 20-2. RECOMMENDED NONSTEROIDAL ANTI-INFLAMMATORY DRUG DOSING

	At-Risk	Low-Risk
Preoperative	1 week	1 to 2 days
Postoperative	1 to several months	1 month

C. Topical Antibiotics

The incidence of endophthalmitis in the United States varies depending on the source but has been reported to be near 0.07% to 0.1%.[38] This low incidence has led to difficulty performing well-controlled randomized, prospective studies evaluating efficacy of topical postoperative antibiotics in endophthalmitis prophylaxis. Several reviews of the current literature have been performed and most concur that there is no significant evidence in the literature supporting the use of postoperative antibiotics to reduce the incidence of endophthalmitis.[24,38] The reviewers raise concerns over the lack of penetration of topically applied antibiotics into the aqueous and vitreous, especially with smaller, self-sealing wounds. The lack of bactericidal levels in the eye and possible emergence of resistance organisms are additional concerns.

Recent studies report a higher incidence of endophthalmitis for clear corneal incisions when compared to scleral tunnel incisions. McDonnell and associates have provided evidence to suggest wound leakage from clear corneal incisions in the early postoperative period with resultant entry of bacteria into the eye.[39] Furthermore, many of these aforementioned studies have not involved the currently available antibiotics moving to the forefront today (ie, fourth-generation fluoroquinolones). Both moxifloxacin (Vigamox) and gatifloxacin (Zymar), fourth-generation fluoroquinolones, have been recognized as having an increased spectrum of coverage and better bioavailability in both the aqueous and vitreous.[40,41] McCulley et al[42] simulated a 5-day postoperative regimen of both moxifloxacin and gatifloxacin in patients with cataracts and found increased aqueous humor levels when compared to prior-generation fluoroquinolones. It remains to be seen if the reported benefits of these new antibiotics will translate into a reduction in endophthalmitis.

A survey by the American Society of Cataract and Refractive Surgeons indicated that 96% of respondent physicians routinely instituted a postoperative antibiotic regimen. The 2011 American Academy of Ophthalmology Preferred Practice Patterns states, "Because of the lack of and impracticality of sufficiently large prospective clinical trials, there is insufficient evidence to recommend a specific antibiotic drug or method of delivery for endophthalmitis prophylaxis. It would appear that antibiotic use on the day of surgery is important rather than waiting until the next day. Any additional prophylactic antibiotic strategy in the perioperative period is up to the ophthalmologist to determine."[43]

IV. CONCLUSION

The administration of medications in the peri- and postoperative periods can improve efficiency, decrease complications, and enhance the visual outcomes after cataract surgery. However, one cannot overemphasize the importance of surgical team diligence in ensuring correct preparation before administering these medications to avoid complications that may result in visual loss. Physicians should review the literature and make evidence-based decisions when instituting these therapies into their practices.

KEY POINTS

1. The administration of medications in the peri- and postoperative periods can improve efficiency, decrease complications, and enhance the visual outcomes after cataract surgery.
2. Despite being useful surgical adjuvants, each therapy needs to be monitored for side effects and ocular toxicity.
3. Therapies should be tailored for each patient based on individual risk factors and a consideration of benefits.
4. One cannot overemphasize the importance of surgical team diligence in ensuring correct preparation before administering these medications to avoid complications that may result in visual loss.
5. Physicians should review the literature and make evidence-based decisions when instituting these therapies into their practices.

References

1. Gills JP, Cherchio M, Raanan MG. Unpreserved lidocaine to control discomfort during cataract surgery using topical anesthesia. *J Cataract Refract Surg.* 1997;23(4):545-550.

2. Kim T, Holley GP, Lee JH, Broocker G, Edelhauser HF. The effects of intraocular lidocaine on the corneal endothelium. *Ophthalmology.* 1998;105(1):125-130.

3. Martin RG, Miller JD, Cox III CC, Ferrel SC, Raanan MG. Safety and efficacy of intracameral injections of unpreserved lidocaine to reduce intraocular sensation. *J Cataract Refract Surg.* 1998;24(7):961-963.

4. Carino NS, Slomovic AR, Chung F, Marcovich AL. Topical tetracaine versus topical tetracaine plus intracameral lidocaine for cataract surgery. *J Cataract Refract Surg.* 1998;24(12):1602-1608.

5. Crandall AS, Zabriskie NA, Patel BC, et al. A comparison of patient comfort during cataract surgery with topical anesthesia versus topical anesthesia and intracameral lidocaine. *Ophthalmology.* 1999;106(1):60-66.

6. Gills JP. Prevention of endophthalmitis by intraocular solution filtration and antibiotics. *J Am Intraocul Implant Soc.* 1985;11(2):185-186.

7. Cionni RJ, Barros MG, Kaufman AH, Osher RH. Cataract surgery without preoperative eyedrops. *J Cataract Refract Surg.* 2003;29(12):2281-2283.

8. Werner L, Pandey SK, Izak AM, Hickman MS, LeBoyer RM, Mamalis N. Evaluation of the cataractogenic effect of viscoanesthetic solutions on the rabbit crystalline lens. *J Cataract Refract Surg.* 2005;31(7):1414-1420.

9. Behndig A, Eriksson A. Evaluation of surgical performance with intracameral mydriatics in phacoemulsification surgery. *Acta Ophthalmol Scand.* 2004;82(2):144-147.

10. Liou SW, Yang CY. The effect of intracameral adrenaline infusion on pupil size, pulse rate, and blood pressure during phacoemulsification. *J Ocul Pharmacol Ther.* 1998;14(4):357-361.

11. Lundberg B, Behndig A. Intracameral mydriatics in phacoemulsification cataract surgery. *J Cataract Refract Surg.* 2003;29(12):2366-2371.

12. Kim JY, Sohn JH, Youn DH. Effects of intracameral carbachol and acetylcholine on early postoperative intraocular pressure after cataract extraction. *Korean J Ophthalmol.* 1994;8(2):61-65.

13. Solomon KD, Stewart WC, Hunt HH, Stewart JA, Cate EA. Intraoperative intracameral carbachol in phacoemulsification and posterior chamber lens implantation. *Am J Ophthalmol.* 1998;125(1):36-43.

14. Mendivil Soto A, Mendivil MP. The effect of topical povidone-iodine, intraocular vancomycin, or both on aqueous humor cultures at the time of cataract surgery. *Am J Ophthalmol.* 2001;131(3):293-300.

15. Barry P, Seal DV, Gettinby G, Lees F, Peterson M, Revie CW. Endophthalmitis Study Group, European Society of Cataract & Refractive Surgeons. Prophylaxis of postoperative endophthalmitis following cataract surgery: results of the ESCRS multicenter study and identification of risk factors. *J Cataract Refract Surg.* 2007;33(6):978-988.

16. Gritz DC, Cevallos AV, Smolin G, Whitcher Jr JP. Antibiotic supplementation of intraocular irrigating solutions. An in vitro model of antibacterial action. *Ophthalmology.* 1996;103(8):1204-1208; discussion 1208-1209.

17. Sakamoto T, Miyazaki M, Hisatomi T, et al. Triamcinolone-assisted pars planavitrectomy improves the surgical procedures and decreases the postoperative blood-ocular barrier breakdown. *Graefes Arch Clin Exp Ophthalmol.* 2002;240(6):423-429.

18. McCuen II, BW, Bessler M, Tano Y, Chandler D, Machemer R. The lack of toxicity of intravitreally administered triamcinolone acetonide. *Am J Ophthalmol.* 1981;91(6):785-788.

19. Burk SE, Da Mata AP, Snyder ME, Schneider S, Osher RH, Cionni RJ. Visualizing vitreous using Kenalog suspension. *J Cataract Refract Surg.* 2003;29(4):645-651.

20. Yamakiri K, Uchino E, Kimura K, Sakamoto T. Intracameral triamcinolone helps to visualize and remove the vitreous body in anterior chamber in cataract surgery. *Am J Ophthalmol.* 2004;138(4):650-652.

21. Cassady JR. Prophylactic subconjunctival antibiotics following cataract extraction. *Am J Ophthalmol.* 1967;64(6):1081-1083.

22. Christy NE, Lall P. Postoperative endophthalmitis following cataract surgery. Effects on subconjunctival antibiotics and other factors. *Arch Ophthalmol.* 1973;90(5):361-366.

23. Colleaux KM, Hamilton WK. Effect of prophylactic antibiotics and incision type on the incidence of endophthalmitis after cataract surgery. *Can J Ophthalmol.* 2000;35(7):373-378.

24. Ciulla TA, Starr MB, Masket S. Bacterial endophthalmitis prophylaxis for cataract surgery: an evidence-based update. *Ophthalmology.* 2002;109(1):13-24.

25. Buxton JN, Smith DE, Brownstein S. Cataract extraction and subconjunctival repository corticosteroids. *Ann Ophthalmol.* 1971;3(12):1376-1379.

26. Corbett MC, Hingorani M, Boulton JE, Shilling JS. Subconjunctival betamethasone is of benefit after cataract surgery. *Eye.* 1993;7 (Pt 6):744-748.

27. Weijtens O, Feron EJ, Schoemaker RC, et al. High concentration of dexamethasone in aqueous and vitreous after subconjunctival injection. *Am J Ophthalmol.* 1999;128(2):192-197.

28. Shah SM, McHugh JD,Spalton DJ. The effects of subconjunctival betamethasone on the blood aqueous barrier following cataract surgery: a double-blindrandomised prospective study. *Br J Ophthalmol.* 1992;76(8):475-478.

29. Fukushima H, Kato S, Kaiya T, et al. Effect of subconjunctival steroid injection on intraocular inflammation and blood glucose level after cataract surgery in diabetic patients. *J Cataract Refract Surg.* 2001;27(9):1386-1391.

30. Bartlett JD, Horwitz B, Laibovitz R, Howes JF. Intraocular pressure response to loteprednol etabonate in known steroid responders. *J Ocul Pharmacol.* 1993;9(2):157-165.

31. Foster CS, Alter G, DeBarge LR, et al. Efficacy and safety of rimexolone 1% ophthalmic suspension vs 1% prednisolone acetate in the treatment of uveitis. *Am J Ophthalmol.* 1996;122(2):171-182.

32. Smith S, Lorenz D, Peace J, McLeod K, Crockett RS, Vogel R. Difluprednate ophthalmic emulsion 0.05% (Durezol) administered two times daily for managing ocular inflammation and pain following cataract surgery. *Clin Ophthalmol.* 2010;7(4):983-991.

33. Srinivasan BD, Kulkarni PS. Inhibitors of the arachidonic acid cascade in the management of ocular inflammation. *Prog Clin Biol Res.* 1989;312:229-249.

34. Flach AJ. Topical nonsteroidal antiinflammatory drugs in ophthalmology. *Int Ophthalmol Clin.* 2002;42(1):1-11.

35. Flach A. Nonsteroidal anti-inflammatory drugs. In: Tasman W, ed. *Duane's Foundation of Clinical Ophthalmology.* Philadelphia: Lippincott, 1994:1-32.

36. McColgin AZ, Heier JS. Control of intraocular inflammation associated with cataract surgery. *Curr Opin Ophthalmol.* 2000;11(1):3-6.

37. Szerenyi K, Sorken K, Garbus JJ, Lee M, McDonnell PJ. Decrease in normal human corneal sensitivity with topical diclofenac sodium. *Am J Ophthalmol.* 1994;118(3):312-315.

38. Liesegang TJ. Use of antimicrobials to prevent postoperative infection in patients with cataracts. *Curr Opin Ophthalmol.* 2001;12(1):68-74.

39. Taban M, Sarayba MA, Ignacio TS, Behrens A, McDonnell PJ. Ingress of India ink into the anterior chamber through sutureless clear corneal cataract wounds. *Arch Ophthalmol.* 2005;123(5):643-648.

40. Hariprasad SM, Shah GK, Chi J, Prince RA. Determination of aqueous and vitreous concentration of moxifloxacin 0.5% after delivery via a dissolvable corneal collagen shield device. *J Cataract Refract Surg.* 2005;31(11):2142-2146.

41. Kim DH, Stark WJ, O'Brien TP, Dick JD. Aqueous penetration and biological activity of moxifloxacin 0.5% ophthalmic solution and gatifloxacin 0.3% solution in cataract surgery patients. *Ophthalmology.* 2005;112(11):1992-1996.

42. McCulley JP, Caudle D, Aronowicz JD, Shine WE. Fourth-generation fluoroquinolone penetration into the aqueous humor in humans. *Ophthalmology.* 2006;113(6):955-999.

43. American Academy of Ophthalmology Cataract and Anterior Segment Panel. Preferred Practice Pattern® Guidelines. *Cataract in the Adult Eye.* San Francisco, CA: American Academy of Ophthalmology; 2011.

21

EXTRACAPSULAR CATARACT EXTRACTION

Maria Aaron, MD; Geoffrey Broocker, MD; Jeff Pettey, MD;
and Geoffrey Tabin, MD

I. INTRODUCTION

Extracapsular cataract extraction (ECCE) is the removal of the anterior lens capsule and extraction of the lens nucleus and cortex, while the peripheral anterior lens capsule, posterior capsule, and zonular attachments remain intact. Traditional ECCE refers to the removal of the intact lens nucleus through a large incision (greater than 6 to 8 mm); however, the strict definition would include phacoemulsification as a form of ECCE. Small incision cataract surgery (SICS) refers to the ECCE procedure through a smaller self-sealing incision, which is typically a 6-mm external incision that is enlarged internally. Traditional ECCE gained popularity over intracapsular cataract extraction in the 1970s and subsequently lost favor to phacoemulsification in the 1990s. According to a survey performed by the American Society of Cataract and Refractive Surgeons, nearly 100% of surgeons who responded were using phacoemulsification in the year 2000.[1] With the advancement of phacoemulsification equipment and technique, fewer cataracts require planned extracapsular surgery. Because of this "shortage" in cases, many residents are graduating without proper training in extracapsular surgery. We feel that graduating residents must be competent in the principles of extracapsular cataract surgery because this skill is valuable when phacoemulsification equipment fails, there is significant endothelial failure, the density of the lens precludes phacoemulsification, or if conversion from phacoemulsification is required. In this chapter, we describe two techniques for extracapsular cataract surgery (traditional ECCE and SICS); however, many variations exist and some of these alternative techniques will also be mentioned.

Henderson BA. *Essentials of
Cataract Surgery, Second Edition (pp 219-233).*
© 2014 Taylor & Francis Group.

II. PREOPERATIVE PREPARATION

The preparation of the patient for ECCE is similar for phacoemulsification. In addition to careful patient selection and education, this procedure also requires a properly signed informed consent, selection of the intraocular lens (IOL), identification of the operative site, adequate pupillary dilation or planned pupil stretch, and proper patient positioning.

III. PERIOPERATIVE PREPARATION

A. Anesthesia

Since ECCE typically requires a larger, sclerocorneal incision, some form of injectional anesthesia is preferred and typically includes retrobulbar, peribulbar, or sub-Tenon's techniques. Both traditional and small incision extracapsular surgeries require the surgeon eliminate posterior pressure. One of the following techniques should be performed for a minimum of 10 minutes prior to the start of the procedure unless there is a known zonular problem:

- Manual: Apply pressure for a few seconds and then release for a few seconds
- Honan balloon: Inflate a Honan balloon to 30 mm Hg and exercise caution when positioning it on the globe
- Super pinky
- Mercury bag

B. Position Surgeon and Microscope

Again, this is similar as for phacoemulsification and discussed in more detail in the preoperative assessment chapter of this text.

IV. PROCEDURE: TRADITIONAL EXTRACAPSULAR CATARACT EXTRACTION

A. Bridle Suture

A bridle suture is often placed to ensure proper positioning of the globe throughout the procedure. To place a bridle suture, the surgeon should rotate the globe inferiorly with a muscle hook in the inferior cul-de-sac or grasp the superior limbus with 0.12 forceps. Then, with the opposite hand, grasp the superior rectus (SR) with 0.3 to 0.5 toothed forceps approximately 10 mm posterior to the limbus and lift the tendon off the globe. Pass a 4-0 silk

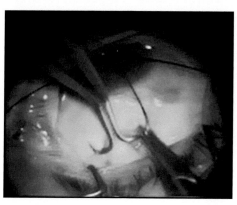

Figure 21-1. Placement of the bridle suture.

suture with a tapered needle under the SR tendon (Figure 21-1). The needle should be flat with the globe to avoid penetration. Cut off the needle and clamp the suture to the drape with a hemostat to rotate the globe down. This suture should be released when the wound is opened to prevent the prolapse of viscoelastic and chamber collapse.

B. Conjunctival Peritomy

This is typically performed by using blunt Wescott scissors to make a radial incision at the 10:00 position (for a right-handed surgeon), 2 mm posterior to the limbus, remembering that Tenon's capsule inserts 1.5 mm posterior to the limbus. Use blunt dissection to remove Tenon's and conjunctiva from the globe. Keep scissor blades parallel to the limbus and insert one blade into the conjunctival pocket. Then pull blades gently toward the cornea and cut to reduce any conjunctival tags present in the field of the wound preparation. Repeat this maneuver until the conjunctival peritomy measures approximately 12 mm (cord length; Figure 21-2).

C. Cautery

Always verify the correct power setting on the machine prior to using the cautery. If using bipolar tips, keep tips approximately 0.5 mm apart. Use a sweeping motion over the sclera and start posteriorly approximately 2 to 3 mm from the limbus to ensure the cautery is not too hot.

D. Incision

1. Groove

Measure the length of the desired wound by marking the sclera with the caliper tips set at 10.5 mm. Use 0.12 forceps to grasp sclera at approximately

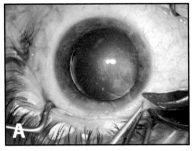
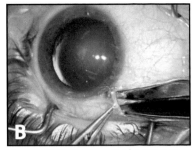

Figure 21-2. Conjunctival peritomy.

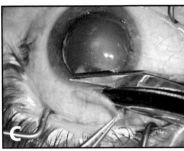

the 2:00 position to stabilize the globe (for a right-handed surgeon). Hold the blade handle perpendicular to the globe and make the incision from left to right approximately 1 mm posterior to the blue line. Consider making the groove more anterior in a blue iris to prevent early entry and iris prolapse. The depth of the groove should be approximately one-half to one-third scleral depth. The length of the groove should be 10.5 mm, beginning at the 10:30 position and ending at approximately the 2:30 position. Attempt to make the groove in one continuous motion by rotating the blade within your fingertips (Figure 21-3A).

2. Tunnel

Use either a #66 or #69 Bard Parker blade to make a scleral tunnel into the cornea. Use a sweeping, circular motion with the blade to enlarge the tunnel for the entire length of the groove (Figure 21-3B). Do not lift the blade to avoid "dog-earring" the flap. The anterior extent of the flap should be at least 1 to 1.5 mm to avoid entering too posteriorly (over the iris root) and risking iris prolapse.

3. Enter anterior chamber

Elevate the anterior lip of the wound with the 0.12 forceps, exposing the apex of the flap, and enter the anterior chamber with a #75 blade parallel to the iris plane. Make a 3-mm incision either to the right side of the wound (right-handed surgeon) or to the left (left-handed surgeon) (Figure 21-3C).

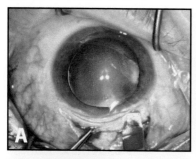
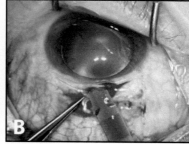

Figure 21-3. Scleral incision.

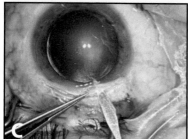

Take care not to lift the flap heavily with the forceps or risk anterior chamber collapse.

E. Viscoelastic Injection

Inject the majority of viscoelastic primarily at the 6:00 position first to push the aqueous out of the eye. Retract the cannula as the anterior chamber fills with viscoelastic.

F. Cystotome

Use a prebent cystotome or use a hemostat to bend a 25-gauge needle (see Chapter 9).

G. Capsulotomy

1. Can-opener

Hold the cystotome with both hands to provide stabilization and penetrate the anterior capsule at the 6:00 position and sweep to the side. Continue making small punctures circumferentially to complete a 6- to 7-mm capsulotomy. With each puncture the surgeon will sweep to the right while going up the left side and to the left while going up the right side. With each puncture, the surgeon will sweep the cystotome toward the previous puncture in order to connect the tears (Figure 21-4).

Figure 21-4. Can-opener capsulotomy.

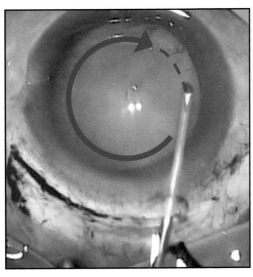

2. Continuous

If a continuous capsulorrhexis is performed, radial tears may be required to facilitate nucleus removal (when the nucleus cannot be hydrodissected and prolapsed out of the bag).

3. Removal of anterior capsule

Use an angled forceps to grasp the central anterior capsule. Ensure that the anterior capsule is free from the peripheral capsule by pulling the capsule gently in all directions and then slowly removing the anterior capsule from the eye. Persistent attachments may require cutting with Vannas scissors or they may tear posteriorly.

H. Enlarge the Wound

Use corneoscleral scissors and enter the anterior chamber with the lower jaw of the scissors and cut toward the opposite side of the wound. Push gently toward the 6:00 position as you cut to ensure that you enlarge the wound at the most anterior aspect of the tunnel. Maintain scissor blades in the groove and keep blades parallel to the iris plane.

I. Nucleus Removal

1. Manual expression

This is achieved by applying external, posterior pressure with forceps or the irrigating lens loop 2 mm posterior to the limbus at the 12:00 position and

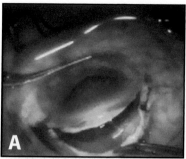

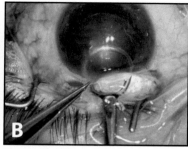

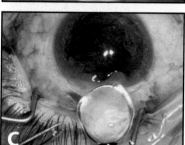

Figure 21-5. (A) Nucleus expression. (B, C) Vectis extraction.

using an assistant to elevate the anterior lip of the wound. When the nucleus begins to prolapse, counter pressure is applied with a muscle hook at the 6:00 position to facilitate removal of the lens. Once the nucleus is partially out of the eye, any pointed instrument may be used to completely rotate the remainder of the lens out of the eye (Figure 21-5A).

2. Lift and extract

Either hydrodissection or manual rotation should be performed to elevate the 12:00 lens into the anterior chamber. To manually rotate the nucleus, use a Sinskey hook, cannula, or cystotome to gently rock the lens in a dialing/ circumferential manner and then lift and rotate. Once the superior portion of the lens is elevated, an irrigating lens loop may be inserted under the lens. The irrigating lens loop is then flattened parallel to the iris plane, lifted toward the cornea, and removed from the eye with the nucleus (Figure 21-5B and C).

J. Suture Placement

To maintain the anterior chamber during cortical removal, it is beneficial to place 2 or 3 10-0 nylon sutures at the 10:00, 12:00, and 2:00 positions. If the iris is light-colored or there is a tendency for iris prolapse, additional sutures may be placed.

K. Cortex Removal

Manual or automated: The cortex may be removed by using either a manual aspirating cannula (eg, Simcoe cannula) or an automated irrigating/aspirating system. This technique is similar to phacoemulsification; however, with a can-opener capsulotomy, care should be taken not to accidentally grasp the anterior capsular leaflets. Strip the cortex toward the center of the pupil and aspirate more aggressively (above the iris plane) only when the port is fully occluded with cortex.

L. Intraocular Lens Implantation

- The capsular bag is reformed with a cohesive viscoelastic prior to implantation of the IOL. It is important to reform the capsular bag and not just deepen the anterior chamber, which pushes the iris and anterior and posterior capsules together. This is achieved by directing the viscoelastic under the anterior capsular leaf of the capsular bag at the 6:00 position.
- If sutures were placed prior to cortical removal, one or more may need to be removed in order to insert a nonfoldable lens. To insert a nonfoldable lens, grasp the lens approximately one-half to one-third onto the optic of the IOL with long-angled forceps (ie, Kelman). Hold the anterior lip of the wound and ease the IOL into the bag by tilting the lens down and pushing the leading haptic into the 6:00 position. When the majority of the IOL is in the capsular bag, the anterior wound is released and the trailing haptic is grasped to prevent extrusion of the IOL when the optic is released. Tap the IOL further into the bag with closed Kelman forceps until the optic is completely behind the pupil. Place or rotate the trailing haptic into the capsular bag as you would with phacoemulsification.

M. Wound Closure

Place a corneal light shield to protect the macula from phototoxicity. Place enough 10-0 nylon sutures to ensure adequate wound closure. With proper wound construction, 4 to 5 sutures should be adequate.

N. Removal of Viscoelastic

One suture should be left untied to allow entry with the automated or manual irrigation/aspiration instrument to completely remove the viscoelastic. Tapping posteriorly on the anterior surface of the IOL will facilitate removal of the viscoelastic retained behind the IOL.

O. Injections

- Pupillary constriction with either intracameral acetylcholine and carbachol is prudent in ECCE to reduce the risk of optic pupillary capture postoperatively.
- Subconjunctival antibiotics and steroids are often used to reduce the risk of infection and lessen inflammation in cases where local anesthesia is performed.

V. PROCEDURE: SMALL INCISION EXTRACAPSULAR CATARACT SURGERY

New surgical techniques for ECCE have dramatically improved the speed and efficiency of traditional ECCE: (1) a well-constructed, self-sealing scleral wound; (2) triangular or envelope capsulotomy, which eliminates the need for capsular staining; and (3) a lens delivery technique that relies on fluidics more than manual forces.

While a superior approach has long been the standard of care in ECCE, a temporal incision has been shown to induce less astigmatism. In one study, the mean induced astigmatic change was 1.28 D following a superior surgical approach due to the effects of gravity and motion of the eyelids on the wound. Following a temporal incision, 0.37 D of astigmatism was induced.[3] While astigmatism may be less with a temporal incision, a superior incision also has some advantages. First, the upper eyelid covers the wound and provides good protection of the superior incision. Additionally, the microscope need not be repositioned between cases. Wound placement should be determined preoperatively based also on any inherent corneal astigmatism that could be ameliorated.

For a superior approach, a bridle suture may be placed if desired. A fornix-based conjunctival peritomy is performed from the 10:00 to the 2:00 position and hemostasis is obtained with cautery. For a temporal approach, the periotomy is made from 7:00 to 11:00.

A. Incision

A straight to slightly frown-shaped scleral incision is made at approximately 30% to 50% depth tangential to the limbus for 6 to 7 mm and approximately 1.5 to 2 mm posterior to the limbus. The crescent blade is then used to create a scleral tunnel, which extends approximately 1 to 1.5 mm into clear cornea. The dissected pocket should then be extended laterally as to create a funnel shape with the interior tunnel being much broader than the exterior opening. The result is a wound much wider in the clear cornea than in the sclera. The external wound will likely be approximately 6 mm in length while the internal wound typically extends 9 mm or more in length.

B. Capsulotomy

With the availability of capsular stains, a continuous curvilinear capsulorrhexis may be preferable. A capsulorrhexis should be large, at least 6 mm in diameter so that the entire nucleus can be easily prolapsed into the anterior chamber. If prolapse of the nucleus is difficult, several radial incisions can be made with the cystotome in the anterior capsule to facilitate prolapse of the nucleus into the anterior chamber.

Alternative capsulotomies may be preferred, especially for cases with poor visibility of the capsule, capsular fibrosis, or very large nuclei. Triangular and envelope capsulotomies allow for delivery of nuclei with low risk of complications.

The triangular capsulotomy is performed using a straight 26-gauge needle attached to a 1-mm syringe filled with BSS. It should be passed through the scleral tunnel with the entry point into the anterior chamber in the scleral, and not the more rigid corneal tissue. Using the bevel tip of the needle with the bevel pointed sideways, a linear cut is made in the capsule. If the wound is superior, the first incision would begin at the 4:00 position and end at 12:00 and a second incision would start at the 8:00 position and meet the other incision at 12:00. This creates a triangular or V-shaped flap of anterior lens capsule that is still attached at its base. Each point of the triangle should be approximately 3 mm from the center of the pupil. The apex of the triangle is then lifted with the needle and then peeled toward what was 6:00 before. If the chamber shallows, a small amount of BSS (or viscoelastic) can be inserted into the anterior chamber to re-deepen the chamber (Figure 21-6).

One advantage of a triangular capsulotomy is that it utilizes a straight needle introduced into the anterior chamber through the unopened scleral wound, maintaining the anterior chamber depth. In addition, the needle can be used to aspirate any liquid lens material that may cause obstruction of the view. Finally, because the triangular capsulotomy is cut and not torn, it creates a reliably consistent triangular shape and minimizes the number of capsular tags.

An envelope capsulotomy can also be created through the unopened scleral wound or following entry into the anterior chamber with the keratome. A 7- to 8-mm cut is made in the anterior capsule 4 to 5 mm from the center of the lens. This straight incision is created using the side of the beveled needle or with the keratome after initial entry into the anterior chamber.

C. Open the Wound

The opening of the internal aspect of the sclerocorneal tunnel is accomplished using the keratome. After initial entry in the center of the tunnel, the sides of the blade are used to open the cornea to the wound's lateral edges. This funnel-shaped wound is internally flared to make the internal wound

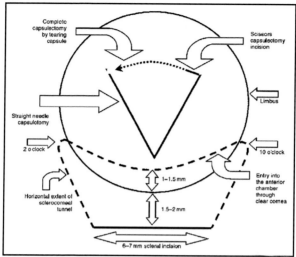

Figure 21-6. Wound construction and Triangular Capsulotomy for SICS. (Reprinted with permission from Ruit S, Paudyal G, Gurung R, Tabin G, Moran D, Brian G. An innovation in developing world cataract surgery: sutureless extracapsular cataract extraction with intraocular lens implantation. *Clin Experiment Ophthalmol.* 2000;28(4):274-279.)

larger than the external scleral portion, which will encourage the nucleus engagement in the tunnel at the time of expression. If available, viscoelastic may be placed in the anterior chamber to facilitate wound creation. A well-constructed internal lip of the wound is the key to it being self-sealing.

D. Nucleus Removal

For both a capsulorrhexis or the triangle capsulotomy, the nucleus is displaced from the capsular bag into the anterior chamber using hydrostatic and gentle mechanical pressure (Figure 21-7). With a large continuous curvilinear capsulorrhexis, hydrodissection will often result in prolapse of the nucleus into the anterior chamber. Irrigating with the Simcoe cannula under the displaced triangular anterior capsule flap as well as under the temporal and nasal edges of the flap will mobilize the lens nucleus. The nucleus is gently directed distal to the wound within the capsular bag, while the irrigation is directed posterior to the nucleus until the superior nuclear pole emerges from the capsular bag into the anterior chamber. It is important not to force the nucleus in any one direction as this will strain and potentially compromise zonules

Figure   21-7.
Expression of lens
during SICS.

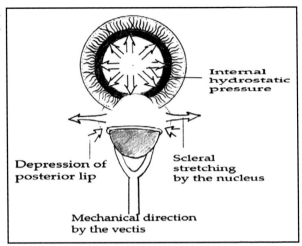

Internal
hydrostatic
pressure

Depression of
posterior lip

Scleral
stretching
by the nucleus

Mechanical direction
by the vectis

and/or extend capsular tears posteriorly. For the envelope capsulotomy, the nucleus is delivered directly from the bag into the mouth of the wound.

While several techniques are available for nucleus removal, one effective technique that is described in this section uses hydrostatic pressure. The vigorously flowing Simcoe cannula is passed posterior to the nucleus until the tip is fully visible beyond the distal pole of the nucleus. The eye is then gently rotated away from the surgeon with the toothed forceps held in the other hand. The curve of the simcoe cannula cups the underside of the nucleus and gently guides the nucleus toward the mouth of the wound. The accumulating irrigation fluid pushes the nucleus further into the wound. Gentle downward pressure using the heel of the Simcoe cannula further opens the wound for nucleus delivery. An irrigating vectus may also be used (see Figure 21-5C).

E. Intraocular Lens Placement

In a standard fashion, the Simcoe cannula can be used to remove all the cortical and epinuclear debris from the anterior chamber and capsular bag. As described under traditional ECCE, the IOL may be placed using viscoelastic. However, if viscoelastic is not available, air is injected into the anterior chamber and a PCIOL inserted into the capsular bag. Once the IOL is in the bag, the triangular capsulotomy flap can be reflected back to cover the IOL.

F. Capsulectomy

If a triangular or envelope capsulotomy was performed, the anterior capsular flap needs to be removed to prevent obstruction of the visual axis. A small incision is made in the anterior capsule at the edge of the base of the triangular flap or the lateral extent of the envelope with fine Vannas scissors while maintaining the AC depth with an irrigating Simcoe cannula or under viscoelastic. The capsular flap is engaged with aspiration using the Simcoe cannula (using low flow irrigation) and used to gently tear the flap entirely across its base, which then should be removed from the AC. Similarly, if viscoelastic is used, an angled forceps can be used to complete the tear at the base (see Figure 21-6).

G. Wound Closure

The Simcoe cannula is used to irrigate and aspirate any residual air or viscoelastic in the AC and the intraocular pressure is restored. The triplanar sclerocorneal tunnel will ideally be self-sealing. Gentle pressure on the globe while observing for wound leak will confirm a water-tight wound. A subconjunctival injection of antibiotic and steroid may be given just superior to the conjunctival wound edge, which balloons the conjunctiva and moves it over the limbus to cover the scleral wound. In the instance of a temporal surgical approach, the conjunctiva is closed over the scleral wound with cauterization or sutures at the wound edges.

H. SICS Outcomes

Utilizing IOLs manufactured in India or Nepal and local pharmaceuticals, the material cost per surgery can be less than $20 per case. Moreover, experienced surgeons routinely perform more than 50 cases per day with an average operating time of minutes per surgery. The results of a prospective, randomized clinical trial in Nepal comparing the manual sutureless extracapsular surgical technique with phacoemulsification demonstrated that at 6 months, 89% of the SICS patients had an uncorrected visual acuity (UCVA) of 20/60 or better and 98% had a best-corrected acuity (BCVA) of 20/60 or better; this outcome was equivalent to the visual acuity outcomes of the phaco patients.[4] Furthermore, SICS is significantly faster, less expensive, and less technology dependent than phacoemulsification and may be the more appropriate surgical procedure for the treatment of advanced cataracts in the developing world. This technique may also benefit our own patient population where cost might drive multitiered care.

VI. POSTOPERATIVE CARE

The postoperative care for the ECCE patient is similar to that for phacoemulsification. Care should be taken to identify any postoperative wound leaks and to treat them when indicated. In addition, tight sutures will create astigmatism that may be managed by cutting sutures when adequate wound healing has been achieved. This may be a minimum of 4 weeks, especially when heavy use of topical corticosteroids had been employed.

VII. CONVERSION FROM PHACOEMULSIFICATION

A. The Indications for Conversion to ECCE

- Mechanical failure of the phacoemulsification machine or hand piece
- Significant capsular injury with sizeable nuclear material still present
- Visualization difficulties making phacoemulsification risky

B. Technique

- Perform a conjunctival peritomy and then enlarge the clear corneal incision by using a #69 blade to create a more limbal corneal or scleral groove that incorporates each side of the corneal incision. Create a tunnel as previously described and enlarge the wound with the corneoscleral scissors beginning with the blade in the original corneal incision.
- After applying a small amount of viscoelastic to protect the endothelium and lift the nuclear remnant, consider the placement of a Sheets lens glide under the nuclear remnants to reduce the risk of nucleus loss into the posterior segment. If the posterior capsule has been violated, dry, manual removal of nuclear fragments is most safe.

VIII. CONCLUSION

ECCE is an essential component of the residents' surgical experience. Each step in the process is important because it provides the foundation for the next step. As beginning surgeons develop competence with traditional ECCE, SICS is a valuable skill, particularly when considering medical missions to third world countries.

KEY POINTS

1. Achieve adequate anesthesia and eliminate posterior pressure.

2. Perform proper construction, placement, and size of the corneoscleral incision, both traditional and small incision.

3. With both the can-opener capsulotomy and triangular capsulotomy, care must be taken to connect the punctures to prevent significant radial tears or capsular leaflets.

4. Carefully remove the lens nucleus using either (1) manual expression, (2) lift and extract, or (3) hydrostatic extraction.

REFERENCES

1. Leaming DV. Practice styles and preferences of ASCRS members—2000 survey. *J Cataract Refract Surg.* 2001;27:948-955.
2. Gohale NS, Sawhney S. Reduction in astigmatism in manual small incision cataract surgery through change of incision site. *Indian J Ophthalmol.* 2005;53:201-203.
3. Ruit S, Tabin G, Chang D A prospective randomized clinical trial of phacoemulsification vs. manual sutureless small-incision extracapsular cataract surgery in Nepal. *Am J Ophthalmol.* 2007;143(1):32-38.

THE SMALL PUPIL

Sherleen H. Chen, MD, FACS and Roberto Pineda II, MD

I. INTRODUCTION

The small pupil presents a common and significant challenge to the beginning phaco surgeon. A miotic pupil impairs visualization of the very structure being removed during cataract surgery. In addition, a diminished red reflex makes capsulorrhexis formation more difficult and interferes with visual cues used to judge sculpting depth. As a result, the small pupil is associated with a higher risk of complications. These include posterior capsular rupture, dropped nuclear fragments, iris trauma, bleeding, and inflammation.

II. CLINICAL SETTING

A small pupil may result from a variety of causes (Table 22-1). At least 2% of phaco cases will have a pupil that dilates maximally to 5 mm or less.

III. MANAGEMENT OF THE SMALL PUPIL

A. Patient Evaluation

1. Examination: Preoperative evaluation includes a careful search for the etiology of the small pupil as this may impact management. For example, synechiae and inflammatory membranes require different techniques than pseudoexfoliation (PXF) or intraoperative floppy iris syndrome (IFIS). Note the pupil diameter after maximal pharmacological dilation in the clinic.

2. Inquire about the use of tamsulosin (also doxazosin, terazosin, alfuzosin, silodosin, and saw palmetto) and anticoagulants (including homeopathic remedies like ginkgo for bleeding).

Henderson BA. *Essentials of Cataract Surgery, Second Edition (pp 235-247).*
© 2014 Taylor & Francis Group.

TABLE 22-1. CAUSES OF SMALL PUPIL

Etiologies of Small Pupil	Mechanism
Pseudoexfoliation syndrome (PXF)	Atrophic changes of dilator and sphincter[1]
Synechiae	Trauma, uveitis, angle closure, and prior surgery
Diabetes	Autonomic dysfunction, rubeosis iridis
Horner syndrome	Sympathetic denervation
Advanced age	Atrophy of iris
IFIS	Selective blockade of α1A of iris dilator muscle
Chronic miotic therapy	Fibrosis of iris sphincter

TABLE 22-2. PREOPERATIVE ANTICOAGULATION MANAGEMENT

Anticoagulants	Discontinued Preoperatively
Coumadin	3 days
Aspirin, NSAIDs	7 to 10 days
Plavix	7 days[2]
Ginkgo	14 days

3. The consent process is crucial to managing patient expectations. Discuss the potential for the following:
   - ¤ Longer surgery
   - ¤ Higher risk for complications
   - ¤ Postoperative issues of longer recovery, cosmesis (especially with a blue iris if the pupil will be mechanically enlarged), and glare due to an atonic dilated pupil

B. Preparation for Surgery

1. Minimize bleeding

If cleared by the primary care physician, consider discontinuing anticoagulants preoperatively to minimize potential bleeding with iris manipulation (Table 22-2).

2. Minimize inflammation

1. If extensive iris manipulation is anticipated or significant posterior synechiae are present, prednisolone 4 times a day for 3 days preoperatively may help to minimize inflammation postoperatively. In patients with a history of uveitis, a 1-week preoperative course of topical steroids is recommended. Oral steroids may be indicated in severe cases.

2. Prophylaxis against cystoid macular edema (CME) and intraoperative miosis should be considered via topical nonsteroidal anti-inflammatory drugs (NSAIDs) taken for 3 days preoperatively and discontinuing any prostaglandin analogs the day before surgery.

3. Maximize dilation

1. Prior to the day of surgery
   - If possible, discontinue miotics (pilocarpine 3 days, phospholine iodide 2 weeks).
   - Consider cyclopegics to maximize pharmacologic dilation (scopolamine 0.25% bid, or atropine 1% qhs × 3 days preoperatively or on the day of surgery).

2. On the day of surgery
   - Topical NSAIDs (suprofen or flurbiprofen) added to the standard mydriatic regimen may reduce intraoperative miosis.
   - Consider placing a pledget soaked with mydriatic and NSAID in the inferior fornix to prolong exposure to the mydriatic and maximize dilation.
   - Avoid phenylephrine 10%, which has been used in the past. Significant concerns about iatrogenic hypertensive crisis, bradycardia (not a misprint), and corneal punctate keratopathy have limited its current use.

3. Intraoperatively
   - Intracameral epi-Shugarcaine[3]
   - Nonpreserved epinephrine placed into the balanced salt solution (BSS) infusion helps minimize intraoperative miosis[4,5] (eg, 0.3 to 0.5 cc of nonpreserved 1:1000 epinephrine into 500 cc BSS).

4. Anesthesia

1. Local injectional or sub-Tenon's anesthesia is preferred in cases of a small pupil, particularly with beginning phaco surgeons or in cases where extensive iris manipulation is anticipated.

2. If topical anesthesia is planned, intracameral supplementation is recommended to minimize pain with iris manipulation.

5. Preoperative orders

1. Order an intraocular lens with a larger diameter optic (6 mm) to minimize the chance of issues with glare should the pupil remain dilated postoperatively.

2. A cohesive viscoelastic (eg, Healon 5, Healon GV by AMO, Provisc by Alcon, and Amvisc Plus by Bausch + Lomb) will hold back iris and maximize viscodilation.

3. Trypan blue or an iris expansion device may be needed; these should be on standby.

C. Surgical Techniques

Specific management techniques will vary according to the etiology of the small pupil, but the basic principles of good surgery remain unchanged. Each step of phacoemulsification serves as the foundation for the next. In complex cases, it is especially important to complete each step well before moving forward. Judicious use of viscoelastics will serve as a helpful surgical aid.

1. Incision

Proper wound construction is even more important. A longer clear cornea incision will decrease iris prolapse if the iris becomes floppy with manipulation or due to α1 blockade (eg, tamsulosin). The longer incision places the corneal entry site more anteriorly and elevated from the iris plane. Similarly, if the corneal entry of a scleral tunnel incision is placed too posteriorly, iris will prolapse more easily than if the entry is more anterior.

2. Enlarge the pupil

1. Choose the simplest method and minimal intervention required to achieve adequate dilation.

2. Perform pupil enlargement only as needed to achieve adequate visualization for capsulorrhexis formation and phacoemulsification. In general, an ideal capsulorrhexis should be 5 to 5.5 mm in diameter for a 6-mm optic IOL. Avoid smaller openings particularly in eyes with pseudoexfoliation due to their tendency toward capsular contraction and zonular dehiscence with anterior capsule fibrosis.

3. Hierarchy

   (a) Viscodilation

      i. A cohesive viscoelastic may enlarge a borderline pupil to a sufficient size.

    ii. May be repeated throughout the remaining steps of phaco-emulsification as needed to maintain pupil dilation and visualization.

(b) Synechiolysis

    i. If synechiae are present, perform synechiolysis under visco-elastic protection. The viscoelastic cannula is used to bluntly lyse synechiae while periodically injecting with viscoelastic. A cyclodialysis spatula may similarly be used to reach under more adherent or distal areas; synechiae are present not only at the pupillary margin, but often are significant under the stroma of the iris itself. A second paracentesis site may provide 360-degree access if the main and side-port incisions are inadequate.

    ii. Strip any fibrotic membranes.

    iii. Complete with viscoelastic injection.

(c) Pupil stretching: If the above maneuvers are inadequate, pupil stretching may be accomplished using either a bimanual technique or with a pupil-stretching instrument. Performed under viscoelastic protection, either method is a fast, simple, gentle, and relatively inexpensive technique to enlarge the pupil with minimal hemorrhage and a typically good cosmetic result. It is probably the first choice for pupil manipulation among most surgeons due to its ease and effectiveness.

    i. Bimanual stretching:[6] Two iris manipulators (Kuglen/Y hooks, Graether collar buttons) are placed at the pupil margin 180 degrees apart. The manipulators are separated in the iris plane in opposite directions toward the iris root slowly and gently over 5 to 10 seconds. Novice surgeons must remember to use the wounds as fulcrums around which to manipulate the instruments, or the wounds will become distorted, with significant corneal striae impairing visualization. One can also aim for approximately 120 degrees of separation, which makes the stretch more effective and may cause less ciliary pain by not having to stretch fully to the iris root.[7] Multiple small foci of hemorrhage at the pupil margin are expected at the end of a stretch. The procedure may be repeated once or twice more in different meridia as needed to achieve further stretch. Viscoelastic is again injected to visualize the maximal result.

      ¤ Advantages: Multiple microsphincter tears, but postsurgical pupil looks round; fast, simple, inexpensive; first choice for many surgeons; but not recommended for IFIS

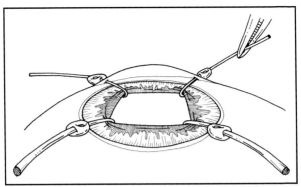

Figure 22-1. Iris hooks. (Reprinted with permission from Pineda R, Espaillat A, Perez VL, Rowe S. *The Complicated Cataract: The Massachusetts Eye and Ear Infirmary Phacoemulsification Practice Hand-book*. Thorofare, NJ: SLACK Incorporated; 2001.)

> ¤ Disadvantages: May not provide sufficient dilation; may cause bleeding, inflammation, permanent mydriasis
>
> ii. Instruments that may be used to stretch the pupil include the Beehler (2 or 3 pronged), Keuch (2 point), and Peters (loop and hook) pupil dilators
>
> ¤ Advantages: Stretches several directions at once relatively fast
>
> ¤ Disadvantages: Requires a special instrument, which is bulkier than the iris manipulators; may tear capsule; may not provide sufficient dilation; may cause bleeding inflammation, permanent mydriasis

(d) Iris retractors provide the advantage of mechanically maintaining stable pupil dilation throughout the case. Pupil expansion can be accomplished with iris hooks or a pupil expansion ring.

i. Iris hooks[8-10] (Figure 22-1)

(a) Two types

1. Disposable nylon, which is more flexible and smaller (5-0)

2. Reusable polypropylene, which is stiffer and larger (4-0)

(b) Hints

1. Place 4 limbal paracenteses (short tract, peripheral cornea parallel to iris plane in a diamond configuration[11]) to prevent iris prolapse through incision and maximize exposure anterior to main incision.

2. A small bolus of viscoelastic injected under the iris focally can help elevate iris from the capsule.

3. Using tying forceps in each hand, the hooks are inserted parallel to the incision, then rotated into position using the plastic donuts.

4. After all the 4 retractors are placed, they are gently retracted to enlarge the pupil and secured with the donut.

   ◻ Advantages: Maintains pupil throughout case; good for floppy iris; smaller profile than expansion rings (better for crowded anterior chamber)

   ◻ Disadvantages: Time-consuming. Needs additional incisions; requires special instruments; excessive dilation may cause sphincter damage

ii. Pupil Expansion Rings

   (a) Single-use rings that retract and protect the pupil margin throughout the case (Figure 22-2)

   (b) Five choices[12-15] (Table 22-3)

   ◻ Advantages: Maintains pupil throughout case; protects iris; gentle, least traumatic

   ◻ Disadvantages: Requires special instruments (ring, inserter); more time to place, extra care removing; added expense

(e) Sphincterotomies

   i. Using long angled Gills or Rappazzo scissors, 8 tiny (0.5 to 0.75 mm) cuts are made at equal intervals in the iris sphincter.[16] This is reserved as a last resort.

   ii. Advantages: No special instruments, fast; permanent mydriasis

   iii. Disadvantages: Permanent mydriasis; can get more bleeding; inflammation, glare, cosmesis

4. Caveat: IFIS[17]

   (a) α1 adrenergic blockers used to treat benign prostatic hypertrophy (BPH) in men and urinary retention in women (relax smooth muscle of bladder neck and prostatic urethra to improve urine outflow)

   i. Examples: tamsulosin (Flomax), doxazosin mesylate (Cardura), terazosin (Hytrin), alfuzosin (Uroxatral), and silodosin (Rapaflo)

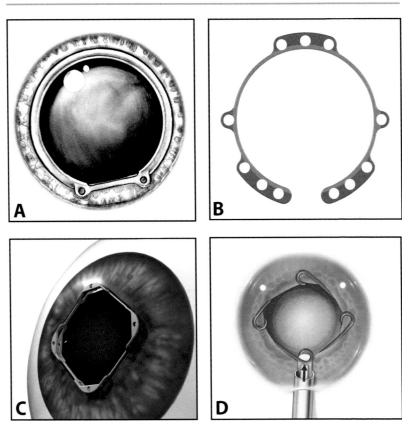

Figure 22-2. Pupil expansion rings. (A) Graether Pupil Expander. (Reprinted with permission from Eagle Vision.) (B) Morcher Pupil Dilator. (Reprinted with permission from FCI Ophthalmics.) (C) Iris Expander. (Reprinted with permission from OASIS.) (D) Malyugin Ring. (Reprinted with permission from MST.)

Minimum incision size: Graether 2.5 mm, Iris Expander 2.2 mm, Malyugin 2.2 mm, Morcher 2.5 mm.

THE SMALL PUPIL   243

Table 22-3. Pupil Expansion Rings

	Graether Pupil Expander	Iris Expander	Malyugin Ring	Morcher Pupil Dilator
Manufacturer	Eagle	OASIS	MicroSurgical Technology	FCI Ophthalmics
Material	Silicone	Polypropylene	Polypropylene (5-0)	PMMA
Insertion method	Preloaded on inserter	Packaged with disposable injector	Packaged with disposable injector	Manual or Geuder injector
Pupil size	6.3 mm	7.0 mm	6.25 or 7.0 mm	5 to 6 mm
Description	Incomplete ring, with 3.5-mm gap bridged by thin strap to allow phaco instrument access	Square with pockets in each corner to support the iris	Scroll in each corner of collapsible square, with 8 points of fixation	Incomplete ring Stiff, may rotate during case
Minimum incision size	2.5 mm	2.2 mm	2.2 mm	2.5 mm

    ii. Tamsulosin and silodosin are the only α1 blockers that are specific to the α1A subtype. The α1A subtype, which predominates in the urethra and iris dilator smooth muscle and is less predominant in peripheral vasculature. Blockade is thought to cause atrophy of iris dilator smooth muscle over time.

  (b) Clinical triad: floppy iris that billows, iris prolapse through wounds, and progressive miosis

  (c) IFIS management

    i. The degree of preoperative dilation may help predict potential difficulty

    ii. Interventions

      (a) Helpful:

        1. Iris hooks

        2. Healon 5 with lowered infusion and vacuum settings

        3. Pupil expansion rings

        4. Preoperative atropine

      (b) Not helpful: pupil stretching and sphincterotomies

    iii. Hints:

      (a) Avoid overinflating AC with viscoelastic or hydrodissection, which promote iris prolapse.

      (b) Viscoelastic over subincisional iris prevents prolapse/phaco tip trauma.

      (c) When eye is filled with viscoelastic, entering dry (without irrigation) will minimize egress of viscoelastic and iris prolapse.

3. Capsulorrhexis

1. Improve visualization with capsular staining if the red reflex is suboptimal.

2. Use a high molecular weight cohesive viscoelastic for maximal control. Maintain control. Consider starting with smaller capsulorrhexis to ensure completion of a continuous capsulorrhexis and enlarge during second pass if too small.

3. A second instrument (eg, Kuglen or Y hook) can help to retract iris.

4. Decrease tendency for capsular contraction and anterior capsule fibrosis (especially in PXF) with a minimum capsulorrhexis diameter of 5 mm.

4. Hydrodissection

1. It is crucial to ensure adequate nuclear rotation before proceeding further.

2. Beware overpressurizing the capsular bag in the setting of a small capsulorrhexis (or risk posterior capsular rupture from capsular block syndrome).

5. Phacoemulsification

1. Technique

   (a) Vertical chop is preferred, as all movements are kept centrally.

   (b) For divide and conquer, remember that the depth of the groove is more crucial for successful cracking than how peripheral the groove extends. Avoid grooving under the iris (without visualization).

2. Lower flow and vacuum settings help prevent inadvertent aspiration of iris and posterior capsule.

3. Be aware of potentially smaller capsulorrhexis.

   (a) Nuclear fragments or the chopper could lacerate the capsulorrhexis.

   (b) Trypan blue staining is helpful for visualization.

6. Cortical clean-up

1. Bimanual irrigation/aspiration (I/A) is often helpful if the view is compromised, especially for subincisional cortex.

2. Consider using a second instrument to peek under iris to ensure complete cortical removal.

3. Remove as much cortex as possible, but avoid heroics.

7. End of case

1. Miotic (eg, miochol E, carbachol)

   (a) Helps reform redundant flaccid pupil and prevents IOL optic capture.

   (b) Helps control intraocular pressure immediately postoperatively.

2. Suturing incision sites may be indicated if iris prolapse occurred intraoperatively.

3. Consider subconjunctival injection of dexamethasone.

D. Postoperative Considerations

1. Manage inflammation.
   i. Watch carefully for a fibrinoid reaction, especially in diabetics, PXF, and uveitis.
   ii. Treat aggressively with steroids.
   iii. CME prophylaxis with topical NSAIDs.
2. Treat glaucoma (due to inflammation, red blood or pigment cells, and retained viscoelastic) as needed (avoid prostaglandin analogs).
3. Consider pilocarpine 1% to 2% for 1 to 2 weeks to help pupil regain its size/shape if inflammation is minimal.

KEY POINTS

1. Prepare yourself and the patient before surgery.
2. A cohesive viscoelastic can help throughout the case.
3. Achieve adequate visualization (trypan blue staining, dilate pupil).
4. Modify the surgical technique for a small pupil.
   - Choose the minimal intervention needed to achieve sufficient dilation.
   - Phacoemulsifcation: use vertical chop or deep grooves in divide and conquer.
   - I/A may require bimanual hand pieces.
5. The general principles of good phaco surgery are even more important in complicated cases.
   - Carefully complete each step adequately before moving to the next.
   - Avoid heroics.

REFERENCES

1. Naumann GOH, Schlötzer-Schrenhardt U, Küchle M. Pseudoexfoliation syndrome for the comprehensive ophthalmologist: intraocular and systemic manifestations. *Ophthalmology.* 1998;105(6):951-968.
2. Davies BR. Combined aspirin and clopidogrel in cataract surgical patients: a new risk factor for ocular haemorrhage? *Br J Ophthalmol.* 2004;88(9):1226-1227.
3. Myers WG, Shugar JK. Optimizing the intracameral dilation regimen for cataract surgery: prospective randomized comparison of 2 solutions. *J Cataract Refract Surg.* 2009;35(2)273-276.

4. Corbett MC, Richards AB. Intraocular adrenaline maintains mydriasis during cataract surgery. *Br J Ophthalmol.* 1994;78(2):95-98.

5. Liou SW, Yang CY. The effect of intracameral adrenaline infusion on pupil size, pulse rate, and blood pressure during phacoemulsification. *J Ocul Pharmacol Ther.* 1998;14(4):357-361.

6. Miller KM, Keener GT. Stretch pupilloplasty for small pupil phacoemulsification. *Am J Ophthalmol.* 1994;117(1):107-108.

7. Dinsmore SC. Modified stretch technique for small pupil phacoemulsification with topical anesthesia. *J Cataract Refract Surg.* 1996;22(1):27-30.

8. deJuan E, Hickingbotham D. Flexible iris retractor. *Am J Ophthalmol.* 1991;111(6):776-777.

9. Mackool RJ. Small pupil enlargement during cataract extraction: a new method. *J Cataract Refract Surg.* 1992;18(5):523-526.

10. Nichamin LD. Enlarging the pupil for cataract extraction using flexible nylon iris retractors. *J Cataract Refract Surg.* 1993;19(6):793-796.

11. Oetting TA, Omphroy LC. Modified technique using iris retractors in clear corneal cataract surgery. *J Cataract Refract Surg.* 2002;28(4):596-598.

12. Graether JM. Graether pupil expander for managing the small pupil during surgery. *J Cataract Refract Surg.* 1996;22(5):530-535.

13. Malyugin B. Small pupil phaco surgery: a new technique. *Ann Ophthalmol (Skokie).* 2007;39(3):185-193.

14. Akman A, Yilmaz G, Oto S Akova YA. Comparison of various pupil dilatation methods for phacoemulsification in eyes with a small pupil secondary to pseudoexfoliation. *Ophthalmol.* 2004;111(9):1693-1698.

15. Kershner RM. Management of the small pupil for clear corneal cataract surgery. *J Cataract Refract Surg.* 2002;28(10):1826-1831.

16. Fine IH. Pupilloplasty for small pupil phacoemulsification. *J Cataract Refract Surg.* 1994;20(2):192-196.

17. Chang DF, Campbell JR. Intraoperative floppy iris syndrome associated with tamsulosin. *J Cataract Refract Surg.* 2005;31(4):664-673.

23

THE MATURE CATARACT
AND CAPSULE DYE

Kenneth L. Cohen, MD

I. INTRODUCTION

The modern cataract operation has progressed to techniques of continuous curvilinear capsulorrhexis (CCC) and phacoemulsification of the nucleus. While these techniques contribute to the excellent outcome of cataract surgery today, the CCC and phacoemulsification can be difficult to perform in eyes with mature and hypermature, white cataracts (Figure 23-1).

Mature and hypermature cataracts are frequent in developing countries and are not uncommon in the immigrant population in the United States.[1,2] When removing a mature cataract, there are multiple operative challenges to the surgeon.[2] Primarily, there is no red reflex. In addition, the characteristics of the capsule are different, making the CCC difficult. The capsule is fragile, less elastic, and may have focal fibrosis, and/or plaques that interfere with the CCC. Due to high intralenticular pressure, the cortex can leak and further obscure the view of the CCC, and the capsulorrhexis can radialize rapidly. The nucleus can be extremely hard, compromising standard phacoemulsification chopping techniques.

While operating on a mature, white cataract is challenging, there are operative techniques that allow for excellent outcome.[3] Of primary importance are achieving a CCC and maneuvers for removal of a hard nucleus. Therefore, the surgeon must appropriately plan the operation. The results of phacoemulsification of the mature, white cataract can be comparable to phacoemulsification of routine cataracts.[2,3]

Henderson BA. *Essentials of Cataract Surgery, Second Edition (pp 249-269).*
© 2014 Taylor & Francis Group.

Figure 23-1. This is a senile, mature, white cataract.

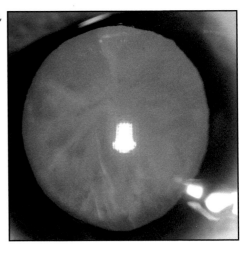

Figure 23-2. The Morgagnian globules are eosinophilic.

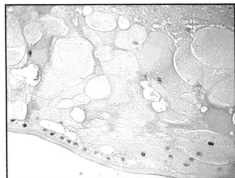

II. WHY DO CATARACTS BECOME WHITE?

The lens develops from the surface ectoderm. The lens cells elongate to become lens fibers, which eventually form the adult nucleus and cortex.[4]

The lens becomes cloudy due to degenerative changes in the lens cortex. Cortical opacities are due to globular degeneration.[4,5] Alterations in the membranes of the lens fibers cause swelling and aggregation of protein. The protein denatures, forming eosinophilic collections of protein, Morgagnian globules (Figure 23-2). Then, the cell membranes break down, releasing the Morgagnian globules, fragments of the lens fibers. The Morgagnian globules and denatured protein cause hyperosmolarity with imbibition fluid. This liquefaction of the cortex causes clouding and a white cortex. When the globules and denatured protein replace the entire cortex, there is a mature, white cataract.

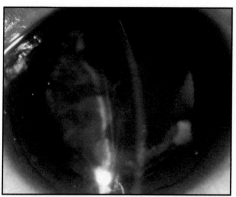

Figure 23-3. This lens has peripheral, wedge-shaped, cuneiform opacities.

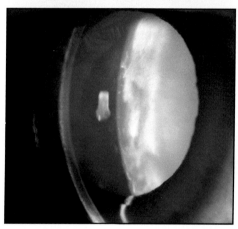

Figure 23-4. The cortex is opacified from the nucleus to the capsule.

III. DEFINING THE STAGE OF MATURITY OF A CATARACT

The state of the cortex determines maturity.[6] An immature senile cataract has partially opacified cortex. The initial characteristic change is that of hydration. Fluid from the aqueous flows into the lens, causing vacuoles and clear clefts. Then, the cortex becomes hazy due to Morgagnian globules and distinct opacities appear. The most common opacity is the cuneiform cataract, peripheral wedge-shaped opacities that extend centrally (Figure 23-3). The immature cataract has a mostly clear cortex.

A mature cataract has a totally opaque cortex that extends to the capsule (Figure 23-4). The lens fibers undergo autolysis, forming a milky-white fluid cortex. This leads to a hyperosmolar cortex. Fluid from the aqueous flows into the lens, and the lens becomes swollen or intumescent (Figure 23-5).

Figure 23-5. This intumescent cataract has a bulging anterior capsule.

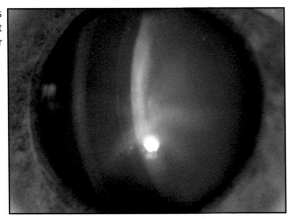

Figure 23-6. This Morgagnian cataract has a floating, sunken nucleus in totally liquefied cortex.

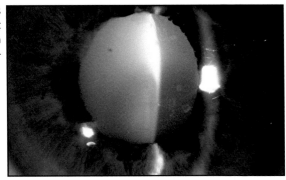

In addition, autolysis of the lens fibers can be extensive such that the entire cortex becomes a milky-white fluid, allowing the nucleus to sink. This is a Morgagnian cataract (Figure 23-6).

If the mature cataract loses fluid into the aqueous, the lens capsule shrinks and wrinkles. When this occurs, the cataract is described as hypermature (Figure 23-7).

IV. White Cataracts Are not all the Same

Many times, even though the cortex is totally cloudy in a mature cataract, the nucleus can be seen. This is possible due to partial liquefaction of the cortex. It is a misconception to assume that a mature, senile cataract always has a dense nucleus. One should attempt to view the nucleus through the liquefied cortex to determine its density. Generally, the nucleus will have color ranging from yellow, moderately dense, to amber, to brown, indicating increasing

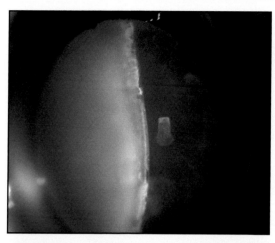

Figure 23-7. This hypermature cataract has a wrinkled anterior capsule due to loss of cortex.

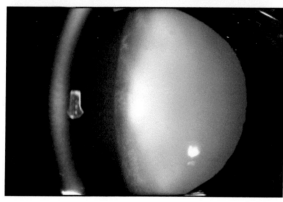

Figure 23-8. This mature, white cataract has a moderately dense, yellow-colored nucleus.

density (Figures 23-8 and 23-9). Determining nuclear density helps with surgical planning.

It is important to identify the special situations of intumescent, hypermature, and Morgagnian cataracts. The intumescent cataract will have a bulging anterior capsule due to high intralenticular pressure causing a shallow anterior chamber. A hypermature cataract will have a wrinkled, irregular anterior capsule associated with a hyper-deep anterior chamber (see Figure 23-7). The Morgagnian cataract will have a floating nucleus in the inferior portion of the lens (see Figure 23-6).

Each of these situations requires specific operative techniques. It is the surgeon's responsibility to clearly identify the clinical characteristics of the white cataract, so that a safe operation can be planned.

Figure 23-9. This mature, white cataract has a hard, dense, amber-colored nucleus.

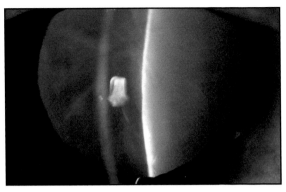

Figure 23-10. This is a senile, mature, white cataract with a dense nucleus.

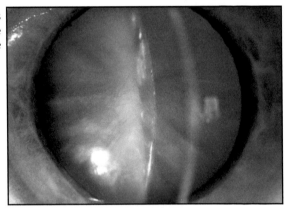

V. CLINICAL ASSOCIATIONS WITH THE WHITE CATARACT

Although uncommon in the United States, mature cataracts are a common initial presentation, 8% to 10%, in developing countries.[7,8] In the United States, it is not uncommon to see mature cataracts in medically underserved populations.

The following figures are clinical associations of mature, white cataracts recently seen at the Kittner Eye Center, University of North Carolina Health Care System. This is not an all-inclusive list (Figures 23-10 to 23-21).

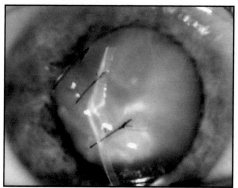

Figure 23-11. This is a white, traumatic cataract due to perforation of the anterior capsule associated with a perforating corneal injury.

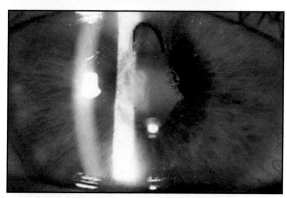

Figure 23-12. This white cataract is associated with sarcoidosis. There are posterior synechiae.

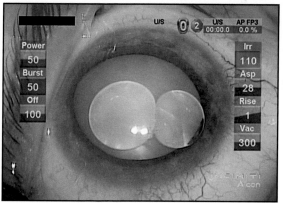

Figure 23-13. This white cataract developed after a pars plana vitrectomy. There is silicone oil in the anterior chamber.

Figure 23-14. This white cataract is associated with a chronic retinal detachment.

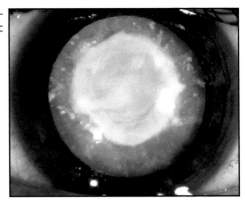

Figure 23-15. This white cataract is associated with retinopathy of prematurity.

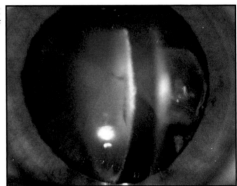

Figure 23-16. This white cataract is associated with sickle cell anemia.

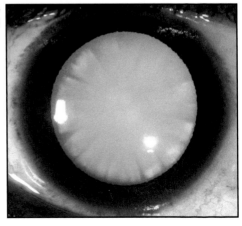

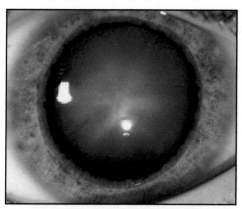

Figure 23-17. This white cataract is associated with intermediate uveitis in a child.

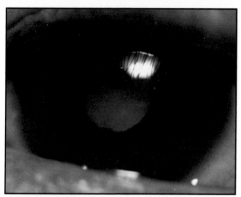

Figure 23-18. This white cataract is associated with uveitic glaucoma due to panuveitis.

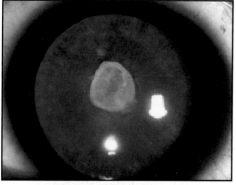

Figure 23-19. This white cataract developed after radiation for rhabdomyosarcoma of the ethmoid sinus.

Figure 23-20. This Morgagnian cataract has a floating, inferiorly displaced brown nucleus. Note the iris sphincter tears.

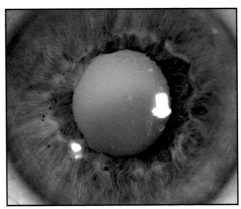

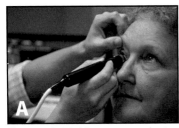
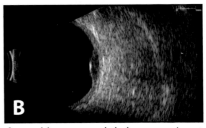

Figure 23-21. Ultrasonography is performed because ophthalmoscopy is not possible due to a white cataract associated with an intraocular tumor (A). B-scan ultrasonography documents the intraocular tumor (B).

VI. A RELATIVE AFFERENT PUPILLARY DEFECT IN THE CONTRALATERAL EYE

An interesting and confusing finding in a patient with a unilateral mature cataract is the presence of an afferent defect in the contralateral eye.[9,10] This is contrary to the common finding of an afferent pupillary defect in the eye with poorer visual acuity. After removal of the mature cataract, the afferent pupillary defect is absent. Although this pupillary defect seems paradoxical, it is hypothesized that in the eye with the mature cataract, there is increased intraocular scatter of light by the mature cataract.[10]

VII. COMPLICATIONS CAUSED BY MATURE CATARACTS

Phacolytic glaucoma is acute onset open angle caused by leaking lens protein obstructing the trabecular meshwork. The lens protein leaks through an

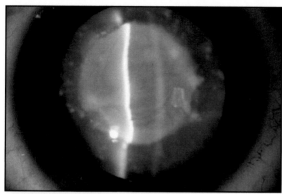

Figure 23-22. This patient has phacolytic glaucoma due to leaking lens protein. The loss of cortex causes a shrunken anterior capsule.

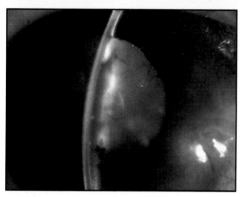

Figure 23-23. This traumatic, white cataract is swollen, with anterior displacement of the lens-iris diaphragm causing phacomorphic glaucoma.

intact lens capsule and is associated with a mature or hypermature cataract. There is an associated macrophage response (Figure 23-22).[11]

Phacomorphic glaucoma is angle-closure glaucoma due to lens intumescence. The swollen cataract causes pupillary block and moves the lens-iris diaphragm anteriorly to block the anterior chamber angle. Phacomorphic glaucoma is usually associated with a traumatic cataract (Figure 23-23).[12]

Phacoanaphylactic endophthalmitis is a rarely diagnosed inflammatory, intraocular condition due to sensitization to lens proteins causing an immune complex disease. Presentation is usually a chronic granulomatous uveitis 1 to 14 days after cataract extraction or trauma to the lens. There is trauma to the lens capsule, mutton-fat keratic precipitates, and synechia formation.[13]

Figure 23-24. This senile, hypermature cataract has calcium plaques and fibrotic folds in the anterior capsule.

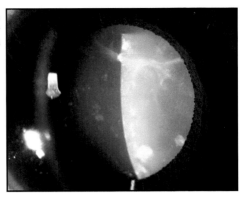

VIII. THE WHITE CATARACT IS A DIFFICULT OPERATION

First and foremost, decreased visualization due to the lack of a red reflex makes the removal of a white cataract challenging. Associated capsule and/or zonular compromise is not uncommon. Ocular and nonocular comorbidities such as previous intraocular surgery, trauma, intraocular inflammation, advanced age, etc add to the operation's complexity.[2,3]

The second major intraoperative issue is dealing with different mechanical forces. An intumescent cataract adds to the outward pull of the zonules, making the capsulorrhexis more difficult. There can be focal calcification, plaques, fibrosis, and decreased elasticity of the anterior capsule adding to the difficulty of performing the capsulorrhexis (Figure 23-24). Alteration of the operative technique is necessary to perform the cataract extraction.[2,3]

When removing the mature, white cataract, the surgeon must be prepared. Preparation is a 3-step planning process.

1. In your mind: This is the thought process to develop the operative plan.
2. In your hands: Make sure the special, key instruments are available.
3. In the eye: Make sure the operative technique is appropriate for the complexities of the mature, white cataract.

IX. PREOPERATIVE CONSIDERATIONS

To evaluate for intraocular pathology, all eyes with a mature cataract should have a preoperative ultrasound evaluation. This allows the surgeon to better inform the patient about visual prognosis and to discuss and plan additional operations as needed. Approximately 9% of eyes with advanced cataract will have posterior segment abnormalities that cause decreased postoperative

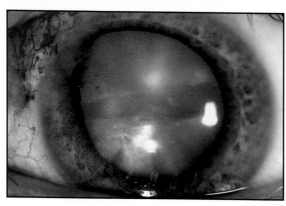

Figure 23-25. This traumatic cataract has zonular weakness in the location of the posterior synechiae.

visual acuity.[14] The most common finding is a retinal detachment, found in 5% of eyes with mature cataracts. Abnormal posterior segment abnormalities detected with ultrasonography tend to occur in patients with diabetes and patients less than 50 years. Ocular abnormalities that should raise suspicion of posterior segment pathology are posterior synechiae, iris colobomas, elevated intraocular pressure, and keratic precipitates.[14] Etiologies for poor postoperative visual acuity are glaucomatous cupping of the optic disc, vitritis, choroidal coloboma, posterior staphyloma, vitreous hemorrhage, and diabetic retinopathy.[14]

When examining a patient with a white, mature cataract, the history is especially important. Is there a history of trauma? If so, look for signs of trauma that could compromise the operation. These signs include iris sphincter tears, asymmetric anterior chamber depth, iridodonesis, phacodonesis, and anterior and posterior synechiae.

Always critically evaluate the status of the capsule and zonules. If there are signs of trauma, be prepared for a compromised capsule and/or zonules during the operation. After trauma, zonular weakness is likely in the location of the posterior synechiae (Figure 23-25). A hole in the capsule is likely after a perforating corneal injury. Similarly, the zonules and posterior capsule are frequently compromised after pars plana vitrectomy (see Figure 23-13).

If there is a history of intraocular inflammation, there may be associated systemic disease (see Figure 23-12). Consultation is necessary to determine the appropriate perioperative anti-inflammatory medical regimen. Iris dilation may be difficult (Figure 23-26).

White cataracts can have calcification and plaques on the anterior capsule. The hypermature, Morgagnian cataract can have fibrotic folds (see Figure 23-24). These findings will make an already difficult capsulorrhexis more difficult. The surgeon must be well versed in the capsulorrhexis tear-out rescue technique.[15]

Figure 23-26. There are extensive posterior synechiae associated with this white cataract due to intraocular inflammation.

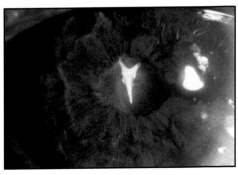

X. CALCULATION OF INTRAOCULAR LENS POWER

The IOLMaster (Carl Zeiss Meditec) is the most commonly used instrument for IOL calculations. However, in an eye with a mature cataract, IOL measurements with the IOLMaster are impossible to obtain. Using partial coherence interferometry, an infrared beam of light measures the distance from the corneal vertex to the retinal pigment epithelium. Obviously, if the cataract is opaque and dense, the beam is blocked, and the axial length cannot be measured. The IOLMaster also measures corneal curvature and anterior chamber depth by measuring the distance between reflected light images. A patient with a mature cataract has difficulty fixating, resulting in erroneous measurements of corneal curvature and anterior chamber depth.

Therefore, alternative techniques to perform biometry for calculation of IOL power must be used. Contact A-scan ultrasonography is perhaps the easiest technique that can be used to perform biometry. Ultrasound measures the axial length and anterior chamber depth. The main problem with contact A-scan ultrasound is avoiding indenting the cornea. Indentation of 0.5 mm will cause approximately a 1.5-D myopic error (too much plus) in the IOL calculation.

Keratometry performed with a manual keratometer can be difficult due to the difficulty controlling fixation in the eye with a mature cataract. The keratometric image is magnified so that only a 3-mm diameter area is viewed. A useful alternative is the handheld keratometer (Figure 23-27). The entire eye is seen through the viewing window, allowing the examiner to easily locate the infrared beam on the center of the cornea.

The gold standard for biometry to measure axial length and anterior chamber depth is immersion ultrasonography (Figure 23-28). Immersion ultrasonography eliminates the issues with the IOLMaster and contact A-scan ultrasonography. The measurements from the IOLMaster are internally adjusted to what the measurements would be if measured using immersion ultrasound. Immersion ultrasound measures from the corneal apex to

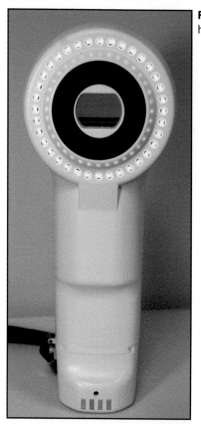

Figure 23-27. This is the NIDEK KM-500 handheld keratometer (NIDEK Co).

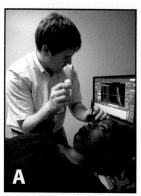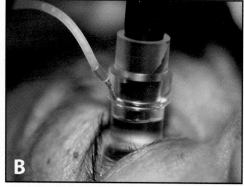

Figure 23-28. Immersion ultrasonography is performed to measure the anterior chamber depth and the axial length (A). The A-scan ultrasound probe is in the Kohn shell for immersion biometry (B).

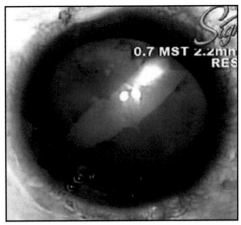

Figure 23-29. This is the Argentinian flag sign. The anterior capsule is stained with 0.06% trypan blue ophthalmic solution. There is a radial tear along the diameter of the anterior capsule.

the internal limiting membrane of the retina. Therefore, measurements from immersion ultrasound biometry and handheld keratometry can be entered into the IOLMaster for use in the desired IOL calculation formula.

XI. PLAN FOR THE OPERATION

The major issue when planning phacoemulsification of the mature cataract is lack of visualization of the anterior capsule making it difficult to perform a CCC. Therefore, most cataract surgeons would plan for the use of trypan blue 0.06% ophthalmic solution (an acid di-azo group dye) to stain the anterior capsule.

Trypan blue instantly stains the anterior capsule. Accepted technique is used at the beginning of the operation. Inject trypan blue through the side-port incision under balanced salt solution, ophthalmic viscosurgical device (OVD), or air. To improve visibility prior to initiation of the capsulorrhexis, irrigate trypan blue out of the anterior chamber. Importantly, trypan blue changes the characteristics of the anterior capsule affecting the creation of the capsulorrhexis. The use of trypan blue causes the capsule to be stiffer, less elastic, and more fragile.[16]

XII. SPECIFIC INSTRUMENTS AND INTRAOCULAR LENSES NEEDED FOR OPERATIVE TECHNIQUES

Are special instruments required for the capsulorrhexis? If the cataract is intumescent, there is an increased chance for radialization of the capsulorrhexis, resulting in the Argentinean flag sign (Figure 23-29).[17] To decrease the chance for radialization of the capsulorrhexis, a highly viscous OVD such as Healon 5 (Abbott Medical Optics) should be used to flatten

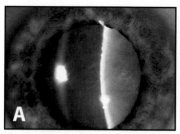 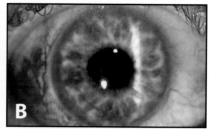

Figure 23-30. This is a mature cataract with an extremely dense, brown-black colored nucleus (A). This is the eye one day after a planned extracapsular cataract extraction (B).

the anterior capsule. If the Argentinean flag sign occurs, intraocular scissors can be used to restart the capsulorrhexis to obtain 2 smooth edges to the capsulorrhexis. In addition, the intraocular scissors can be used to restart the capsulorrhexis in the 2-stage capsulorrhexis technique.[18] Intraocular scissors may be necessary to cut through or around fibrotic folds or plaques in the anterior capsule.

Different choppers should be available. The appropriate nucleus dismantling technique used will depend on the density, thickness, hardness, and brittleness of the nucleus. For example, a longer horizontal chopper will be needed to place around a large nucleus of moderate density. A vertical chopper may be needed to chop a more dense nucleus.

If the nucleus is brown-black in color, phacoemulsification of this very hard nucleus may not be possible (Figure 23-30). Therefore, instruments for an extracapsular cataract extraction (ECCE) should be available. Conversion from a phacoemulsification to an ECCE will require sclerocorneal scissors. Planning an ECCE as the initial technique for removal of a very dense large nucleus requires blades and instruments for performing a sclerocorneal tunnel incision. Basic forceps and needle holder for suturing with 10-0 nylon are necessary.

Other situations regarding operative technique and instruments abound. If the cataract is due to trauma and is soft, there is likely an associated defect in the capsule and/or zonules. Intraocular scissors may be necessary for initiation of the capsulorrhexis. Have an endocapsular tension ring available and know to place the ring's opening 180 degrees from the area of zonular weakness. When aspirating a soft, traumatic cataract, a safer operative technique may be a bimanual approach separating the irrigation and aspiration to 2 instruments placed through two 1.2 mm × 1.4 mm trapezoidal incisions rather than a coaxial approach through a relatively larger incision. The bimanual approach allows the aspirating and irritating instruments to switch locations and easily access lens material. Especially when removing a traumatic cataract, have an anterior segment vitrectomy probe available. Use triamcinolone acetonide injectable suspension, 40 mg/mL, to identify vitreous in the anterior segment.

Availability of instruments to deal with iris abnormalities is a must, especially when mature cataracts are associated with either trauma or inflammation. Injection of an OVD posterior to the iris may be all that is needed to lyse posterior synechiae. Alternatively, a Barraquer sweep can be used to lyse anterior and/or posterior synechiae. If the pupil is small, use a pupil snapper to stretch the iris sphincter in all quadrants. If the pupil is still not large enough, iris hooks or an iris dilating ring should be used.

IOL calculations for placement of a 1-piece and a 3-piece posterior chamber IOL should be on hand. The IOLs selected should be for both placement in the ciliary sulcus and in the capsular bag. Zonular and/or capsular problems warrant consideration of a 3-piece IOL placed in the capsular bag or ciliary sulcus with proper adjustment of IOL power. In these situations, a 3-piece IOL should be more stable. When there is a zonular dehiscence, placement of a 3-piece IOL is in the bag, with the haptics in the meridian of dehiscence. This helps to support the area of zonular weakness. If there is a radial tear of the anterior capsule, place the haptics of the 3-piece IOL 90 degrees to the tear. A 3-piece IOL, not a 1-piece IOL, can always be placed in the ciliary sulcus, if there is enough anterior capsular support. Adjust IOL power for sulcus placement.[19]

XIII. PITFALLS OF THE WHITE CATARACT OPERATION

In summary, the most important pitfall of the mature, white cataract operation is performing the capsulorrhexis. There is no red reflex against which to view the edges of the capsulorrhexis. Creating the capsulorrhexis can be complicated by fibrotic folds, calcified plaques, leakage of white cortex, high intralenticular pressure, and undiagnosed capsule/zonular abnormalities. The second most important pitfall is the undiagnosed intraocular pathology which may cause a poor postoperative visual outcome and require medical and/or operative therapy.

ACKNOWLEDGMENTS

I gratefully acknowledge the expertise of the ophthalmic photographers, Sarah Moyer, CRA, OCT-C; Debra Cantrell, COA; and Rona Lyn Esquejo-Leon, CRA at the Kittner Eye Center.

KEY POINTS

1. Challenging operation
   a. No red reflex
   b. Different mechanical forces
   c. Physical changes in capsule make capsulorrhexis difficult
   d. Intumescent cataract
   e. Hypermature cataract
   f. Morgagnian cataract
   g. Hard, dense, large nucleus with little or no epinucleus and cortex to protect the posterior capsule
   h. Weak zonules and/or zonular dehiscence
2. Associated pathology
   a. Preoperative B-scan ultrasonography to evaluate for posterior segment pathology
   b. History and signs of trauma
   c. Systemic disease and/or intraocular inflammation
   d. Previous pars plana vitrectomy
3. Trypan blue
   a. Inject under air or viscoelastic
   b. Instantly stains anterior capsule
   c. Makes capsule more fragile
   d. Makes capsule less elastic
4. Plan
   a. In your mind: Thought process to develop the operative plan
      i.   Immersion ultrasonography for biometry
      ii. Fibrotic folds and calcium plaques in anterior capsule
      iii. Prevention of Argentine flag sign with intumescent cataract
      iv. Pupil abnormalities
      v.   Zonular weakness
      vi. Chopping technique
      vii. Medical consultation
      viii. Select OVDs
      ix. Vitrectomy
      x.   Fold or load into injector 3-piece IOL

(continued)

KEY POINTS (CONTINUED)

b. In your hands: Availability of special, key instruments and supplies
   i. Trypan blue
   ii. Specific chopper for chopping technique
   iii. Viscous OVD
   iv. Endocapsular tension ring
   v. Instruments to correct iris and pupil abnormalities
   vi. Iris retractors
   vii. Iris dilating ring
   viii. Capsule support system
   ix. Bimanual instruments for cortex removal
   x. 1-piece IOL and 3-piece IOL
   xi. Contingency instruments for conversion to extracapsular cataract extraction
   xii. Vitrectomy probe
   xiii. Triamcinolone acetonide suspension injectable 40mg/mL

c. In the eye: Operative technique appropriate for the complexities with the mature, white cataract
   i. Be prepared for the unexpected
   ii. Capsulorrhexis gone awry
   iii. Conversion to extracapsular cataract extraction
   iv. Vitrectomy
   v. Placement of 3-piece IOL with posterior capsule and/or zonular abnormalities

REFERENCES

1. Shahit E, Sheikh A, Fasih U. Complications of hypermature cataract and its visual outcome. *Pak J Ophthalmol.* 2011;27:58-62.
2. Ermis SS, Ozturk F, Inan UU. Comparing the efficiency and safety of phacoemulsification in white mature and other types of senile cataracts. *Br J Ophthalmol.* 2003;87:1356-1359.
3. Vasavada A, Singh R, Desai J. Phacoemulsification of white mature cataracts. *J Cataract Refract Surg.* 1998;24:270-277.
4. Yanoof M, Sassani JW. *Lens in Ocular Pathology.* 6th ed. Philadelphia: Mosby Elsevier; 2009:361-392.
5. Spencer TS, Mamilis N. The pathology of cataracts. In: *Cataract Surgery.* Steiner RR, ed. Philadelphia: Saunders Elsevier; 2012:3-10.
6. Duke-Elder S. Diseases of the lens and vitreous, glaucoma and hypotony. In: *System of Ophthalmology.* Vol XI. St. Louis: C. V. Mosby; 1969:145-146, 160-163.

7. Salem MA, Ismail L. Factors influencing visual outcome after cataract extraction among Arabs in Kuwait. *Br J Ophthalmol.* 1987;71:458-461.
8. Ilavska M, Kardos L. Phacoemulsification of mature and hard nuclear cataracts. *Bratigl Lek Listy.* 2010;111:93-96.
9. Lam BL, Thompson HS. A unilateral cataract produces a relative afferent pupillary defect in the contralateral eye. *Ophthalmology.* 1990;97:334-338.
10. Miki A, Tijima A, Takagi M, Usui T, et al. Pupillography of relative afferent pupillary defect of contralateral to monocular mature cataract. *Can J Ophthalmol.* 2006;41:469-471.
11. Richter C. Lens-induced open angle glaucoma: phacolytic glaucoma (lens protein glaucoma). In: Ritch R, Shields MB, Kiupin T, eds. *The Glaucomas.* 2nd ed. St. Louis: Mosby;1996:1023-1026.
12. McKibbin M, Gupta A, Atkins AD. Cataract extraction and intraocular lens implantation in eye with phacomorphic or phacolytic glaucoma. *J Cataract Refract Surg.* 1996;22:633-636.
13. Marak GE. Phacoanaphylactic endophthalmitis. *Surv Ophthalmol.* 36;1992:325-339.
14. Salman A, Parmar P, Vanila CG, Thomas PA, Nelson JC, Sudasan A. Is ultrasonography essential before surgery in eyes with advanced cataracts? *J Postgrad Med.* 2006;52:19-22.
15. Little BC, Smith JH, Packer M. Littlecapsulorhexis tear-out rescue. *J Cataract Refract Surg.* 2006;32:1420-1422.
16. Wollensak G, Sporl E, Pham D-T, Biomechanical changes in the anterior lens capsule after trypan blue staining. *J Cataract Refract Surg.* 2004;30:1526-1530.
17. Mehndra M. Phacoemulsification in intumescent mature cataract: Managing a run-out capsulorhexis. Symposium on Cataract, IOL and Refractive Surgery, Boston MA, April 9-14, 2010. http://ascrs2010.abstractsnet.com/handouts/000105_PHACOEMULSIFICA-TION_IN_INTUMESCENT_MATURE_CATARACT.ppt, Retrieved May 17, 2013.
18. Figueiredo CG, Figueiredo J. Figueiredo GB. Brazilian technique for prevention of the Argentinean flag sign in white cataract. *J Cataract Refract Surg.* 2012;38:1531-1536.
19. Hill W. Doctor-hill.com IOL power calculations bag vs. sulcus IOL power. http://doctor-hill.com/iol-main/bag-sulcus.htm Published December 27, 2012. Retrieved May 17, 2013.

24

ZONULAR INSTABILITY AND ENDOCAPSULAR TENSION RINGS

John C. Hart, Jr, MD, FACS

I. INTRODUCTION

Cataract surgery in the presence of poor lens support is one of the most challenging situations faced by the cataract surgeon. Failure to recognize and appropriately compensate for poor lens support can result in vision-threatening complications. Endocapsular tension rings (ECTRs) are devices that help compensate for poor lens support and thereby decrease the risk of both intraoperative and postoperative complications. ECTRs were first described by Hara et al in 1991.[1]

II. ANATOMY

The lens is supported equatorially by zonular fibers that originate from basal laminae of the nonpigmented epithelium of the pars plana and pars plicata of the ciliary body.

- Zonular fibers insert on the lens capsule at the equator, 1.5 mm onto the anterior lens capsule and 1.25 mm onto the posterior lens capsule.
- The equatorial fibers regress with age, leaving anterior and posterior zonular insertions.
- The lens is supported posteriorly by the vitreous.[2]

III. HISTORY

In all cataract cases, a history of trauma should be sought. The trauma may have been recent or remote in time and could be blunt or sharp in nature. In any case where there is ectopia lentis with no history of trauma, a systemic disorder such as Marfan syndrome, homocystinuria, or Weill-Marchesani syndrome should be ruled out.[3]

Henderson BA. *Essentials of Cataract Surgery, Second Edition (pp 271-280).*
© 2014 Taylor & Francis Group.

IV. EXAMINATION

Preoperative examination of the patient with suspected zonular weakness or loss requires techniques that accentuate the mismatch between eye movement and movement of the lens and iris.

- Preoperative signs of zonular weakness are most commonly visible at the slit lamp and may include pseudoexfoliation syndrome, iridodonesis, phacodonesis, subluxation of the crystalline lens, vitreous prolapse into the anterior chamber, or an overt zonular dialysis.

- Phacodonesis is best seen through a maximally dilated pupil. The larger the pupil the better; therefore, use cyclopentolate 1% in addition to standard dilating drops and allow more time for the eye to dilate.

- To most easily visualize phacodonesis, use low magnification and focus on the anterior capsule. Ask the patient to look left or right and then back directly toward the light. Do not move the slit beam when the eye moves. Watch for movement of the lens when the eye moves back to the primary position.

- To best visualize a zonular dialysis, have the patient look in the direction of the suspected dialysis. Rotate the microscope away from the dialysis, allowing an oblique view of the suspicious area. This will overcome some of the total internal reflection of the cornea and allow a more peripheral view of the lens. This works best for nasal or temporal zonular dialyses because the patient is positioned upright in the slit lamp.

- Any patient with suspected zonular weakness should be examined in the supine position with an indirect ophthalmoscope (without an additional condensing lens). This position allows gravity to pull the lens posteriorly and will frequently uncover an otherwise occult zonular dialysis. Instruct the patient to look in the cardinal positions while the examiner observes the lens obliquely.

- Iridodonesis, or iris movement, will frequently be focal and located over the area of zonular weakness or loss. The iris appears to billow like a sheet in the wind. This finding is best seen at the pupil margin just after the patient blinks.

- The iridolenticular gap sign, first described by Robert Osher, MD, is an increased space between the pupil margin and the anterior lens capsule. This sign indicates a partial subluxation of the crystalline lens.[4]

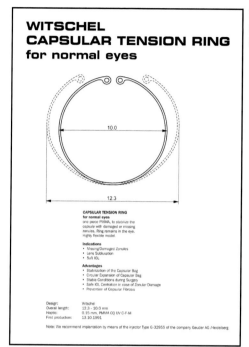

WITSCHEL CAPSULAR TENSION RING for normal eyes

Figure 24-1. Standard ECTR. (Reprinted with permission of FCI Ophthalmics.)

V. ENDOCAPSULAR TENSION RING DESIGNS AND BENEFITS

A. Standard Endocapsular Tension Ring

A standard ECTR is an open loop polymethylmethacrylate (PMMA) ring with eyelets on each end (Figure 24-1).[5] Standard ECTRs are available from several companies and come in various sizes. The majority of cases do well with an 11 mm ECTR (compressed diameter) because the capsular bag diameter is typically just larger than 10 mm. A slight overlap of the ends of the ECTR within the capsule has no ill effect. When positioned within the capsule, the ECTR expands, placing the capsule on stretch. Outward pressure exerted by the ECTR on the capsular bag distributes support from areas with normal zonules to areas of zonular weakness or loss. This redistribution of support also corrects decentration of the capsular bag. Improved support for the capsular bag and zonules decreases the risk of iatrogenic worsening of the zonular damage during surgery and allows stable in-the-bag intraocular lens fixation. Expansion and centration of the capsular bag helps to maintain

Figure 24-2. Cionni ECTR for 2-point fixation. (Reprinted with permission of FCI Ophthalmics.)

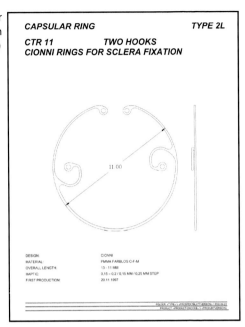

separation between the anterior chamber and vitreous cavity. Separation of these chambers helps tamponade vitreous from entering the anterior chamber and decreases the risk for loss of nuclear fragments into the vitreous; therefore, the risk of both intra- and postoperative retinal complications is decreased.[6] The capsulorrhexis and posterior capsule must be intact to ensure safe implantation of an ECTR.

B. Cionni Modified Endocapsular Tension Rings

Designed by Robert Cionni, MD, Cionni modified ECTRs (Morcher Ghmb) are modifications of a standard ECTR that feature one or two fixation eyelets that extend in a plane anterior to the main ECTR (Figure 24-2). The fixation eyelets are positioned anterior to the capsulorrhexis for suture fixation to the sclera. A 9-0 Prolene (Ethicon) suture is used in a double-armed fashion to provide transscleral support to the center of the zonular dialysis. The knot is typically covered by a scleral flap. There are 2 single fixation element Cionni ECTRs available, one for manual insertion and one for insertion with an injector. There is also a Cionni ECTR with 2 fixation elements. Cionni ECTRs are indicated for profound zonular damage (> 4 clock hours) with or without progressive zonulopathy (eg, pseudoexfoliation syndrome, Marfan syndrome).[7]

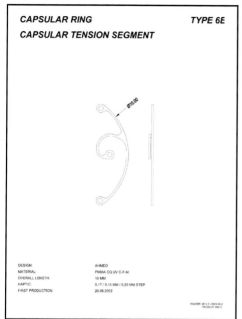

CAPSULAR RING   TYPE 6E

CAPSULAR TENSION SEGMENT

Ø10.00

DESIGN: AHMED
MATERIAL: PMMA CQ UV C-F-M
OVERALL LENGTH: 10 MM
HAPTIC: 0.17 / 0.15 MM / 0.25 MM STEP
FIRST PRODUCTION: 20.06.2002

FOLDER: 6E V 3 / 2003-04-2
PRODUCT: 6NE V

Figure 24-3. Ahmed endo-capsular tension segment. (Reprinted with permission of FCI Ophthalmics.)

C. Henderson Modified Endocapsular Tension Ring

Designed by Bonnie An Henderson, MD, the Henderson ECTR (Morcher Gmbh) is a modification of a standard ECTR that features 8 equally spaced indentations of 0.15 mm. The indentations are intended to ease the removal of cortical material trapped between the ECTR and the capsule while maintaining expansion of the capsular bag (cortex trapped between a standard ECTR and the capsule can be extremely difficult to remove safely without further zonular damage). Like a standard ECTR, the Henderson ECTR should be used in cases with less than 4 clock hours of zonular loss in the setting of an intact capsulorrhexis and posterior capsule.

D. Ahmed Capsular Tension Segment

Designed by Iqbal (Ike) Ahmed, MD, the Ahmed ECTR segment (Morcher Ghmb) (Figure 24-3) is a modification of a Cionni ECTR. Like a Cionni ECTR, the Ahmed capsular tension segment (CTS) has a suture fixation eyelet for scleral fixation but instead of a complete ECTR, the portion of the device that is inserted within the capsule is a 10 mm segment of an ECTR.[8] This device does not require an intact capsulorrhexis or posterior capsule because it does not expand within the capsular bag. Multiple Ahmed ECTR segments may be used as necessary. Unlike a standard ECTR, the Ahmed CTS can be implanted without dialing the device into the capsule, thereby minimizing the risk of trauma to the remaining zonules.[9]

E. Coloboma Shield

Designed by Dr. Rasch (Morcher types L and G, Morcher Gmbh) this is a tinted ECTR with an integrated 60- or 90-degree shield. The Coloboma Shield can be used in the setting of iris and zonular coloboma or after trauma with zonular and iris damage. By filling the iris defect, the integral opaque shield protects against intraocular lens (IOL) edge glare and/or monocular diplopia from polycoria. This device is not currently FDA approved but permission for use can be obtained from the FDA on a compassionate use basis.

VI. INDICATIONS FOR ENDOCAPSULAR TENSION RINGS

Standard or Henderson ECTRs are indicated in the setting of mild-to-moderate zonular weakness or a zonular dialysis of 4 clock hours or less. Cionni modified ECTRs are indicated for zonular dialyses of 4 or more clock hours in size or in the setting of progressive zonulopathy.[10]

It is important to understand that some causes of zonulopathy are progressive and will tend to affect all zonules. Other causes of zonulopathy are stationary and tend to spare some zonules. Zonulopathy caused by systemic disease is commonly progressive, while zonulopathy caused by trauma is typically stationary. Zonules that remain after trauma are typically normal as long as there is no further damage to the eye.[11]

A. Pseudoexfoliation Syndrome

Pseudoexfoliation syndrome is one of the most common indications for standard ECTRs. In this syndrome, there is a spectrum of zonular damage that will dictate which ECTR is most appropriate. A standard or Henderson ECTR may be used unless there is severe phacodonesis or overt zonular dialysis greater than 4 clock hours, in which case a Cionni ECTR with transscleral fixation is more appropriate to ensure long-term capsular support. Numerous cases of late onset subluxation of an IOL fixated within the capsular bag, with or without an ECTR, have been reported in patients with pseudoexfoliation syndrome. Close long-term follow-up is indicated in this subset of patients with progressive zonulopathy.[12]

B. Trauma

If the patient has a traumatic cataract or a history of previous ocular trauma, an ECTR should be available during cataract surgery. Iatrogenic zonular damage should always be suspected in patients with a past ocular history of vitrectomy, trabeculectomy, ruptured globe repair, or radial keratotomy. With these surgeries, there can be a prolonged period of hypotony in the early post-operative period that can damage the zonular complex.[13]

C. Intraoperative Zonulopathy

Intraoperative zonulopathy is zonular damage seen or caused during cataract surgery. Segmental loss of both the anterior and posterior zonules results in a zonular dialysis. The zonules on either side of a zonular dialysis are especially susceptible to breakage from further trauma. Prompt recognition of intraoperative zonulopathy is critical because delay in diagnosis typically results in worsening of the zonular damage. A number of signs reflect the spectrum of possible zonular injuries.

- The earliest sign is a focally bright red reflex seen at the edge of the dilated pupil. This sign is due to a focal area of stretched zonules with minimal subluxation of the lens away from the area of zonular damage.

- Radiating folds in the anterior capsule and difficulty puncturing the anterior capsule during capsulorrhexis indicate zonular laxity and weakness.

- Phacodonesis is due to diffuse damage to all zonules and is usually associated with systemic disease (eg, pseudoexfoliation syndrome or Marfan syndrome). Phacodonesis may not be evident on preoperative examination; however, the forces placed on the lens and zonules during surgery are far greater than those generated during normal eye movements. Standard or Henderson ECTRs may not be sufficient for long-term support of the IOL in patients with preoperative phacodonesis due to systemic disease. A suture-fixated Cionni ECTR would provide better long-term IOL support.[10]

- Capsular fold sign represents a partial zonular dialysis. Ordinarily, the lens capsule is supported internally by the lens. If there is segmental loss of the posterior zonules, the posterior capsule will billow focally and be thrown into folds after lens removal.

D. High Myopia

High myopia (axial length >26 mm) is a relative indication for standard or Henderson ECTRs because these patients frequently have lax zonules and floppy lens capsules. ECTRs aid in this setting primarily by stretching the capsule to decrease the risk of inadvertent aspiration.[13]

VII. CONTRAINDICATIONS FOR ENDOCAPSULAR TENSION RINGS

- A continuous curvilinear capsulorrhexis and intact posterior capsule are necessary for implantation of an ECTR. If there is a defect in either the anterior rhexis or posterior capsule, then insertion of the ring could extend the defect when the ECTR expands within the capsular bag. This may worsen the capsular defect and possibly result in loss of the ECTR into the vitreous. An Ahmed capsular ring segment would be more appropriate in either of these settings.[9]
- If the zonular dialysis is greater than 4 clock hours, a standard or Henderson ECTR is contraindicated. A Cionni ECTR or Ahmed CTS would be more appropriate.

VIII. TIMING OF ENDOCAPSULAR TENSION RINGS IMPLANTATION: TWO LINES OF THOUGHT

Many surgeons implant the ECTR immediately after hydrodissection to take advantage of the extracapsular support provided during phacoemulsification of the lens. Others routinely implant the ECTR only after removal of the lens. These surgeons stabilize the lens capsule prior to phacoemulsification with disposable iris or capsule retractors affixed to the capsulorrhexis. This method allows easier cortical cleanup, since cortex is not trapped by the ring and may be less traumatic to the zonules.[14]

IX. ENDOCAPSULAR TENSION RINGS INSERTION PEARLS

- Allow sufficient surgical time for cases with weak zonules because these cases typically are more complex than standard cataract surgery.
- Stabilize the anterior chamber with a dispersive ophthalmic viscosurgical device (OVD) prior to capsulorrhexis. A dispersive OVD tamponades vitreous if there is a zonular dialysis and tends to remain in the anterior chamber better than a cohesive OVD. Often, iris or pupillary abnormalities prevent a thorough preoperative evaluation of zonular injury. In these cases, after the anterior chamber is stabilized with a dispersive OVD, the iris can be retracted with a Kuglen hook and the zonules can be directly visualized. The operative plan may then be altered if necessary.
- Beware of vitreous! Vitreous in the anterior chamber must be removed prior to insertion of the ECTR.

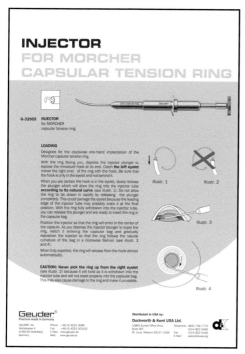

Figure 24-4. Instructions for use of Geuder ECTR injector. (Reprinted with permission of FCI Ophthalmics.)

- Begin the capsulorrhexis 180 degrees away from the center of the zonular dialysis. The capsulorrhexis should be initiated with a sharp instrument. In patients with severe zonular instability, iris retractors or a second instrument may be necessary for counter tension during capsulorrhexis. The capsulorrhexis should be large enough to prolapse the lens into the anterior chamber, if possible.

- Hydrodissection should completely separate the cortex from the capsule so that the lens can spin freely in the capsular bag.

- Inject a cohesive OVD beneath the rhexis to create space.

- Most surgeons find using an inserter significantly easier than using a manual technique. Inserters may be disposable or reusable. The most commonly used inserter is made by Geuder. Carefully follow the directions for use of the ECTR inserter (Figure 24-4).

- Prior to inserting the ECTR, sharply focus the microscope on the capsulorrhexis edge. This allows for clear visualization of the ring as it is positioned within the capsular bag.

- Phacoemulsification should be performed under low flow settings with the irrigation bottle height significantly lowered to decrease the risk of vitreous prolapse into the anterior chamber.

KEY POINTS

1. If a patient has a history suggestive of previous ocular trauma, a physical finding of zonular instability, or a history of a systemic disease that could impair the zonules, be prepared to alter your surgical technique to compensate for zonular weakness.

2. Allow sufficient surgical time for cases with zonular weakness. These cases typically take significantly more operating room time than a typical case. Allot the time these cases deserve.

3. Maintain positive pressure in the anterior chamber with a dispersive OVD. Never allow collapse of the anterior chamber in a patient with weak zonules because this will stress the zonules and increase the risk of vitreous prolapse into the anterior chamber.

4. Do not use an ECTR if there is a tear in the capsulorrhexis or posterior capsule.

5. Choose the appropriate ECTR for the patient. Standard or Henderson ECTRs are indicated for zonular dialyses of 4 clock hours or less. For dialyses 4 clock hours or larger, a Cionni ECTR or an Ahmed CTS with scleral fixation is appropriate.

REFERENCES

1. Hara T, Hara T, Yamada Y. "Equator ring" for maintenance of the completely circular contour of the capsular bag equator after cataract removal. *Ophthal Surg.* 1991;22:358-359.

2. Rosenfeld SI, Blecher MH, Bobrow JC, et al. *2005-2006 Basic and Clinical Science Course (BCSC) Section 11: Lens and Cataract.* San Francisco, CA: American Academy of Ophthalmology; 2006.

3. Chang DF. IOL selection for the weakened capsular bag. *Cataract Refract Surg Today.* 2004;May:52-54.

4. Osher RH. The CTR's US debut. *Cataract Refract Surg Today.* 2004;January:27-28.

5. Menapace R, Findl O, Georgopoulos M, et al. The capsular tension ring: designs, applications and techniques. *J Cataract Refract Surg.* 2000;26:898-912.

6. Gimbel HV, Sun R. Clinical applications of capsular tension rings in cataract surgery. *Ophthalmic Surg Lasers.* 2002;333:44-53.

7. Cionni RJ, Osher RH. Management of profound zonular dialysis or weakness with a new endocapsular ring designed for scleral fixation. *J Cataract Refract Surg.* 1998;24:1299-1306.

8. Ahmed IK, Kranemann C. Morcher CTR segment. *Video J Cataract Refractive Surg.* 2003;14(2).

9. Ahmed IK. Rings versus segments. *Cataract Refract Surg Today.* 2004;January:42-45.

10. Cionni RJ, Osher RH, Marques DM, et al. Modified capsular tension ring for patients with congenital loss of zonular support. *J Cataract Refract Surg.* 2003;29:1668-1673.

11. Cionni RJ, Osher RH. Endocapsular ring approach to the subluxed cataractous lens. *J Cataract Refract Surg.* 1995;21:3:245-249.

12. Crandall A. Late bag dislocation in pseudoexfoliation. Paper presented at *American Academy of Ophthalmology Annual Meeting,* October 21, 2002; Orlando, FL.

13. Fine IH, Hoffman RS. Phacoemulsification in the presence of pseudoexfoliation: challenges and options. *J Cataract Refract Surg.* 1997;23:160-165.

14. Ahmed IK, Cionni RJ, Kranemann C, Crandall AS. Optimal timing of capsular tension ring implantation: Miyake-Apple video analysis. *J Cataract Refract Surg.* 2005;31:1809-1813.

25

CAPSULAR COMPLICATIONS AND MANAGEMENT

Evan Waxman, MD, PhD

I. INTRODUCTION

Rupture of the posterior capsule with or without vitreous prolapse is the most common intraoperative complication of cataract surgery. Estimates of its occurrence range from 1% to 3%. Studies show that the occurrence is higher for beginning surgeons but that it remains a significant risk even for experienced surgeons. It is important for every cataract surgeon to be familiar with the techniques needed to manage this complication.

II. WHY YOU SHOULD NOT BREAK THE POSTERIOR CAPSULE

Rupture of the posterior capsule with or without vitreous loss results in an increased incidence of secondary intraoperative and postoperative complications that can result in poor visual outcomes. These complications include the following:

- Cystoid macular edema
- Retinal tears and detachment
- Glaucoma
- Corneal decompensation
- Endophthalmitis
- Retained lens material
- Prolonged postoperative inflammation
- Prolonged case time and patient discomfort

Henderson BA. *Essentials of Cataract Surgery, Second Edition (pp 281-291).*
© 2014 Taylor & Francis Group.

Figure 25-1. (A) Anterior capsule. (B) Anterior capsular notch.

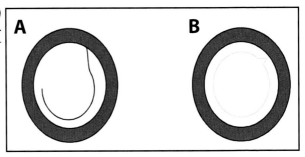

Figure 25-2. Rupture with hydrodissection.

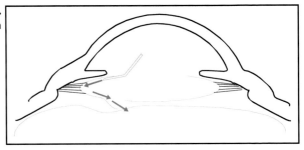

III. WAYS TO BREAK THE CAPSULE: THINGS NOT TO DO

Capsular complications can be initiated during many stages of cataract surgery.

A. Incision Construction

While it is unlikely that posterior capsular rupture would occur during incision creation, any technique that results in leakage around the incision during subsequent steps results in an unstable eye in which the posterior capsule is more likely to be damaged.

B. Capsulorrhexis

Losing the capsulorrhexis peripherally or creation of a V-shaped notch in the capsular rim can cause the capsular tear to extend to the posterior capsule (Figure 25-1).

C. Hydrodissection

Overvigorous hydrodissection especially in the presence of an anterior chamber filled with hyperviscous viscoelastic can create sufficient pressure to rupture the posterior capsule (Figure 25-2).

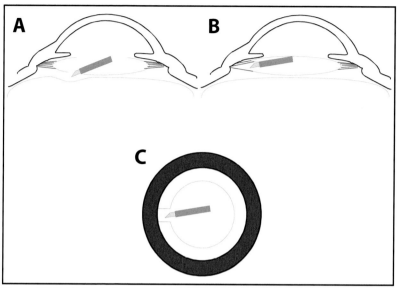

Figure 25-3. (A) Sculpting too deep. (B) Sculpting too peripherally. (C) Sculpting the anterior capsule.

D. Nuclear Sculpting

It is possible to use the phacoemulsification hand piece to sculpt too deeply and directly break the capsule with the phaco tip. More commonly, the capsule is broken when sculpting too peripherally especially when the surgeon is using the iris as a landmark in a case with a widely dilated pupil (Figure 25-3).

E. Turning, Chopping, and Cracking

Placing a second instrument through the anterior capsular rim, through the posterior capsule, or peripherally around the outside of the lens can result in capsular tears or zonular dehiscence (Figure 25-4).

F. Nuclear Fragment Removal

Capsular rupture during this stage can result from failure to keep the posterior capsule back with a second instrument or continued aspiration after the phaco tip has fully penetrated a nuclear fragment. A complication becomes more likely in the setting of anterior chamber instability caused by a poorly constructed incision or incisional stress due to "heavy hands."

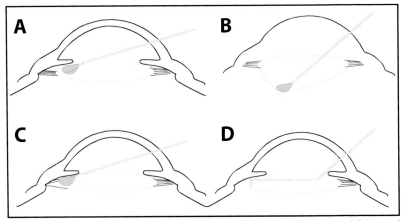

Figure 25-4. (A) Second instrument through the anterior capsular rim. (B) Second instrument through the posterior capsule. (C) Second instrument too peripheral. (D) Chopping around the equator.

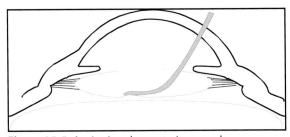

Figure 25-5. Aspirating the posterior capsule.

G. Cortical Removal

It is possible to aspirate and tear the capsule during cortical removal. The maneuvers necessary to remove subincisional cortex can make this a particularly difficult step (Figure 25-5).

IV. SIGNS THAT YOU HAVE BROKEN THE CAPSULE

There are a number of intraoperative signs that can lead the surgeon to suspect that the posterior capsular has been broken. Early recognition of capsular rupture is important for minimizing the risk of secondary complications. Unfortunately, the following early signs are often missed:

- Deepening of the anterior chamber: There is, at the time when the capsule is broken, a sudden change in the eye as pressures between chambers equalize. This can result in a sudden and sometimes transient deepening of the anterior chamber and an increase in pupil size.

- Movement of the lens away from the phaco tip and loss of followability: The coaxial irrigation of the phaco tip can push the nuclear pieces backward because there is now no barrier to posterior movement. In addition, the pieces may be knotted up in vitreous and not easily aspiratable.
- Vitreous in the phaco or aspiration tip: In many cases, the first sign the cataract surgeon has of vitreous prolapse is the presence of strands of material in the phaco or aspiration tip that do not behave the way nucleus or cortex would.
- The sudden appearance of an area at the level of the posterior capsule that is "too clear."
- The absence of lens material that has not yet been removed.

V. WHAT TO DO WHEN YOU SUSPECT YOU HAVE BROKEN THE CAPSULE

There are a number of steps that should be taken when the surgeon first suspects a capsular rupture.

A. Stop Phacoemulsification and Aspiration

Continued phacoemulsification and aspiration can enlarge a capsular tear, push lens material into the vitreous, and result in the aspiration of vitreous and retinal traction. It is important to resist the impulse to immediately remove all the instruments from the eye. Removal of the phacoemulsification hand piece before stabilizing the anterior chamber can increase the size of a capsular tear and create a vacuum that pulls the vitreous forward. Initially, irrigation should be continued to maintain a stable eye.

B. Inject Viscoelastic

Injecting a viscoelastic, ideally a dispersive viscoelastic, into the anterior chamber and over the area of suspected capsular break could stabilize the eye to allow more safe removal of the instruments and further assessment.

C. Stop Irrigation

Once viscoelastic has been injected, the surgeon can stop irrigation.

D. Inspect and Assess

Once the eye has been stabilized, the surgeon can further assess for the presence of a capsular complication. At this point, simple observation is often enough to determine the state of the capsule. In some cases, it will be useful to use a second instrument or viscoelastic to retract the iris or touch the lens

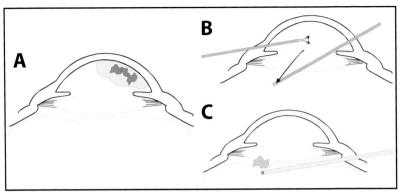

Figure 25-6. (A) Trapping fragments with viscoelastic. (B, C) Pars plana lift from below.

capsule. A dry Weck cell placed at an incision site can be used to assess for the presence of vitreous at the incision.

VI. WHAT TO DO WHEN THE CAPSULE IS BROKEN

The surgical goals in the presence of a capsular complication are as follows:
- Removal of the remaining lens material
- Removal of all vitreous from the anterior chamber while preserving the remaining capsule for a lens implant
- Minimizing trauma to the retina

A. Removing the Remainder of the Nucleus

Nuclear pieces may be lifted using viscoelastic or a second instrument. Pieces should be trapped once in the anterior chamber with viscoelastic. These maneuvers may be accomplished through a limbal side port. In some cases, it may be easier to approach pieces through a pars plana incision. The technique chosen for the removal of the trapped pieces will depend on the size, number, and location of the nuclear pieces; the presence of vitreous; the size of the capsular tear; and personal preference. Possible techniques are shown in Figure 25-6 and are described as follows.

1. Expression of remaining pieces

For this technique, the incision must be enlarged to allow for the expression of the largest remaining piece. An irrigating vectis attached to a viscoelastic syringe is placed under the piece. Injecting viscoelastic as the vectis applies pressure on the posterior lip of the incision expresses the nuclear piece.

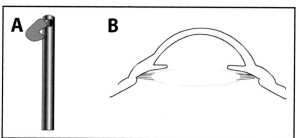

Figure 25-7. (A) Removing nuclear fragment with the vitrector. (B) Do not chase a lost fragment.

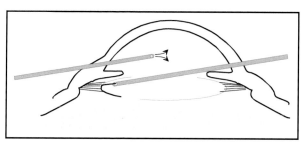

Figure 25-8. Bimanual I/A with vitrector.

2. Continued phacoemulsification

Medium-sized fragments trapped in viscoelastic may be emulsified with the phacoemulsification hand piece. Reasonable fluidic settings are aspiration 20 mL/min, vacuum 100 mm Hg, and bottle height set just high enough to keep the anterior chamber pressurized. Twenty centimeters above eye height is a good starting point. It is important to use additional viscoelastic as necessary and to avoid aspirating vitreous.

3. Nuclear fragment removal with the vitrector

Small- to medium-sized pieces can be cut and aspirated by the vitrectomy unit (Figure 25-7). A bimanual technique is used. The machine is set to "irrigation/aspiration (I/A) cut" mode so that pieces enter the tip prior to cutting. The cut rate is slowed to 300 cuts/second to allow molding of the fragment into the tip. Aspiration, vacuum, and bottle height should be set as above.

Regardless of which technique is used, it is important to avoid chasing a fragment into the vitreous cavity. It is safer to abandon a piece to be recovered later via a pars plana vitrectomy than to proceed and possibly create a retinal tear.

B. Removing the Remainder of the Cortex

Cortex can be removed using the vitrector as a bimanual I/A device (Figure 25-8). Two side-port paracenteses are used. A handheld irrigation cannula can be placed through one side port. The vitrector is placed through the other. The machine is set to "I/A/cut" or "I/A" to avoid damaging the remaining capsule.

Cortex can be stripped off the capsule in the usual way except that it should be pulled toward the capsular tear to avoid extending it. For this same reason, the cortex at the site of the capsular tear should be removed last. As cortex is removed, it is necessary to watch for vitreous prolapse and proceed with vitrectomy and injection of additional viscoelastic as needed.

While it would be ideal to remove the entire cortex, it is sometimes better to leave a small amount behind rather than risk retinal complications or further compromise the capsule.

C. Removing Vitreous From the Anterior Chamber

The goal of the limited anterior vitrectomy required for managing vitreous prolapse during complicated cataract surgery is the removal of vitreous from the anterior chamber. While some vitreous is removed from the eye, it is desirable to remove as little as is necessary to clear the anterior chamber. The coaxial vitrector is a poor tool for this goal. Irrigation from a coaxial vitrector irrigates fluid into the vitreous at the same location that vitreous is being cut and aspirated. This creates unwanted turbulence and creates fluid pockets. The hydrodisplaced vitreous is forced up into the anterior segment, worsening the vitreous prolapse. It is therefore strongly recommended that the entire vitrectomy be performed using a bimanual technique. The irrigation line should be held in the anterior chamber through a limbal side port away from the capsular tear and the vitreous. The vitrector can be placed through another side port in a position at which it can cut and aspirate vitreous while pulling it down into the vitreous cavity. The larger main incision should not be used. Leakage around the vitrector encourages vitreous flow toward the incision.

The vitrector should be set in the I/A cut mode in which cutting starts before aspiration. It is important to remember that this also means that vitreous will not be removed until the foot pedal is depressed into position 3. Reasonable settings include bottle height at about 20 cm above the eye and adjusted to the height needed to keep the eye stable, aspiration rate of 18 cc/min, and vacuum at 100 mm Hg. The cut rate should be set to the maximum the machine is capable of to minimize vitreous traction.

Other important points regarding vitrectomy for capsular complications are as follows:

- Complete removal of vitreous from the eye is unnecessary and can cause the eye to collapse and "square off" at the site of rectus muscle insertion. This makes subsequent steps more difficult.
- The tip of the vitrector should remain visible at all times during the procedure. A vitrector hidden by the iris can quickly cause damage to the iris, ciliary body, or retina.

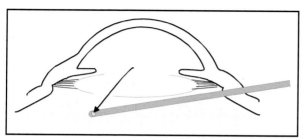

Figure   25-9. Pars plana vitreous removal from below.

- Vitreous cleanup can be facilitated by labeling strands with 4 mg/mL Kenalog (Bristol-Myers Squibb), using a technique described by Burk et al in 2003.[1]

Using the vitrector through the limbal side port is an ungainly way of pulling vitreous into the vitreous cavity. The angle of approach is awkward and any leakage around the side-port incision will cause vitreous to flow toward and into the incision. If the vitrector is instead placed through a pars plana incision, it is in a more natural position to pull vitreous back. Furthermore, an instrument in this position is in a natural place to float or push lens fragments up. Pars plana management of vitreous loss begins with a small peritomy.

An incision is created 3.5 mm back from the limbus with an microvitreoretinal (MVR) blade. A Viscoat cannula (Alcon, Inc) can be used to push or float pieces up. The same vitrector that would be used through the limbal side port can now be inserted through the pars plana incision. The incision is sutured closed when the vitrectomy is complete. While straightforward in theory, this technique can put the anterior segment surgeon in unfamiliar territory. In addition, just as in a planned pars plana vitrectomy, there is a real risk of creating a retinal tear. As a result, some surgeons have suggested that a cataract surgeon should not perform a pars plana cleanup unless he or she is also skilled at detecting and treating retinal tears (Figure 25-9).

D. Placing an Implant

A complete discussion of implant choice and techniques for implant placement are outside the scope of this chapter. Briefly, the surgeon will choose among a capsule-supported sulcus intraocular lens (IOL), an anterior chamber IOL, and an iris- or scleral-sutured sulcus IOL. The choice will be made based on the amount of capsular support as well as surgeon experience and personal preference.

E. Completing the Case

Once the implant is placed, a few steps remain. The main incision should be sutured closed. This will create a more stable eye for the remaining steps. A miotic agent can be instilled to constrict the pupil. This helps to keep vitreous back and can make any vitreous strands more visible by peaking the pupil. Additional Kenalog can be used to identify any errant strands of vitreous. Vitreous strands may be swept out of incisions using an iris sweep or a viscoelastic cannula through a side port. The final vitrectomy and removal of viscoelastic are performed with the vitrector through the side ports. The side ports may then be sutured to help ensure that they do not attract vitreous through the pupil.

F. Postoperative Management

Capsular rupture and vitreous prolapse carry an increased risk of postoperative inflammation, infection, and glaucoma. While subconjunctival and oral antibiotics have not been shown to be helpful in reducing endophthalmitis in routine cataract surgery, they may be considered in the case of complicated surgery. In addition, the use of postoperative topical glaucoma agents or oral acetazolamide may be considered.

It is helpful to see the patient with a complicated case more often postoperatively. It is important to inform the patient of any complications after surgery. This should be done using terms that the patient will understand and should be done in a way that does not cause undue anxiety. The majority of cataract surgery complicated by vitreous loss results in a good outcome. Generally, the patient should be informed that the odds are still good for a favorable outcome.

KEY POINTS

1. The salvage of a complicated case should be done in a calm, considered fashion. It will take longer than an uncomplicated case. It is important to consider patient comfort in these cases. Additional systemic or local anesthesia should be considered to keep the patient comfortable and maintain a calm, controlled operative experience.

2. Surgical complications can be stressful for the surgeon. Intraoperative stress can lead to further mistakes and additional complications. Stress can be minimized by preparing in advance for complications. Preparation can include the following:

   ¤ Mentally rehearsing for the management of a complication as if it were a planned part of the case.

   ¤ Recognizing and preparing in advance for a case that is more likely to be difficult.

   ¤ Assuring that all instruments, sutures, and material necessary to manage the complication are in the operating room before every case.

REFERENCE

1. Burk SE, Da Mata AP, Snyder ME, et al. Visualizing vitreous using Kenalog suspension. *J Cataract Refract Surg.* 2003;29(4):645-651.

FURTHER READING

Astbury, N. Management of capsular rupture and vitreous loss in cataract surgery. *Community Eye Health.* 2008;21(65): 6-8.

Eye Movies Ltd. Vitreous loss: principles of management phaco 3.5 complications [Video]. YouTube. http://www.youtube.com/watch?v=tdHksE-73X0. Published 2009.

Reeves, SW, Kim, T. How to perform an anterior vitrectomy. *EyeNet Magazine,* from http://www.aao.org/publications/eyenet/200604/pearls.cfm

BIBLIOGRAPHY

Chang DF. Strategies for managing posterior capsular rupture. In: Chang DF, ed. *Phaco Chop: Mastering Techniques, Optimizing Technology, and Avoiding Complications.* Thorofare, NJ: SLACK Incorporated; 2004.

Coombes A, Gartry D. *Cataract Surgery.* Malden, Mass: Blackwell BMJ Books; 2003.

Lisa Brothers Arbisser, MD Focal Points 2009 Module: Anterior Vitrectomy for the Anterior Segment Surgeon Volume XXVII, Number 2, March 2009, (Module 2 of 3), from http://store.aao.org/2009-focal-points-module-anterior-vitrectomy-for-the-anterior-segment-surgeon.html

Nichamin LD. Posterior capsular rupture and vitreous loss. In: Chang DF, ed. *Phaco Chop: Mastering Techniques, Optimizing Technology, and Avoiding Complications.* Thorofare, NJ: SLACK Incorporated; 2004.

Nordlund ML, Marques DM, Marques FF, et al. Techniques for managing common complications of cataract surgery. *Curr Opin Ophthalmol.* 2003;14(1):7-19.

Cystoid Macular Edema

Ryan Fante, MD and Shahzad I. Mian, MD

I. Introduction

Cystoid macular edema (CME) is a significant complication after cataract surgery. In a systematic review of 43 studies that investigated the incidence of CME following cataract surgery, 1.4% of eyes had CME after cataract extraction. In fact, CME is a more frequent complication after cataract surgery than endophthalmitis, retinal detachment, vitreous hemorrhage, and choroidal hemorrhage.[1,2]

II. History

A. Vogt

In 1918, Alfred Vogt first recognized that CME occurs secondary to multiple ocular conditions.[3]

B. Irvine

In 1953, Irvine gave the Francis I. Proctor lecture, in which he discussed a "vitreous syndrome" that occurred in some patients after intracapsular cataract extraction (ICCE).[4] He speculated that the formation of vitreous adhesions to the wound was the cause of patients' postoperative vision loss and scotomas. Irvine associated these symptoms with clinically evident macular edema that seemed to be completely and spontaneously reversible.[5]

C. Nichols

Nichols later observed a similar type of reversible macular edema that was not associated with vitreous adhesions.[5]

Henderson BA. *Essentials of Cataract Surgery, Second Edition (pp 293-303).*
© 2014 Taylor & Francis Group.

D. Gass and Norton

In 1966, Gass and Norton became the first to describe the fundoscopic and angiographic findings of CME, which was later termed the *Irvine-Gass syndrome*.[6]

III. DEFINITION AND EPIDEMIOLOGY

CME is the most frequent visual complication following otherwise uncomplicated cataract surgery; the peak incidence is at 6 to 8 weeks postoperatively.[7] CME can be defined clinically (associated with visual acuity <20/40) or by angiography (detected on fluorescein angiogram). Given recent improvements in optical coherence tomography (OCT), this modality has become the standard method for diagnosis and monitoring of CME.[8]

The incidence of CME following ICCE is up to 60%, while that following extracapsular cataract extraction (ECCE) is 15% to 30%.[9] In the setting of modern phacoemulsification techniques, angiographic CME occurs in 19% of patients[10]; the rate of clinical CME is much lower, occurring in 1% to 2% of cases.[7]

IV. PATHOPHYSIOLOGY

Pseudophakic CME results from increased permeability of perifoveolar capillaries, leading to formation of cystoid spaces and lacunar cavities in the Henle's and outer plexiform layers.[6] With disruption of the blood-ocular barrier, Henle's layer serves as a reservoir as it absorbs and accumulates large quantities of fluid. The fovea is relatively avascular with limited capillary reabsorption, so fluid that leaks out of nearby vessels has a propensity to collect in this region. In addition, the internal limiting membrane is thinnest at the macula, increasing foveal susceptibility to inflammatory exudates and toxic products. The excess fluid produces traction and mechanical stress on the Müller cells, a type of neuronal glial cell within the retina, causing cell degeneration.[5] This leads to symptoms of decreased central vision and scotomas.

V. RISK FACTORS

Risk factors for CME include preoperative, intraoperative, and postoperative conditions (Table 26-1).

A. Preoperative

Preoperative risk factors include diabetes, particularly in those patients who have preexisting diabetic retinopathy,[11] hypertension, presence of an epiretinal membrane, history of chronic anterior or posterior uveitis,[12] and previous history of CME.[7]

TABLE 26-1. RISK FACTORS ASSOCIATED WITH PSEUDOPHAKIC CYSTOID MACULAR EDEMA	
Preoperative	Diabetes
	Hypertension
	Epiretinal membrane
	Chronic uveitis
	Previous CME
Intraoperative	ICCE versus ECCE versus phacoemulsification
	Vitreomacular traction
	UV light exposure
	Posterior capsular rupture
	Vitreous loss
	Iris prolapse
	IOL type
Postoperative	Epinephrine
	Dipivefrin
	Prostaglandin analogs
	Inflammation
	Hypotony

B. Intraoperative

Intraoperative risk factors include the type of cataract surgery performed (ICCE > ECCE > phacoemulsification), ultraviolet light exposure, vitreomacular traction, posterior capsular rupture, vitreous loss (incarceration to the wound or adhesion to the iris), iris prolapse, and intraocular lens (IOL) type (iris-supported > closed-loop anterior chamber IOL). Posterior capsular rupture seems to be the most significant operative risk factor for CME.[7]

C. Postoperative

Postoperative risk factors include the use of certain medications (epinephrine, dipivefrin, and prostaglandin analogs), inflammation, and hypotony.[7]

VI. DIAGNOSIS

The diagnosis of CME is based on the patient's symptoms, clinical findings, and imaging findings.

Figure 26-1. Clinical findings of CME. The fundus photo reveals a yellowish foveal reflex and perifoveal hemorrhages. (Reprinted with permission of Kellogg Eye Center, University of Michigan.)

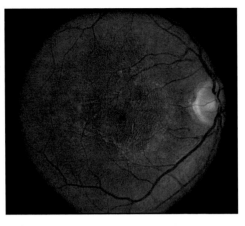

A. Symptoms

Patients with CME may experience symptoms of decreased visual acuity, pain, redness, and photophobia. They may also have decreased contrast sensitivity, metamorphopsia, and central scotoma.[7]

B. Clinical Findings

Ophthalmologic examination of patients with CME may show surgical complications of the anterior segment, including altered pupil shape, anterior chamber reaction with ciliary flush, abnormalities of the lens, or vitreous adhesions. Other clinical findings include loss of the foveal reflex or a yellowish spot on the retina. Perifoveal cystoid spaces along with honeycomb lesions, perifoveal hemorrhages, capillary microaneurysms, and optic disc edema may also be visible using red-free light (Figure 26-1).[6]

C. Imaging

1. Fluorescein angiography

Historically, the gold standard in diagnosis of CME, fluorescein angiography, typically shows a petaloid pattern of the macula with feathery margins, occasionally associated with optic disc edema (Figure 26-2).[6] Characteristics of the perifoveal fluid leakage visualized by fluorescein angiography, however, have not been found to correlate with the degree of visual acuity loss in patients with CME.

2. Optical coherence tomography

Macular thickening and cystoid spaces can be easily visualized and measured on images obtained by OCT (Figure 26-3). Macular thickness measured

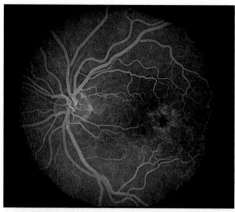

Figure 26-2. Fluorescein angiography in CME. Late leakage from perifoveal vessels produces a classic petaloid pattern around the fovea. (Reprinted with permission of Kellogg Eye Center, University of Michigan.)

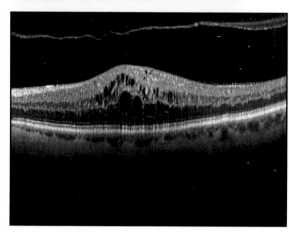

Figure 26-3. Optical coherence tomography in CME. Cystic intraretinal spaces are visible in the macula in a patient who developed CME following cataract extraction. (Reprinted with permission of Kellogg Eye Center, University of Michigan.)

by OCT has also been shown to correlate with postoperative visual acuity.[13] Due to improvements in OCT resolution and greater ease of use, OCT is frequently used to diagnose and monitor CME.[14]

VII. TREATMENT

CME most often resolves spontaneously. After 3 to 12 months, up to 80% of symptomatic pseudophakic CME patients note resolution without treatment.[8] Due to lack of long-term randomized controlled trials, there is currently no standard of care for CME prophylaxis or treatment. However, in multiple case series and smaller trials, agents targeting mediators of inflammation and vascular permeability have been found to improve the rate of CME resolution.[9]

TABLE 26-2. TREATMENT OPTIONS FOR PSEUDOPHAKIC CYSTOID MACULAR EDEMA	
Medication	Corticosteroids NSAIDs Corticosteroid/NSAID combination Carbonic anhydrase inhibitors Anti-VEGF agents
Surgical procedure	Pars plana vitrectomy IOL exchange Nd:YAG laser vitreolysis Grid laser

Current treatment of CME consists of corticosteroids, nonsteroidal anti-inflammatory drugs (NSAIDs), carbonic anhydrase inhibitors, and/or anti-vascular endothelial growth factor (VEGF) agents. There are also several surgical options available for treatment of CME (Table 26-2).

A. Corticosteroids

Corticosteroids can be administered by many routes including topical, periocular (retrobulbar or sub-Tenon's), intravitreal, systemic, or sustained-release devices.

1. Topical corticosteroids

A typical regimen for topical corticosteroids includes prednisolone acetate 1% QID followed by a slow taper. This slow taper is required, as studies have found a high rate of CME recurrence when steroids are discontinued abruptly.[15]

2. Intravitreal triamcinolone

While intravitreal triamcinolone has been found to be effective in treatment of diabetes-related CME, recent studies evaluating effectiveness of triamcinolone in the treatment of pseudophakic CME have reported mixed results. Sorensen et al found no significant improvement in CME with this treatment, while Boscia et al found only temporary reduction in CME in refractory cases.[16,17] Since triamcinolone has been found to last for 6 to 9 months in the vitreous cavity, there is concern for the possible ocular side effects caused by this long duration of steroid exposure.[18]

3. Sustained drug delivery devices

A phase II study is currently enrolling patients to investigate an intravitreal dexamethasone implant for CME after cataract surgery.[19]

B. NSAIDs

A systematic review of studies examining the effectiveness of NSAIDs in treating CME after cataract surgery found that topical NSAIDs, particularly ketorolac 0.5%, are effective in treatment of chronic CME. There is not enough evidence, however, to determine the effectiveness of NSAIDs in treating acute CME.[20]

1. Types

Several NSAIDs have been studied in the treatment of acute CME. Ketorolac, diclofenac, bromfenac, and nepafenac are approved for the treatment of pain and inflammation following cataract surgery. Rho reported that both diclofenac and ketorolac are equally effective in reducing CME and restoring visual acuity following uncomplicated cataract surgery.[21] Another study found that prednisolone 1% administered QID in addition to ketorolac can have a synergistic effect on the treatment of CME.[22]

2. Corneal permeation

Studies have also investigated the ability of various NSAIDs to permeate the cornea. Nepafenac has the greatest corneal permeation, followed by diclofenac, bromfenac, and ketorolac, respectively.[23]

3. Adverse effects

Adverse effects associated with the use of NSAIDs include burning and irritation of the eyes, superficial punctate keratitis, and delayed wound healing. This can result in thinning and perforation of the cornea.

C. Carbonic Anhydrase Inhibitors

Carbonic anhydrase inhibitors act on carbonic anhydrase bound to retinal pigment epithelium.[7] Limited data exist regarding efficacy in treatment of CME; however, Curkovic et al found that after 8 weeks of treatment, patients given oral acetazolamide had faster resorption of macular edema and obtained ultimate visual acuity that was significantly better. This study also showed a benefit in treating patients with anti-inflammatory drugs and acetazolamide simultaneously.[24]

D. Anti-VEGF Agents

Arevalo et al reported that intravitreal bevacizumab monotherapy significantly improved visual acuity and macular thickness measurements in a series of 28 patients with chronic CME.[25]

E. Surgical Treatment

In select cases, there are surgical options for treating CME, including pars plana vitrectomy to remove incarcerated vitreous, IOL exchange, Nd:YAG laser vitreolysis to remove vitreous adhesions to the corneal wound, and grid laser for diabetic macular edema.[7]

VIII. PROPHYLAXIS

Several studies have investigated the optimal regimen for CME prophylaxis; high-risk patients appear to benefit from topical NSAIDs. Small comparative trials evaluating efficacy show superiority of topical NSAIDs to corticosteroids in prevention of angiographic CME, although the effect on long-term visual outcome is uncertain.[9]

A. Nepafenac

A retrospective review of 450 patients who received nepafenac prophylaxis for cataract surgery found that no one developed clinical CME while 5 in the control group developed clinical CME ($P = 0.0354$).[26]

B. Indomethacin

Yavas et al reported a significant reduction in CME in postcataract surgery patients who received indomethacin (0% CME in patients receiving pre- and postoperative indomethacin, 15% CME in postoperative indomethacin only group, 33% CME in controls).[27]

C. Flurbiprofen

In a study by Solomon et al, the use of prophylactic flurbiprofen 0.03% resulted in a reduced rate of angiographic CME after 21 days but not after 60 days. It also resulted in 20/40 vision 2 weeks earlier than placebo. There was no long-term effect of flurbiprofen 0.03% on the incidence of clinical CME or visual acuity.[28]

D. Diclofenac

Studies by McColgin et al and the Italian Diclofenac Study Group found that diclofenac 0.1% decreased the incidence of angiographic CME at 36 days and 140 days but did not result in any improvement in visual acuity.[29]

E. Ketorolac

Ketorolac 0.5% reduced the rate of angiographic CME after 40 days in studies conducted by Flach et al[30] and Rho.[31]

IX. CONCLUSION

CME is one of the most common complications of cataract surgery. The most important risk factor for CME is intraoperative rupture of the posterior capsule. OCT imaging is an essential tool for diagnosing and monitoring CME. Topical NSAIDs and corticosteroids remain the first-line treatment of clinical and angiographic CME; simultaneous administration of corticosteroids and NSAIDs seems to result in quicker resolution of clinical symptoms. For high-risk patients, prophylaxis with topical NSAIDs decreases the incidence of early angiographic CME and may also help with faster visual recovery postoperatively. While current treatments clearly show temporary benefit and shorten the clinical course of CME, the effect on long-term visual outcomes is unclear; larger trials will be needed to further clarify optimal treatment.

KEY POINTS

1. CME is the most frequent visual complication after uncomplicated cataract surgery with incidence rates as high as 1% to 19%. Peak incidence is 6 weeks to 8 weeks postoperatively.

2. Pseudophakic CME results from increased permeability of perifoveolar capillaries, leading to the formation of cystoid spaces and lacunar cavities in the Henle's and outer plexiform layers.

3. Risk factors include diabetes, hypertension, uveitis, intraoperative complications, and postoperative medications such as epinephrine or prostaglandin analogs.

4. The diagnosis of CME is based on the patient's symptoms, clinical findings, and imaging findings.

5. Treatment of CME consists of corticosteroids, NSAIDs, carbonic anhydrase inhibitors, and surgery.

REFERENCES

1. American Academy of Ophthalmology Cataract and Anterior Segment Panel. Preferred Practice Pattern Guidelines. Cataract in the Adult Eye. San Francisco, CA: American Academy of Ophthalmology; 2011. Available at: www.aao.org/ppp

2. Powe NR, Schein OD, Geiser SC, et al. Synthesis of the literature on visual acuity and complications following cataract extraction with intraocular lens implantation. Cataract Patient Outcome Research Team. *Arch Ophthalmol.* 1994;112:239-252.

3. Wolfensberger TJ. The historical discovery of macular edema. *Doc Ophthalmol.* 1999;97:(3-4):207-16.

4. Irvine SR. A newly defined vitreous syndrome following cataract surgery. *Am J Ophthalmol.* 1953;36:599-619.

5. Irvine AR. Cystoid maculopathy. *Surv Ophthalmol*. 1976;21:1-17.

6. Gass JD, Norton EW. Cystoid macular edema and papilledema following cataract extraction: a fluorescein fundoscopic and angiographic study. *Arch Ophthalmol*. 1966;76:646-661.

7. Ray S, D'Amico DJ. Pseudophakic cystoid macular edema. *Semin Ophthalmol*. 2002;17:167-180.

8. Shelsta HN, Jampol LM. *Pharmacologic therapy of pseu*dophakic cystoid macular edema: 2010 update. *Retina*. 2011;31:4-12.

9. Yonekawa Y, Kim IK. Pseudophakic cystoid macular edema. *Curr Opin Ophthalmol*. 2012;23(1):26-32.

10. Ursell PG, Spalton DJ, Whitcup SM, Nussenblatt RB. Cystoid macular edema after phacoemulsification: relationship to blood-aqueous barrier damage and visual acuity. *J Cataract Refract Surg*. 1999;25(11):1492-1497.

11. Pollack A, Leiba H, Bukelman A, Abrahami S, Oliver M. The course of diabetic retinopathy following cataract surgery in eyes previously treated by photocoagulation. *Br J Ophthalmol*. 1992;76:228-231.

12. Estafanous MF Lowder CY, Meisler DM, Chauhan R. Phacoemulsification cataract extraction and posterior chamber lens implantation in patients with uveitis. *Am J Ophthalmol*. 2001;131:620-625.

13. Kim SJ, Belair ML, Bressler NM, et al. A method of reporting macular edema after cataract surgery using optical coherence tomography. *Retina*. 2008;28:870-876.

14. Lobo C. Pseudophakic cystoid macular edema. *Ophthalmologica*. 2012;227(2):61-67.

15. Rosetti L. Medical prophylaxis and treatment of pseudophakic cystoid macular edema after cataract surgery. The results of meta-analysis. *Ophthalmology*. 1998;105:397-405.

16. Sorensen TL, Haamann P, Villumsen J, Michael. Intravitreal triamcinolone for macular oedema: efficacy in relation to aetiology. *Acta Ophthalmol Scand*. 2005;83(1):67.

17. Boscia F, Furino C, Dammacco R, Ferreri P, Sborgia L, Sborgia C. Intravitreal triamcinolone acetonide in refractory pseudophakic cystoid macular edema: functional and anatomic results. *Eur J Ophthalmol*. 2005;15(1):89-95.

18. Jonas JB. Intravitreal triamcinolone acetonide for treatment of intraocular oedematous and neovascular diseases. *Acta Ophthalmol Scand*. 2005;83(6):645-663.

19. United States National Institutes of Health. Ozurdex for combined pseudophakic cystoid macular edema and diabetic macular edema after cataract surgery. http://clinicaltrials.gov.

20. Sivaprasad S, Bunce C, Wormald R. Non-steroidal anti-inflammatory agents for cystoid macular edema following cataract surgery: a systematic review. *Br J Ophthalmol*. 2005; 89(11):1420-1422.

21. Rho DS. Treatment of acute pseudophakic cystoid macular edema: diclofenac versus ketorolac. *J Cataract Refract Surg*. 2003;29(12): 2378-2384.

22. Heier JS, Topping TM, Baumann W, et al. Ketorolac vs. prednisone vs. combination. *Ophthalmology*. 2000;107:2034-2039.

23. Lindstrom R, Kim T. Ocular permeation and inhibition of inflammation: an examination of data and expert opinion on the clinical utility of nepafenac. *Curr Med Res Opin*. 2006;22(2):397-404.

24. Curkovic T, Vukojevic N, Bucan K. Treatment of pseudophakic cystoid macular oedema. *Coll Antropol*. 2005;29(suppl 1):103-105.

25. Arevalo JF, Garcia-Amaris RA, Roca JA, et al. Primary intravitreal bevacizumab for the management of pseudophakic cystoid macular edema: pilot study of the Pan-American Collaborative Retina Study Group. *J Cataract Refract Surg*. 2007;33:2098-2105.

26. Wolf EJ, Braunstein A, Shih C, Braunstein RE. Incidence of visually significant pseudophakic macular edema after uneventful phacoemulsification in patients treated with nepafenac. *J Cataract Refract Surg*. 2007;33:1546-1549.

27. Yavas GF, Ozturk F, Kusbeci T. Preoperative topical indomethacin to prevent pseudophakic cystoid macular edema. *J Cataract Refract Surg*. 2007;33:804-807.

28. Solomon LD. Efficacy of topical flurbiprofen and indomethacin in preventing pseudophakic CME. Flurbiprofen-CME study group I. *J Cataract Refract Surg.* 1995;21:73-81.
29. Efficacy of diclofenac eyedrops in preventing postoperative inflammation and long-term cystoid macular edema. Italian Diclofenac Study Group. *J Cataract Refract Surg.* 1997;23:1183-1189.
30. Flach AJ, Jampol LM, Weinberg D, Kraff MC, Yannuzzi LA, Campo RV, et al. Improvement in visual acuity in chronic aphakic and pseudophakic cystoid macular edema after treatment with topical 0.5% ketorolac tromethamine. *Am J Ophthalmol.* 1991 Nov 15;112(5):514-519.
31. Rho DS. Treatment of acute pseudophakic cystoid macular edema: Diclofenac versus ketorolac. *J Cataract Refract Surg.* 2003 Dec;29(12):2378-2384.

27

ENDOPHTHALMITIS

Francis S. Mah, MD

I. INTRODUCTION

Endophthalmitis is a serious condition that can result in permanent and dramatic loss of vision.[1] Early diagnosis and treatment are 2 of the most important factors related to good visual outcomes in cases of endophthalmitis.[2]

This chapter is intended as an overview of postoperative endophthalmitis (POE), a complication resulting from bacterial or fungal infection following cataract surgery. POE can occur as an acute infection, presenting up to 6 weeks postsurgery, or as a chronic condition, occurring months or even years after initial surgery.

II. OVERVIEW OF INCIDENCE AND SEQUELAE

- Even with modern sterile techniques for cataract surgery, the eye is not a sterile environment. The periocular flora can be introduced into the eye during and/or after surgery, and this may result in endophthalmitis, the most devastating outcome of cataract surgery (Figure 27-1).[3]

- The true incidence of POE is not known, but published reports indicate the incidence ranges from 1 in 350 to 1 in 1000 patients.[4]

- There are several factors that may influence the risk of developing POE. When the incidence of culture-proven endophthalmitis is compared to the length and complexity of the surgical procedure, there appears to be a correlation. It is clear that the risk of infection increases as more instruments are introduced into the eye. If a secondary

Henderson BA. *Essentials of Cataract Surgery, Second Edition* (pp 305-317).
© 2014 Taylor & Francis Group.

Figure 27-1. Endo-
phthalmitis.

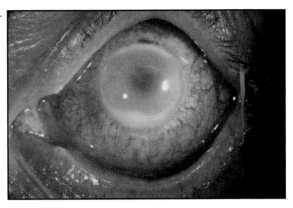

surgery must be performed on an eye, the risk of postoperative
infection also rises dramatically.[1,5]

- Most POE occurs in the first 6 weeks following surgery; these are
  considered acute cases. However, between 10% and 20% of cases occur
  after 6 weeks and are considered chronic POE. [1,5]
- Confirming a diagnosis remains an issue in the treatment of POE.

III. DIAGNOSIS

A. Physical Presentation: Signs and Symptoms

- While prevention of POE is the critical component in achieving
  better visual outcomes, once a problem develops, it is urgent that the
  diagnosis be made early.[2]
- Bacterial endophthalmitis usually presents with acute symptoms.
  The most common are decreased visual acuity, redness, lid swelling,
  and pain in the eye beyond what was experienced immediately
  postsurgery.[2]
- Current diagnostic guidelines recommend a complete ophthalmic
  evaluation, including ophthalmoscopy and posterior segment
  ultrasonography, if needed.
- The Endophthalmitis Vitrectomy Study (EVS) reported that for
  all treatment groups, initial visual acuity at presentation was a key
  predictor of visual outcome: for eyes with worse initial acuity, worse
  final vision results regardless of the treatment.[2]

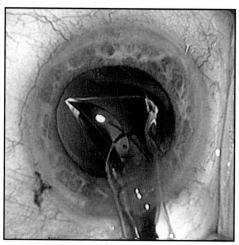

Figure 27-2. Injection of foldable IOL.

B. Laboratory Studies

The most important laboratory studies are Gram stain and culture of the aqueous and vitreous humors. Intraocular cultures can confirm the diagnosis.

C. Polymerase Chain Reaction

- Polymerase chain reaction (PCR) technology is a molecular technique that utilizes the ability of enzymes to amplify DNA from small amounts of clinical specimens.
- PCR technology has been used successfully to detect bacteria and fungi in ocular samples and has significantly increased the number of intraocular samples from which a confirmed diagnosis can be made. Currently, PCR technology is primarily available in large research hospitals.[6,7]

IV. SURGICAL PROCEDURES IN CATARACT SURGERY

- In the past 10 years, cataract surgery has undergone tremendous advances in almost all aspects of the procedure:
  - The size and location of the incision have changed.
  - There are new phacoemulsification (PE) techniques.
  - The use of foldable intraocular lens (IOL) materials of different types with injectable systems has been introduced (Figure 27-2).
  - Sutureless wounds are now standard practice.
- Extracapsular cataract extraction (ECCE) using PE and phaco chop has become a widely used procedure for cataract removal.

- Since 1996, when the majority of surgeons working in institutional settings switched to sutureless temporal clear corneal incisions, the increase in clear corneal incisions has been associated with an increased incidence of endophthalmitis.[4,8,9]
- Scleral tunnel incision: A scleral lamellar dissection is carried forward into the clear cornea so that the entrance into the anterior chamber forms a watertight internal closure. This incision has a posterior placement and a narrow profile. Advantages follow[4,8,9]:
  - Sutureless incision
  - Reduced postoperative astigmatism
  - Potentially, a reduced rate of POE
- Clear corneal incision: A tiny incision is made into the perimeter of the cornea on the side of the eye closest to the temple (temporal clear corneal incision). Advantages follow[4,8,9]:
  - Easier access to the eye without obstruction by the brow
  - Less early postoperative inflammation relative to scleral incisions
  - Less subconjunctival erythema and hemorrhage in the first several weeks after surgery
  - Potentially, an increased risk of POE. This is not an advantage

V. PERIOPERATIVE RISK FACTORS

A. Patient Risk Factors

1. Periocular infection

- The primary source of bacteria in culture-positive cases of POE is believed to be the ocular surface and the periocular area of the patient.[3,10]
- Reducing the bacterial load both prior to and during surgery is essential.

2. Patient characteristics

- Some characteristics (eg, diabetes and compromised immune system) are believed to put certain patients at higher risk for developing endophthalmitis; however, no conclusive data have been reported.[1,5,11,12]
- There are no universally agreed upon criteria for identifying or targeting high-risk patients for specific prophylactic procedures.

B. Surgical Risk Factors

Risk factors associated with the surgical procedure may also lead to the development of POE[1,5,11,12]:

- ¤ Increased operative time with repeated introduction and reintroduction of surgical tools into the eye
- ¤ Complicated procedure
- ¤ Posterior capsule rupture/vitreous loss
- ¤ Retained lens fragments
- ¤ Inadequate sterilization of the operative field
- ¤ Contamination of surgical instruments and/or solutions
- ¤ Consideration of IOL material may become an issue. A prospective POE study has suggested an increased risk with silicone versus acrylic IOLs

C. Postoperative Complications

Wound architecture as a risk factor[1,4,5,8,9,11,12]:

- ¤ Wound leaks or wounds that easily leak are related to the size of the incision.
- ¤ A microleak after surgery clearly puts the eye at significant risk of infection.
- ¤ Microcontamination caused by contamination at the time of surgery and by microleaks in the wound is a serious risk factor, particularly in the first 24 hours postsurgery.

VI. MICROBIOLOGY OF ENDOPHTHALMITIS

The organisms being recovered from the vitreous and the aqueous of endophthalmitis cases are the same organisms present on the conjunctiva and the periocular area.[3,10]

A positive Gram stain and infection with species other than gram-positive, coagulase-negative micrococci are significantly associated with poor visual outcome.[2,10]

A. Gram positive

1. The EVS determined that the majority of bacteria found in acute POE, 94.2%, were gram positive (Figure 27-3).[2]
2. The most commonly cultured microorganism is *Staphylococcus epidermidis*, which is less virulent than the others normally present in the periocular flora.[2,3,10]

Figure 27-3. *Staphylo-coccus aureus.*

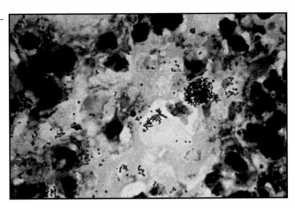

B. Gram negative

1. The EVS reported 6% of the bacteria found were gram-negative species.[2]
2. *Pseudomonas aeruginosa*, *Proteus*, and *Haemophilus* species are the most common gram-negative organisms isolated in patients with POE.[2]
3. Although gram-negative organisms are less frequent, they cause more severe infection.[2]

C. Fungi

POE caused by fungus is very rare and may be caused by many species, including *Candida*, *Aspergillus*, and *Penicillium*.[1,2,5,10]

VII. PROPHYLAXIS: THERAPEUTIC OPTIONS AND CONSIDERATIONS

- Given the potential for a devastating outcome, there is urgent need to prevent the occurrence of endophthalmitis following cataract surgery.
- Efforts are focused in 2 key areas: (1) eradicating bacteria on the surface of the conjunctiva and the eyelids and (2) reducing the incidence of intraocular contamination.[4,13-18]

A. Spectrum of Activity

- When choosing an anti-infective for reducing the ocular flora prior to surgery, there are several factors to be considered (Figure 27-4):
  - Spectrum of activity of the anti-infective against specific bacteria and the susceptibility pattern of the bacteria to that drug.

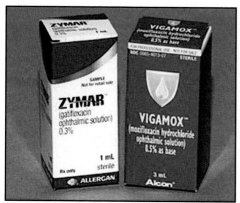

Figure 27-4. Fourth-generation fluoroquinolone antibiotics.

- Ability of the anti-infective to penetrate the tissue, achieve a therapeutic level, and maintain that level over a period of time sufficient to eradicate the bacteria.
- Effectiveness in reducing ocular flora. The fluoroquinolones offer the best coverage of bacteria likely to be found in the periocular area.

B. Antisepsis

1. Povidone-iodine, used at 1% to 10% solution (most commonly used at 5%), is generally agreed to be an effective measure to reduce bacteria in the eye prior to surgery (Figure 27-5).[13-15]
2. Although it clearly reduces the number of bacteria on the surface of the eye and the evidence is the strongest for its use as a prophylactic agent, there is still no definitive, prospective, randomized study confirming that it decreases the rate of endophthalmitis.[13-15]

C. Anti-Infectives

1. Anti-infectives are currently being used pre-, intra-, and/or postoperatively.
2. The question of efficacy in decreasing the rate of POE has not been definitively answered, and as yet, there is no widely accepted protocol for use of anti-infectives in cataract surgery.
3. Anti-infectives are used topically, as intracameral or subconjunctival injection, and systemically, either orally or intravenously.[14]
4. Of the topical anti-infectives currently available commercially, the fluoroquinolones have the highest potency for use in the ocular area. They have a broad spectrum of activity against the most frequent

Figure 27-5. Povidone-iodine.

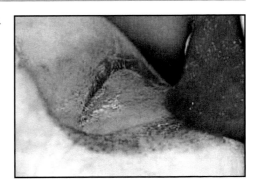

gram-positive and gram-negative organisms found in the ocular area. One area of increasing concern is the increase in bacterial resistance to fluoroquinolones, therefore, a review of the most common pathogens in the area in addition to the susceptibility profile of the region should be considered when choosing a prophylactic agent.[16]

5. Recent prospective studies suggest that the use of intracameral agents are beneficial in the reduction of POE. Although various agents have been described in the literature, including vancomycin, gentamicin, moxifloxacin, and cefazolin to name a few, the evidence is the strongest for cefuroxime.[4]

D. Issues of Resistance

When considering issues of resistance, multiple factors include spectrum of activity, low minimum inhibitory concentrations, local resistance patterns, penetration into key ocular tissues, length and frequency of use, patient compliance, and exposure of agent to environment. In general, bacterial resistance will always be an issue.

E. When to Initiate Therapy

1. One inherent advantage to using prophylaxis in cataract surgery is that the antiseptic or anti-infective can be placed directly on the potential site of infection (ie, in/on the eye).

2. There is an opportunity to utilize these drugs exactly where they are needed prior to, during, and after surgical intervention.

3. While there are no definitive studies on the question of which anti-infective or which delivery method, antibiotic prophylaxis is widely practiced in cataract surgery.

4. It is recommended that a combination of antiseptic and anti-infective be used. Antiseptics, such as povidone-iodine, work immediately

(within 2 minutes of contact) to kill bacteria, whereas anti-infectives require more time to get to the site of action and eradicate bacteria. The combination of anti-infectives and antiseptics shows a significantly greater reduction of bacterial colony counts than either applied alone.[4,14,16]

F. Mechanical Protection

1. A brief survey of the Internet reveals that the majority of physician-sponsored Web sites inform patients that they will have both a patch and a metal or plastic shield or only a shield over the affected eye after surgery.

2. There is a good deal of latitude in the use of both the patch and the shield.

VIII. FOLLOW-UP

• The schedule of postoperative follow-up visits is a subject of considerable debate and varies from country to country, from site to site, and within sites.

• The purpose of the first follow-up visit is not primarily to detect endophthalmitis, although 10% of endophthalmitis cases develop within the first 24 hours postsurgery.[1,2,5,11,12] The objective is to look for unusual inflammation, to determine if the wound is leaking, and to check the intraocular pressure and any other sign of possible complication.

• The frequency of the visits should be designed to support the optimal outcome of surgery, quickly identifying and managing complications. This requires timely and accurate diagnosis and appropriate treatment of complications of surgery, providing satisfactory optical correction and clear instructions to the patient.

IX. TREATMENT

• To date, the EVS is the only large, prospective, randomized study on the management of endophthalmitis.

• Early results showed that vitrectomy had a significant advantage in those patients whose visual acuity was limited to perception of light. When visual acuity was perception of hand movements or better, then vitrectomy showed no advantage over vitreous biopsy or tap and intravitreal anti-infective injection.[19]

• The EVS has simplified the approach to treatment, which should start immediately once the diagnosis is made. As a result of its findings, most patients are now treated in an office setting with vitreous tap and intravitreal injection rather than with vitrectomy and are managed on an outpatient basis without hospitalization for intravenous anti-infectives.

A. Acute Postoperative Endophthalmitis

1. Vitrectomy

- The EVS showed that patients who presented with vision of light perception only had much better visual results with immediate pars plana vitrectomy than with tap/biopsy.
- Vitrectomy has the obvious benefit of debulking the vitreous, removing virulence factors, and decreasing organism load.
- Vitrectomy may also enhance fluid circulation in the vitreous cavity, allow for an increase of anti-infectives to the infection site, and provide ample material for laboratory analysis.

2. Vitreous biopsy/tap

- In all cases where visual acuity is better than light perception, a single-port vitreous biopsy or tap should be performed.
- The specimen should be smeared for Gram stain and plated for culture.
- Once the procedure is completed, the intraocular injection can be given.
- Intravitreal anti-infective injection.
  - The vitreous is usually the location of the infecting pathogens in POE.
  - Since the eye is an enclosed cavity and is further isolated by a blood-ocular barrier, direct intravitreal injection is an effective way to deliver anti-infectives directly to the site of infection.[2,19]

B. Chronic POE

1. Chronic or delayed-onset endophthalmitis can begin weeks, months, or years after cataract surgery.
2. In chronic POE, the inflammation may occur with only mild pain and often responds initially to topical corticosteroids.
3. Chronic endophthalmitis may be caused by fungal organisms (such as *Candida parapsilosis*), *Propionibacterium acnes*, and nonvirulent forms of *S epidermidis*.
4. Culturing these organisms can be difficult and usually requires a vitrectomy to obtain an adequate specimen.

5. The causative organisms may be slow growing, and sterilization might be more likely with vitrectomy than with intraocular anti-infectives alone.

6. For these cases that were not included in the EVS and for which no standard protocol exists, decisions about the use of vitrectomy should be based on the severity of the vitreous involvement or the difficulty in obtaining a positive culture rather than on initial visual acuity.[20]

X. COUNSELING PATIENTS

- An important component of achieving good visual outcome after cataract surgery is patient education.

- Patients should be instructed on how to care for the eye after surgery, protect the eye, avoid inappropriate activities, properly use medications, keep required follow-up visits, and recognize symptoms that require immediate medical attention.

- The most serious complication of cataract surgery is the development of POE. Patients should be informed about the signs and symptoms of endophthalmitis, which include increasing pain, excessive redness, decreasing vision, periocular swelling, and/or heavy tearing. If these signs are present, the ophthalmologist should be contacted immediately.

- Prompt diagnosis and treatment provide the best chance for a positive outcome, and patient responsibility should be strongly emphasized during the postoperative phase.

KEY POINTS

1. Even with modern sterile techniques for cataract surgery, the eye is not a sterile environment. Periocular flora can be introduced into the eye during and/or after surgery, and this may result in endophthalmitis, the most devastating outcome of cataract surgery.

2. Early diagnosis and treatment are 2 of the most important factors related to good visual outcomes in cases of endophthalmitis.

3. Since 1996, when the majority of surgeons working in institutional settings switched to sutureless temporal clear corneal incisions, the increase in clear corneal incisions has been associated with an increased incidence of endophthalmitis.

4. Povidone-iodine, used as 1% to 10% solution (most commonly used as 5%), is generally agreed to be an effective measure to reduce bacteria on the eye prior to surgery. It is recommended that a combination of anti-septic and anti-infective be used. Antiseptics, such as povidone-iodine, work immediately to kill bacteria, whereas anti-infectives require more time to get to the site of action. The combination of anti-infectives and antiseptics shows a significantly greater reduction of bacterial colony counts than either applied alone.

5. The most serious complication of cataract surgery is the development of POE. Patients should be informed about the signs and symptoms of endophthalmitis, which include increasing pain, excessive redness, decreasing vision, periocular swelling, and/or heavy tearing. If these signs are present, the ophthalmologist should be contacted immediately.

6. Early results showed that vitrectomy had a significant advantage in those patients in whom visual acuity was limited to perception of light. When visual acuity is perception of hand movements or better, then vitrectomy showed no advantage over vitreous biopsy or tap and intravitreal anti-infective injection.

REFERENCES

1. Aaberg Jr TM, Flynn Jr HW, Schiffman J, Newton J. Nosocomial acute-onset post-operative endophthalmitis survey: a 10-year review of incidence and outcomes. *Ophthalmology*. 1998;105:1004-1010.

2. Endophthalmitis Vitrectomy Study Group. Results of the Endophthalmitis Vitrectomy Study: a randomized trial of immediate vitrectomy and of intravenous antiinfectives for the treatment of postoperative bacterial endophthalmitis. *Arch Ophthalmol*. 1995;113: 1479-1496.

3. Speaker MG, Milch FA, Shah MK, et al. Role of external bacterial flora in the pathogenesis of acute postoperative endophthalmitis. *Ophthalmology*. 1991;98:639-650.
4. Barry P, Seal DV, Gettinby G, et al. ESCRS study of prophylaxis of postoperative endophthalmitis after cataract surgery. *J Cataract Refract Surg*. 2006;32(3):407-410.
5. Kattan HM, Flynn Jr HW, Pflugfelder SC, et al. Nosocomial endophthalmitis survey: current incidence of infection after intraocular surgery. *Ophthalmology*. 1991;98:227-238.
6. Barza M, Pavan PR, Doft BH, et al. Evaluation of microbiological diagnostic techniques in postoperative endophthalmitis in the Endophthalmitis Vitrectomy Study. *Arch Ophthalmol*. 1997;115:1142-1150.
7. Okhravi N, Adamson P, Lightman S. Use of PCR in endophthalmitis. *Ocular Immunol Inflammation*. 2000;8:189-200.
8. Bohigian G, Cooper B, Holekamp N. Endophthalmitis after cataract surgery: clear cornea versus scleral tunnel wounds. The Charles T. Campbell Eye Microbiology Lab. UPMC Health System. Available at: http://eyemicrobiology.upmc.com/2001Abstracts/2001Abs10. htm. Accessed 14.11.02.
9. Nagaki Y, Hayasaka S, Kadoi C, et al. Bacterial endophthalmitis after small incision cataract surgery: effect of incision placement and intraocular lens type. *J Cataract Refract Surg*. 2003;29:20-26.
10. Han DP, Wisniewski SR, Kelsey SF, et al. Microbiologic yields and complication rates of vitreous needle aspiration versus mechanized vitreous biopsy in the Endophthalmitis Vitrectomy Study. *Retina*. 1999;19:98-102.
11. Schmitz S, Dick HB, Krummenauer F, Pfeiffer N. Endophthalmitis in cataract surgery: results of a German survey. *Ophthalmology*. 1999;106:1869-1877.
12. Fisch A, Salvanet A, Prazuck T, The French Collaborative Study Group on Endophthalmitis: epidemiology of infective endophthalmitis in France. *Lancet*. 1991;338:1373-1376.
13. Speaker MG, Menikoff JA. Prophylaxis of endophthalmitis with topical povidone-iodine. *Ophthalmology*. 1991;98:1769-1775.
14. Ciulla TA, Starr MB, Masket S. Bacterial endophthalmitis prophylaxis for cataract surgery: an evidence-based update. *Ophthalmology*. 2002;109:13-24.
15. Ferguson AW, Scott JA, McGavigan J, et al. Comparison of 5% povidone-iodine solution against 1% povidone-iodine solution in preoperative cataract surgery anti-sepsis: a prospective randomized double blind study. *Br J Ophthalmol*. 2003;87:163-167.
16. Masket S. Preventing, diagnosing, and treating endophthalmitis. *J Cataract Refract Surg*. 1998;24:725-726.
17. Montan PG, Wejde G, Setterquist H, Rylander M, Zetterstrom C. Prophylactic intracameral cefuroxime: evaluation of safety and kinetics in cataract surgery. *J Cataract Refract Surg*. 2002;28:982-987.
18. Jensen MK, Fiscella RG. *Comparison of Endophthalmitis Rates Over 4our Years Associated with Topical Ofloxacin vs. Ciprofloxacin (Poster)*. Ft. Lauderdale, Fla: Association for Research in Vision and Ophthalmology; 2002.
19. Sternberg P, Martin D. Management of endophthalmitis in the post-endophthalmitis Vitrectomy Study era. Editorial. *Arch Ophthalmol*. 2001;119:754-755.
20. Clark WL, Kaiser PK, Flynn Jr HW, Belfort A, Miller D, Meisler DM. Treatment strategies and visual acuity outcomes in chronic postoperative Propionibacterium acnes endophthalmitis. *Ophthalmology*. 1999;106:1665-1670.

28

Surgical Management of Cataract in the Glaucoma Patient

Jack Manns, MD; Sandra M. Johnson, MD;
and Peter A. Netland, MD, PhD

I. Introduction

Cataract is the leading cause of reversible blindness in the world, while glaucoma is the leading cause of age-related irreversible vision loss.[1] Due to increasing age of the population and changes of demographics, the prevalence of glaucoma is increasing in the United States, and the coexistence of cataracts and glaucoma will likewise increase.[2] The surgical management of a cataract in a patient with glaucoma will become an increasingly prevalent clinical situation confronting the cataract surgeon. Moreover, cataract may affect monitoring of glaucoma progression, medical or surgical therapy for glaucoma may affect cataract, and patients with glaucoma may have risk factors for cataract surgery.[3]

II. Preoperative Considerations

The preoperative cataract history and examination in a patient with glaucoma requires careful assessment of cataract as well as consideration of factors related to the coexistence of glaucoma.

A. History

The history includes the number of medications required to control the patient's glaucoma, because in some cases, cataract and glaucoma surgery can be an opportunity to decrease the need for glaucoma medications.[4]

Henderson BA. *Essentials of
Cataract Surgery, Second Edition (pp 319-328).*
© 2014 Taylor & Francis Group.

1. Prostaglandin analogs

Prostaglandin analogs have been associated with cystoid macula edema (CME) following cataract surgery (especially when the posterior capsule has been compromised) and with prolonged uveitis. Although still a controversial topic, some evidence suggests that discontinuing prostaglandin analog in patients with reasonable control of intraocular pressure (IOP) prior to surgery and pretreating with topical ketorolac may decrease occurrence of CME.[5]

2. Cholinergic drugs

Although cholinergic drugs are now less commonly used, occasional use of these drugs occurs in glaucoma patients. Cholinergic drugs may impair pupillary dilation and can be discontinued prior to cataract surgery, if possible. Long-acting cholinergic drugs such as echothiophate and demecarium may decrease plasma concentrations or activity of pseudocholinesterase, the enzyme that metabolizes succinylcholine, thereby enhancing the neuromuscular blockade effect of depolarizing muscle relaxants. Use of muscle relaxants such as succinylcholine should be avoided in these patients.

3. Corticosteroids

Glaucoma suspects, patients with primary open-angle glaucoma (POAG), or patients with first-degree relatives with POAG have been found to have a significant increase in IOP following topical steroid use.[6] In these patients, lower potency steroids could be considered due to a reduced occurrence of an IOP response.[7] The need for postoperative steroids may be an indication for a combined procedure if the patient is already on multiple glaucoma medications and has a history of being a steroid responder.

B. Examination

1. Cornea

Guttata representative of endothelial loss may play a role in the decision of performing a one-site phacotrabeculectomy versus a two-site procedure. Two-site phacotrabeculectomy surgery may be associated with more endothelial loss.[8] Severe endothelial cell loss may result in the need for partial or full thickness corneal transplantation, which can be performed, if needed, after cataract and glaucoma surgery.

2. Gonioscopy

Visualization of the angle structures can identify occludable angles, plateau iris, pseudoexfoliation, or secondary angle closure. Narrow and occludable angles may deepen with cataract extraction alone. When present, peripheral anterior synechiae should be quantified and localized, as this can help to identify causes of secondary angle closure and may provide useful information if an anterior chamber IOL needs to be placed. The angle should be also assessed for angle recession if there is a history of trauma, as this is difficult to diagnose after cataract extraction. Neovascularization may prompt treatment with anti-VEGF therapy to lessen bleeding in the anterior chamber at surgery. Sampaolesi line may be seen in patients with pseudoexfoliation or pigmentary glaucoma.

3. Lens capsule

Pseudoexfoliation syndrome is an independent risk factor for vitreous loss.[9,10] Pseudoexfoliation material deposition may be seen most easily on the anterior lens capsule. It is important to check for phacodonesis (best performed undilated) in patients with pseudoexfoliation or a history of trauma. In patients with significant loss of zonular support, it may be helpful to have a capsular tension ring available for the procedure.

4. Optic nerve

The optic nerve should be evaluated for cupping, correlated to visual field loss, and appropriately staged. Patients with advanced glaucomatous optic nerve damage are usually treated with combined surgery rather than cataract surgery alone.

5. Iris

The amount of dilation should be noted to appropriately plan for management of inadequate dilation at the time of surgery. Options include stretching, hooks, rings, or other procedures or devices to produce adequate pupil size for safe cataract surgery.

III. SURGICAL TECHNIQUE

A. Anesthesia Choices and "Wipe-Out"

Wipe-out is a term used to describe unexplained visual loss following surgery in advanced glaucoma patients. Although multiple causes may contribute to "wipe-out," risk factors include postoperative hypotony, choroidal effusions, and advanced visual field defects prior to surgery.[11,12] In some instances, damage to the optic nerve could result from the increase in IOP from peribulbar and retrobulbar anesthesia. Color Doppler ultrasound studies have shown that retrobulbar, peribulbar, and sub-Tenon's anesthesia cause a reduction of blood flow to the optic nerve, especially if epinephrine is used in the mixture.[13,14] The anterior application of anesthesia (topical, subconjunctival, anterior sub-Tenon's, and intracameral) avoids this unwanted effect on the optic nerve perfusion but may not achieve akinesia as effectively as would retrobulbar, peribulbar, and sub-Tenon's anesthesia.

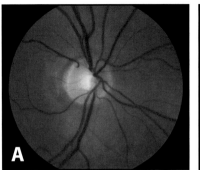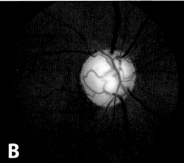

Figure 28-1. Surgical approaches vary depending on the stage of the disease. These 2 patients have primary open-angle glaucoma. The patient with the disc shown on the left would be a candidate for cataract surgery alone or combined surgery, whereas the patient with the disc shown on the right would likely be treated with combined or staged surgery. The status of the disc may be determined from the examination prior to surgery or, after removal of the cataract, during surgery.

B. Surgical Approaches

Cataract surgery in the glaucoma patient involves 3 major surgical approaches:

1. Cataract surgery alone
2. Combined cataract and glaucoma surgery
3. Staged, glaucoma surgery followed by cataract surgery or *vice versa*

The stage of the glaucoma and other factors may influence the choice of procedure (Figure 28-1).

1. Cataract surgery alone

Cataract surgery alone can be considered when visual function is impaired by cataract, if glaucoma damage is mild to moderate, and IOP is controlled on medical therapy. Cataract surgery alone has been used successfully in patients with POAG, narrow-angle glaucoma, phacolytic and phacomorphic glaucomas, and patients with pseudoexfoliation.

Evidence-based review has shown an overall trend toward an IOP decrease of 2 to 4 mm Hg at 1 to 2 years after cataract extraction.[15] Cataract extraction by phacoemulsification lowers the IOP in glaucomatous and nonglaucomatous eyes proportional to the presurgical IOP. Poley et al demonstrated that cataract surgery by phacoemulsification in normotensive and eyes with ocular hypertension and primary open-angle glaucoma resulted in greater IOP reduction in the eyes with the highest IOPs prior to surgery, showing reduction of IOP up to 27% to 34%.[16] He did not report preoperative gonioscopy findings and there may have been patients with narrow angle glaucoma in his population.

Eyes with narrow-angle glaucoma may show a widening of the anterior chamber angle and deepening of the anterior chamber following cataract extraction.[17,18] Thus, patients with chronic angle-closure glaucoma and mild synechial angle closure may be treated with cataract surgery alone. With a shallow anterior chamber, generous use of a dispersive viscoelastic is useful to protect the corneal endothelium and deepen the anterior chamber.

Phacolytic glaucoma is initially managed medically with the goals of reducing the IOP and inflammation prior to surgery. If further IOP reduction is required before surgery, and if there are no medical contraindications, intravenous mannitol or acetazolamide should be considered. Intraoperatively, if the IOP remains elevated, a paracentesis could be performed initially to prevent rapid decompression of the eye. Staining of the anterior capsule is usually required. If the cortex is liquefied, hydrodissection is not necessary and if there is positive pressure from the cortex, the liquid cortex can be aspirated after opening the capsular bag.[19] Although extracapsular cataract extraction (ECCE) is considered the surgical technique of choice in phacolytic glaucoma, there are reports demonstrating the safety and efficacy of phacoemulsification and manual small incision extracapsular cataract surgery.[15,20]

Phacomorphic glaucoma is treated initially in the same fashion as phacolytic glaucoma, with IOP lowering and anti-inflammatory medications. Laser iridotomy may relieve any component of pupillary block,[21] and osmotic drugs may help deepen the anterior chamber prior to surgery. Ultrasonography should be performed on eyes with phacomorphic glaucoma and opaque ocular media to allow timely detection of any mass lesion and to guide appropriate surgical management.[22] As with narrow-angle glaucoma, generous use of a dispersive viscoelastic is useful to protect the corneal endothelium and to deepen the anterior chamber. Many of these patients have some deepening of the anterior chamber with preoperative cycloplegia. A vitreous tap or small gauge vitrectomy can be used for additional deepening of the anterior chamber.[23,24] Initiating a capsulorrhexis predisposes to a radial tear due to intralenticular pressure associated with the intumescent lens. This can be avoided by aspirating the cortex[15] or using a bent needle attached to a syringe of balanced salt solution introduced through the paracentesis to perform the capsulorrhexis.[25]

Patients with pseudoexfoliation glaucoma showed a greater reduction of IOP following cataract extraction compared to those with POAG (−3.15 mm Hg versus -1.54 mm Hg, respectively) 2 years after surgery.[26] The presence of pseudoexfoliation increases the chance of having an inadequately dilated pupil and weak zonules. Postoperatively, patients with pseudoexfoliation are prone to IOP spikes, capsular opacification, capsular phimosis, and intraocular lens decentration.[27]

Intraoperative management of small pupil is relatively common in glaucoma patients compared with the general population and is discussed in Chapter 23.

Elevation of IOP during the immediate postoperative period following cataract surgery is thought to be multifactorial. The major factors are thought to be retained ophthalmic viscosurgical devices (OVDs) and compromise of outflow facility. Increased IOP occurs in as many as 18% to 45% of eyes after phacoemulsification, peaking at 8 to 12 hours after surgery.[28] Patients with glaucoma have a higher peak IOP in comparison to those without glaucoma.[29] Therefore, many surgeons attempt to minimize the postoperative IOP spike by attempting to remove as much OVD as possible, and treating patients prophylactically and postoperatively with IOP-lowering medications. Patients who develop increased IOP after cataract surgery may be treated with anterior chamber decompression by depressing the posterior lip of the paracentesis postoperatively. The IOP can be measured in patients with glaucoma later in the same operative day, closer to the 8- to 12-hour peak in IOP.

2. Combined cataract and glaucoma filtering procedure

Combined surgery can be considered in patients with a cataract who demonstrate one of the following:

- Likelihood for the cataract to progress and become visually significant (if not already) following a glaucoma procedure
- Poor control of glaucoma with medications or after laser trabeculoplasty
- Use of multiple medications or those who require maximally tolerated glaucoma medication
- Poor compliance with medications
- Advanced glaucoma
- Narrow angle with permanent synechial angle closure
- Unlikelihood to tolerate multiple surgical procedures

The main advantages of a combined cataract and glaucoma filtering procedure include elimination of the need for a second operation, reduced likelihood of transient increased IOP during the postoperative period,[30] and improved visual acuity associated with cataract extraction. The main disadvantages of combined surgery versus cataract surgery alone include longer operating time, more complex postoperative care, slower visual recovery, possibly less IOP control versus trabeculectomy alone, and long-term bleb problems.

The most commonly employed combined cataract and glaucoma filtering procedure is a phacoemulsification technique combined with trabeculectomy. Evidence-based literature review indicates a benefit from the use of mitomycin-C in combined surgery, producing lower mean postoperative IOP.[31] Most surgeons perform a fornix-based conjunctival flap for combined

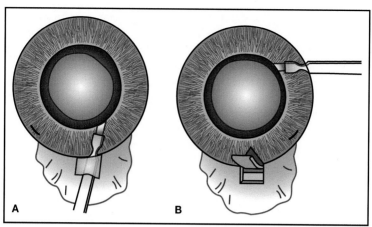

Figure 28-2. One-site (A) and two-site (B) combined cataract and trabeculectomy show similar efficacy for lowering of IOP, and are chosen depending on surgeon preference.

trabeculectomy and cataract surgery, rather than a limbus-based flap, because of lack of evidence for difference in efficacy[32] and convenience of the fornix-based flap. When the fornix-based flap is performed, a useful water-tight vertical mattress wound closure has been described.[33] Surgeons may choose to perform trabeculectomy through the same site as cataract surgery (one-site surgery) or perform cataract surgery at one location, with trabeculectomy at a different location (two-site surgery). Randomized, prospective studies demonstrate that one-site surgery is equally effective for controlling IOP compared with two-site surgery.[8,34] Although one-site surgery may take less intraoperative time,[34] the decision to perform one- versus two-site surgery is based on surgeon preference at this time (Figure 28-2).

Newer alternatives for combined cataract and glaucoma filtering procedures have emerged. In recent years, phacoemulsification has been combined with the EX-PRESS glaucoma filtration device implanted under a scleral flap (Alcon, Inc),[35] Trabectome (NeoMedix, Inc),[36] viscocanalostomy, deep sclerectomy, canaloplasty, endoscopic cyclophotocoagulation, and tube-shunt devices.[37] Although these procedures have advantages, evidence is insufficient to indicate that alternative procedures are superior to trabeculectomy for combined surgery.

3. Staged procedure

A staged procedure, with trabeculectomy first followed by a cataract extraction, can be considered in a patient who can tolerate 2 separate procedures, in which the glaucoma is the prevailing condition. In addition, a staged procedure can be used if the IOP is very high and one wants to minimize the risk of a suprachoroidal hemorrhage, decreasing the operative time by performing the cataract extraction in the future. Performing a trabeculectomy prior to cataract surgery is known to accelerate cataract formation.[38] It should be noted that decreased bleb function has been observed after cataract surgery in patients with functioning filters, which can result in a significant increase of IOP requiring treatment with additional medication or surgery.[15,39] Some surgeons have advocated use of 5-fluorouracil or needling after cataract surgery in patients with blebs.

IV. CONCLUSION

Coexisting cataract and glaucoma is a common clinical problem. Surgical options include cataract surgery alone, combined surgery, and staged surgery, with the choice of treatment individualized to each patient. Understanding the key ideas involved in the surgical management of a cataract in a patient who also has glaucoma is an important consideration for all cataract surgeons.

KEY POINTS

1. As the population ages and demographics change, the surgical management of a cataract in a patient with glaucoma will become an increasingly prevalent clinical situation that the cataract surgeon must be comfortable handling.

2. The preoperative cataract history and examination in a patient with glaucoma requires the same careful assessment as those without glaucoma but additional considerations should be given to prostaglandin analog use preoperatively, history of a steroid response, gonioscopy, signs of compromised zonules, and stage of glaucoma.

3. Cataract extraction alone can be considered in patients with mild or well-controlled POAG or those with narrow-angle glaucoma, phacolytic and phacomorphic glaucomas, and pseudoexfoliation.

4. A combined surgery can be considered in patients who have a cataract with moderate to advanced glaucoma, poor control of glaucoma after medications or laser trabeculoplasty, require maximal medical therapy, or use multiple glaucoma medications. Other candidates for combined surgery may include patients who are likely to experience visually significant cataract progression, poorly compliant patients, those with narrow angles and synechial angle closure, and patients who are unlikely to tolerate multiple surgical procedures.

5. A staged procedure can be considered in a patient who can tolerate 2 separate procedures when glaucoma is the prevailing clinical problem.

REFERENCES

1. Pascolini D, Mariotti SPM. Global estimates of visual impairment: 2010. *Br J Ophthalmol.* 2012;96:614-618.
2. Friedman DS, Wolfs RC, O'Colmain BJ, et al. Prevalence of open-angle glaucoma among adults in the United States. *Arch Ophthalmol.* 2004;122:532-538.
3. Johnson SM. *Cataract Surgery in the Glaucoma Patient.* New York, NY: Springer, 2009.
4. Bobrow JC. Prospective intrapatient comparision of extracapsular cataract extraction and lens implantation with and without trabeculectomy. *Am J Ophthamol.* 2000;129:291-296.
5. Wittpenn JR, Silverstein S, Heier J, Kenyon KR, Hunkeler JD, Earl M. A randomized, masked comparison of topical ketorolac 0.4% plus steroid vs steroid alone in low-risk cataract surgery patients. *Am J Ophthalmol.* 2008;146:554-560.
6. Becker B, Hahn KA. Topical corticosteroids and heredity in primary open angle glaucoma. *Am J Ophthalmol.* 1964;54:543-551.
7. Mindel JS, Tavitian HO, Smith Jr H, Walker EC. Comparative ocular pressure elevation by medrysone, fluorometholone, and dexamethasone phosphate. *Arch Ophthalmol.* 1980;98:1577-1578.
8. Buys YM, Chipman ML, Zack B, et al. Prospective randomized comparison of one- versus two-site Phacotrabeculectomy two-year results. *Ophthalmology.* 2008;115:1130-1133.
9. Scorolli L, Scorolli L, Campos EC, Bassein L, Meduri RA. Pseudoexfoliation syndrome: a cohort study on intraoperative complications in cataract surgery. *Ophthalmologica.* 1998;212:278-280.
10. Lumme P, Laatikainen LT. Risk factors for intraoperative and early postoperative complications in extracapsular cataract surgery. *Eur J Ophthalmol.* 1994;4:151-158.
11. Costa VP, Smith M, Spaeth GL, Gandham S, Markovitz B. Loss of visual acuity after trabeculectomy. *Ophthalmology.* 1993;100:599-612.
12. Francis BA, Hong B, Winarko J, Kawji S, Dustin L, Chopra V. Vision loss and recovery after trabeculectomy: risk and associated risk factors. *Arch Ophthalmol.* 2011;129:1011-1017.
13. Netland PA, Siegner SW, Harris A. Color Doppler ultrasound measurements after topical and retrobulbar epinephrine in primate eyes. *Invest Ophthalmol Vis Sci.* 1997;38:2655-2661.
14. Eke T. Anesthesia for glaucoma surgery. *Ophthalmol Clin North Am.* 2006;19:245-255.
15. Friedman DS, Jampel HD, Lubornski LH, et al. Surgical strategies for coexisting glaucoma and cataract: an evidence-based update. *Ophthalmology.* 2002;109:1902-1913.
16. Poley BJ, Lindstrom RL Samuelson TW. Long-term effects of phacoemulsification with intraocular lens implantation in normotensive and ocular hypertensive eyes. *J Cataract Refract Surg.* 2008;34:735-742.
17. Hayashi K, Hayashi H, Nakao F, Hayashi F. Changes in the anterior chamber angle width and depth after intraocular lens implantation in eyes with glaucoma. *Ophthalmology.* 2000;107:698-703.
18. Kurimoto Y, Park M, Sakaue H, Kondo T. Changes in the anterior chamber configuration after small-incision cataract surgery with posterior chamber intraocular lens implantation. *Am J Ophthalmol.* 1997;124:775-780.
19. Venkatesh R, Tan CS, Kumar TT, Ravindran RD. Safety and efficacy of manual small incision cataract surgery for phacolytic glaucoma. *Br J Ophthalmol.* 2007;91:279-281.
20. Chakrabarti A, Singh S, Krishnadas R. Phacoemulsification in eyes with white cataract. *J Cataract Refract Surg.* 2000;26:1041-1047.
21. Tomey KF, al-Rajhi AA. Neodymium:YAG laser iridotomy in the initial management of phacomorphic glaucoma. *Ophthalmology.* 1992;99:660-665.
22. Al-Torbak A, Karcioglu ZA, Abboud E, Netland PA. Phacomorphic glaucoma associated with choroidal melanoma. *Ophthalmic Surg Lasers.* 1998;29:510-513.
23. Chang DF. Pars plana vitreous tap for phacoemulsification in the crowded eye. *J Cataract Refract Surg.* 2001;27:1911-1914.

24. Dada T, Kumar S, Gafia R, Aggarwal A, Gupta V, Sihota R. Sutureless single-port transconjunctival para plana limited vitrectomy combined with phacoemulsification for management of phacomorphic glaucoma. *J Cataract Refract Surg.* 2007;33:951-955.

25. Chan DDN, Ng ACK, Leung CKS, Tse KKR. Continuous curvilinear capsulorhexis in intumescent or hypermature cataract with liquefied cortex. *J Cataract Refract Surg.* 2003;29;431-434.

26. Damji KF, Konstas AG, Liebmann JM, et al. Intraocular pressure following phacoemulsification in patients with and without exfoliation syndrome: a 2 year prospective study. *Br J Ophthalmol.* 2006;90(8):1014-1018.

27. Conway RM, Schlötzer-Schrehardt U, Küchle M, Naumann GO. Pseudoexfoliation syndrome: pathological manifestations of relevance to intraocular surgery. *Clin Exp Ophthalmol.* 2004;32:199-210.

28. Hildebrand GD, Wickremasinghe SS, Tranos PG, et al. Efficacy of anterior chamber decompression in controlling early intraocular pressure spikes after uneventful phacoemulsification. *J Cataract Refract Surg.* 2003;29:1087-1092.

29. Shingleton BJ, Gamell LS, O'Donoghue MW, et al. Long-term changes in intraocular pressure after clear corneal phacoemulsification: normal patients versus glaucoma suspect and glaucoma patients. *J Cataract Refract Surg.* 1999;25:885-890.

30. Hopkins JJ, Apel A, Trope GE, et al. Early intraocular pressure after phacoemulsification combined with trabeculectomy. *Ophthalmic Surg Lasers.* 1998;29:273-279.

31. Jampel HD, Friedman DS, Lubomski LH, et al. Effect of technique on intraocular pressure after combined cataract and glaucoma surgery: an evidence-based review. *Ophthalmology.* 2002;109:2215-2224.

32. Solus JF, Jampel HD, Tracey PA, et al. Comparison of limbus-based and fornix-based trabeculectomy: success, bleb-related complications, and bleb morphology. *Ophthalmology.* 2012;119:703-711.

33. Wise JB. Mitomycin-compatible suture technique for fornix-based conjunctival flaps in glaucoma filtration surgery. *Arch Ophthalmol.* 1993;111:992-997.

34. Cotran PR, Roh S, McGwin G. Randomized comparison of 1-site and 2-site phacotrabeculectomy with 3-year follow-up. *Ophthalmology.* 2008;115:447–454.

35. Kanner EM, Netland PA, Sarkisian Jr SR, Du H. Ex-PRESS miniature glaucoma device implanted under a scleral flap alone or combined with phacoemulsification cataract surgery. *J Glaucoma.* 2009;18:488-491.

36. Francis BA, Minckler D, Dustin L, et al. Combined cataract extraction and trabeculotomy by the internal approach for coexisting cataract and open-angle glaucoma: initial results. *J Cataract Refract Surg.* 2008;34:1096-1103.

37. Francis BA, Singh K, Lin SC, et al. Novel glaucoma procedures: a report by the American Academy of Ophthalmology. *Ophthalmology.* 2011;118:1466-1480.

38. Mitchell P, Smith W, Attebo K, Healey PR. Prevalence of open-angle glaucoma in Australia. The Blue Mountains Eye Study. *Ophthalmology.* 1999;106:2144-2153.

39. Klink J, Schmitz B, Lieb WE, et al. Filtering bleb function after clear cornea phacoemulsification: a prospective study. *Br J Ophthalmol.* 2005;89:597-601.

29

PRESBYOPIA AND FUTURE
INTRAOCULAR LENSES

Jessica B. Ciralsky, MD and Priyanka Sood, MD

I. INTRODUCTION

Advances in cataract surgery have afforded ophthalmologists the ability to restore visual acuity. Improved intraocular lens (IOL) technology and lens calculations have led to more accurate, reproducible postoperative results, and less dependence on glasses for distance visual acuity. The remaining challenge of cataract surgery is to restore the accommodative ability of the young crystalline lens. Multifocal and accommodating lenses are the present response to this challenge, with newer models and technologies on the horizon. Success with these premium lenses often requires surgical experience and diligent surgical planning. Patient selection, expectation management, accurate biometry, and skilled cataract surgery are all necessary to achieve patient satisfaction.

II. THE PRESENT

A. Monovision

Using monofocal lenses, patients can overcome presbyopia by aiming the nondominant eye for near vision (mild myopia) and the dominant eye for distance vision (emmetropia). Monovision is not tolerated by all patients due to the loss of depth perception and asthenopia caused by anisometropia. A trial of monovision contact lenses should be performed prior to lens implantation to ensure patient acceptance. Monovision can be performed without incurring any extra costs for the patient.

Henderson BA. *Essentials of Cataract Surgery, Second Edition (pp 329-339).*
© 2014 Taylor & Francis Group.

Figure 29-1. Crys-
talens. (Reprinted
with permission from
Bausch & Lomb.)

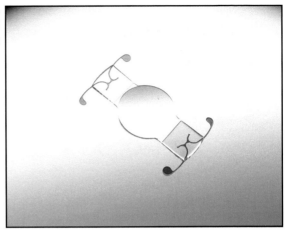

B. Accommodating Lenses

Accommodating lenses generally work by utilizing the accommodative properties of the eye to provide axial movement, change the curvature of the IOL, or alter the refractive index of the IOL for presbyopia correction.[1]

C. Multifocal Lenses

Multifocal lenses split incoming light rays into separate near and distance images. The brain interprets these simultaneously received images, allowing for a range of vision.

III. CURRENT PRESBYOPIC INTRAOCULAR LENSES

A. Crystalens

Crystalens (Bausch & Lomb) is the only FDA-approved accommodating lens in the United States (Figure 29-1). It was first introduced in 2003 as the AT-45 model. Several changes in the design of the lens have resulted in improved lens stability, improved near visual acuity, and decreased spherical aberrations. The Crystalens evolution includes the Crystalens 5-0 in 2006, Crystalens HD in 2008, and finally, the Crystalens AO in 2009.[2]

The Crystalens AO is an aspheric silicone biconvex 5.0 mm optic with hinged plate haptics with polyimide foot loops at the ends of each haptic. The mechanism of action is not fully understood. The proposed mechanism involves contraction of the ciliary muscle with accommodative effort. This leads to a redistribution of the ciliary muscle causing an increase in vitreous pressure, which subsequently causes the Crystalens to vault the optic forward.[3]

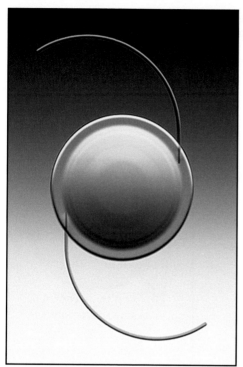

Figure 29-2. ReZoom. (Reprinted with permission from Abbott Medical Optics Inc.)

A more recent theory, accommodative arching, proposes that the optic also tilts or flexes with ciliary body contraction, providing additional near vision.[4]

Crystalens recipients have high quality vision and contrast sensitivity similar to traditional monofocal lens recipients with the added benefit of improved range of vision. Disadvantages of the Crystalens include unpredictable refractive outcomes, variable accommodation of the lens, and Z-syndrome. Z-syndrome is an asymmetric capsular contraction syndrome that causes optic tilt and leads to astigmatism and reduced visual acuity. Nd:YAG capsulotomy can be used to treat Z-syndrome.[5]

B. The Multifocals

In 1997, the first multifocal IOL debuted as the Array lens (Abbott Medical Optics). The Array lens has zonal refractive technology consisting of 5 refractive zones of alternating near and far vision. Excessive photic phenomena, halos, and glare made this lens fall out of favor. The second generation of the zonal refractive design, the ReZoom lens (Abbott Medical Optics Inc), was released in 2005 with novel Balanced View Optics technology (Figure 29-2). The ReZoom lens is a foldable 3-piece acrylic lens with a 6-mm optic containing 5

Figure 29-3. ReSTOR lens. (Reprinted with permission from Alcon Laboratories, Inc.)

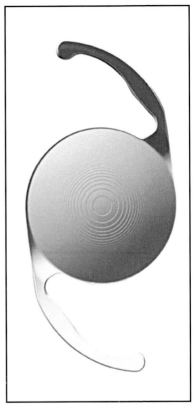

alternating refractive zones. Zones 1, 3, and 5 are dedicated to distance vision whereas zones 2 and 4 are near dominant. ReZoom is extremely sensitive to pupil size due to the configuration of the refractive zones.[6]

The more recent multifocal platforms feature diffractive technology, using small steps on the optical surface to direct light to different focal points. The two FDA-approved multifocal lenses that rely on diffractive technology are the ReSTOR lens (Alcon Laboratories, Inc) and the TECNIS multifocal (Abbott Medical Optics Inc).

The ReSTOR (Figure 29-3) is a foldable, single-piece acrylic lens with a 6-mm biconvex optic that utilizes apodization, a gradual reduction of diffractive step heights from the center to the periphery of the optic. The lens has a central apodized, diffractive 3.6-mm zone surrounded by concentric rings (12 rings in the +4.00 model and 9 rings in the +3.00 model) on the anterior surface of the optic. The peripheral portion of the optic is a refractive optic dedicated to distance vision. The original ReSTOR IOL +4.0 was introduced in 2005 with a +4.00 power at the lenticular plane. In 2008, the

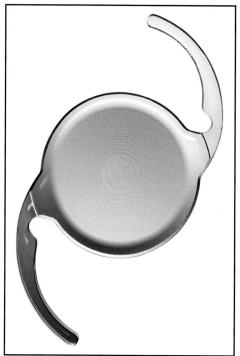

Figure 29-4. TECNIS multifocal lens. (Reprinted with permission from Abbott Medical Optics Inc.)

aspheric ReSTOR IOL +3.0 debuted, providing +3.00 D at the lenticular plane (+2.5 D at the spectacle plane) for improved intermediate distance.[7]

The TECNIS multifocal (Figure 29-4) is an aspheric UV-blocking lens with a 6-mm optic offered in both a 1- and 3-piece design. Silicone and acrylic versions of the multifocal lens are FDA approved. Uniquely, the posterior surface of the optic is fully diffractive, making the lens completely pupil independent. Other advanced features include the frosted 360-degree posterior square edge, designed to limit posterior capsular opacification and glare, and the high Abbe number optic material to limit chromatic aberrations. The add power is a +4.00 at the lenticular plane.[7]

Advantages of the multifocals include improved range of vision, especially near vision, and decreased dependence on spectacle correction. Disadvantages include glare, halos, decreased contrast sensitivity, and "waxy" vision.[7]

IV. PATIENT SELECTION

Achieving good outcomes with presbyopia-correcting IOLs starts with appropriate patient selection. It is crucial to spend time with the patient preoperatively to get to know a patient's personality, hobbies, and expectations.

Several screening questionnaires have been devised and are commonly used to aid the process of selection.

A. Visual Expectations

Expectations need to be set in advance of surgery. Hypercritical patients with unrealistic expectations should be avoided. Presbyopia-correcting IOLs do not guarantee spectacle independence. Surgery will only limit one's dependence on corrective lenses.

B. Compromise

Side effects are inherent to many of the newer IOL designs. Patients must be willing to accept potential side effects in exchange for improved range of vision. Photic phenomena, glare and halos, and reduced contrast sensitivity are often seen after multifocal lens implantation. Patients who often drive at night may want to avoid multifocal lenses.

C. Visual Potential

Patients undergoing presbyopia-correcting IOLs should have the potential for good vision to reap the full benefits of the new technology. Patients with advanced glaucoma, macular pathology, and corneal guttae should be avoided.

D. Astigmatism

Astigmatism (≥ 0.75) should be addressed either intraoperatively or post-operatively through on-axis corneal incisions, limbal relaxing incisions, or refractive laser surgery.

E. Need for Enhancements

Patients with presbyopia-correcting lenses are very sensitive to residual refractive errors. Residual refractive errors should be treated with refractive laser surgery for symptomatic patients.

F. Cost

Patients must be willing to pay extra for the novel technology.

V. SPECIAL REQUIREMENTS OF PREOPERATIVE ASSESSMENT

The evolving IOL technology has led to rising patient expectations when undergoing cataract surgery. Successful outcomes are possible with diligent preoperative planning. Presbyopia-correcting lenses are very sensitive to small refractive errors, making accurate biometry essential. A healthy ocular surface and reliable instrumentation can provide reproducible results. Additionally, a thorough examination should be performed to identify other ophthalmic pathology preoperatively that could result in suboptimal outcomes.

A. Biometry

1. Keratometry

Keratometry can be obtained through many different methods. Manual keratometry is optimal when obtained on a reliable, regularly calibrated keratometer. Surgeons often verify readings with a second modality, commonly the autokeratometer on the IOLMaster (Carl Zeiss Meditec) or the LENSTAR LS 900 (Haag-Streit AG).

2. Axial length

Immersion A-scan or automated biometry on the IOLMaster or the LENSTAR LS 900 can be used to obtain axial length measurements.

3. IOL formula

Two-variable formulas (Holladay I, Hoffer Q, and SRK/T) or newer generation formulas (Holladay II or Haigis) can be utilized.

B. Other Testing

1. Topography

Corneal topography is recommended to rule out corneal pathology, including keratoconus, irregular astigmatism, and pellucid marginal degeneration. Additionally, topography can guide astigmatism-correcting procedures.

2. Optical coherence tomography

Screening for macular pathology with optical coherence tomography (OCT) preoperatively is commonly advised.

3. Ocular surface

Optimizing the ocular surface is critically important. A healthy ocular surface allows for accurate biometry and improved refractive outcomes. A compromised tear film leads to compromised vision and an unhappy patient. Patients should be pretreated for dry eyes and blepharitis.

4. Pupil size

Pupillary size should be considered when selecting an IOL as many presbyopia-correcting lenses are sensitive to pupil size.

VI. SURGICAL CONSIDERATIONS

Surgical considerations for presbyopia-correcting IOLs vary based on the particular lens being implanted. The surgeon should be aware of lens-specific surgical nuances involving wound construction and stability, capsulorrhexis size and centration, cortical clean-up, and IOL centration and positioning. Optimal surgical techniques help achieve ideal postoperative results.[8]

VII. PATIENT SATISFACTION

Many patients are satisfied after presbyopia-correcting IOL surgery. FDA and independent studies have shown good visual acuity, less dependence on spectacle correction, and patient satisfaction after implantation. Patient bias may play a role in some of these reported findings; patients often believe out-of-pocket expenses buy a better product and a better outcome. Setting expectations preoperatively and addressing common sources of dissatisfaction postoperatively are important steps to ensure successful surgery.

Before explanting a presbyopia-correcting IOL in an unhappy patient, perform a detailed examination for common, correctable problems. Residual refractive errors should be addressed with refractive laser surgery; even small refractive errors can be visually significant. Optimize the ocular surface, as an unhealthy tear film can degrade the quality of vision. Treat any OCT-evident cystoid macular edema, another common cause of discontentment. Lens centration should be checked and addressed if decentration has occurred. Patients with presbyopic-correcting IOLs are also very sensitive to posterior capsular opacification. Nd:YAG capsulotomy should only be performed after a long discussion with the patient; once a capsulotomy has been completed, explantation of the IOL becomes much more difficult and ill advised.[9]

VIII. FUTURE LENSES

Presbyopic lens design continues to evolve. Many new IOLs are being developed and several are already being implanted abroad. Here are some of the more promising lenses that will hopefully be available in the near future:

- Tetraflex (Lenstec Inc) is an anteriorly vaulted accommodating lens composed of a flexible acrylic 5.75-mm single-optic lens with 2 haptics. It vaults forward with accommodative effort to provide approximately 2.4 D of accommodation. The Tetraflex is currently available in Europe.[10]
- 1CU (HumanOptics AG) is a one-piece foldable acrylic lens with a 5.5-mm single optic attached to 4 flexible haptics. With accommodative effort, there is anterior movement of the lens. The 1CU is currently available in Europe.[11]

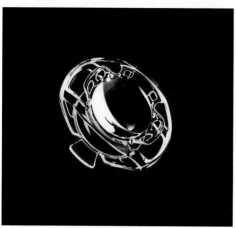

Figure 29-5. Synchrony lens. (Reprinted with permission from Abbott Medical Optics Inc.)

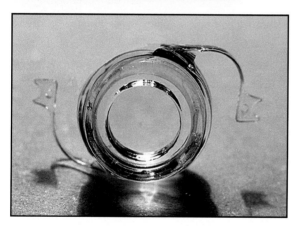

Figure 29-6. Dynacurve. (Reprinted with permission from NuLens Ltd.)

- Synchrony (Abbott Medical Optics Inc) is a foldable accommodating lens that uses a dual-optic system. It consists of a high plus-powered anterior lens connected to a minus-powered posterior lens by a spring haptic (Figure 29-5). With accommodative effort, the zonules release tension on the capsular bag, allowing the front optic to move anteriorly and provide approximately 3 D of accommodation. The Synchrony is currently available in Europe.[10]

- Dynacurve (NuLens Ltd) is a sulcus-based lens that achieves accommodation by altering the curvature of the lens (Figure 29-6). Dynacurve is composed of silicone gel between 2 rigid plates. The back plate acts like a piston to push the gel through a central opening in the front plate. The Dynacurve is still under investigation but is theoretically able to achieve large amounts of accommodation (>40 D).[10]

- Light Adjustable Lens (LAL; Calhoun Vision Inc) is a foldable, photosensitive, 3-piece silicone lens with PMMA haptics designed to achieve emmetropia after implantation. Approximately 1 to 4 weeks after surgery, UV light is used to activate polymerization of silicone macromers embedded in the lens matrix to adjust and subsequently lock in residual refractive errors. The LAL is available in Europe; multifocal patterns of the LAL are still under investigation.[12]

IX. CONCLUSIONS

Surgical restoration of accommodation remains an elusive target. Current technology, however, has made great strides toward this goal and IOL design continues to evolve at an exciting pace. Good results and happy patients require the surgeon to set realistic expectations, perform accurate preoperative testing, execute skillful cataract surgery, and address postoperative concerns thoroughly. Future designs will inevitably provide more accurate results, less unwanted visual phenomenon, and a wider range of vision.

KEY POINTS

1. Options for correcting presbyopia with current technology include monovision, accommodating lenses, and multifocal lenses. Each modality has specific advantages and disadvantages.

2. Patient selection and counseling are paramount to achieving good results and happy patients. Preoperative considerations include patient expectations, specific visual needs, and cost.

3. Exclusion criteria include hypercritical patients and patients with eye pathology that limits visual outcomes. Moderate and high amounts of astigmatism need to be addressed and adequately treated.

4. Accurate biometry and keratometry readings need to be obtained preoperatively.

5. Several new promising presbyopia-correcting lenses are on the horizon with the promise of presbyopia reversal.

REFERENCES

1. Pepose J. New accommodating IOLs. *Advanced Ocular Care*. Oct 2011. Available at: http://bmctoday.net/advancedocularcare/2011/.

2. Dell S. Evolution and functionality of the Crystalens IOL. *Cataract Refractive Surg Today*. March 2011 supplement. Available at: http://bmctoday.net/crstoday/2011.
3. Wiles S. Crystalens—What is the mechanism? In: Chang DF, Dell SJ, Hill WE, et al. eds. *Mastering Refractive IOLs: The Art and Science*. Thorofare, NJ: SLACK Incorporated; 2008:189-190.
4. Waltz K. Crystalens–What is the mechanism? In: Chang D, Dell S, Hill W, Lindstrom R, Waltz K eds. *Mastering Refractive IOLs: The Art and Science*. Thorofare, NJ: SLACK Incorporated; 2008:186-188.
5. Whitman J. Managing Crystalens complications. In: Chang D, Dell S, Hill W, Lindstrom R, Waltz K eds. *Mastering Refractive IOLs: The Art and Science*. Thorofare, NJ: SLACK Incorporated; 2008:817-820.
6. Lane SS, Morris M, Norda L, et al. Multifocal intraocular lenses. *Ophthalmol Clin N Am*. 2006;19:89-105.
7. Davis EA, Donnenfeld ED, Barsam A, Starr CE. How to get the most out of the three premium IOLs. *Cataract Refractive Surg Today*. Jan 2012. Available at: http://bmctoday.net/crstoday/2012/.
8. Hill WE. Round 4: the one-two punch. *Cataract Refractive Surg Today*. Jan 2011 Supplement. Available at: http://bmctoday.net/crstoday/2011/.
9. Donnenfeld ED. Patients unhappy with presbyopia-correcting IOLs. *Cataract Refractive Surg Today*. May 2007. Available at: http://bmctoday.net/crstoday/2007/.
10. Lichtinger A, Rootman DS. Intraocular lenses for presbyopia correction: past, present, and future. *Curr Opin opthalmol*. 2012; 23(1):40-46.
11. Dick HB. Refractive IOL selection—European perspective. In: Chang D, Dell S, Hill W, Lindstrom R, Waltz K, eds. *Mastering Refractive IOLs: The Art and Science*. Thorofare, NJ: SLACK Incorporated; 2008:504-518.
12. Chayet A, Badala F, Sandstedt C, et al. Calhoun light adjustable lens—Presbyopia Correction. In: Chang D, Dell S, Hill W, Lindstrom R, Waltz K, eds. *Mastering Refractive IOLs: The Art and Science*. Thorofare, NJ: SLACK Incorporated; 2008:229-231.

30

CATARACT SURGERY AFTER REFRACTIVE SURGERY

Nisha V. Shah, MD; Jessica Chow, MD; and Sonia H. Yoo, MD

I. INTRODUCTION

With a rising popularity of refractive surgery, the number of patients with a history of laser ablative surgery that will need cataract surgery will only continue to grow. This chapter pertains to those patients undergoing cataract surgery with a history of surgical refractive correction, particularly laser in situ keratomileusis (LASIK), photorefractive keratectomy (PRK), and radial keratotomy (RK). These cases have specific complexities that we hope to address. The top 2 issues are IOL selection and minimizing complications.

II. INTRAOCULAR LENS

A. Selection

While most optic lens designs are for monofocal vision (usually targeting distance only), multifocal designs reduce the need for reading glasses. However, multifocal lenses may introduce a greater amount of glare and halos, particularly in postrefractive surgery patients. Toric intraocular lenses (IOLs) may also be an option to eliminate the need for astigmatism correction. Overall, postrefractive surgery patients may have a greater amount of higher-order aberrations, and may thus benefit from IOLs that decrease spherical aberration to result in better visual acuity and contrast sensitivity.[1] Cataract surgery in patients with any history of refractive surgery are generally more complex cases, and the surgeon should be aware of details such as incision type, location of prior incisions, visualization, chamber stability, the need for sutures, and further ammetropia management. Good communication with the patient is important, and these patients should be educated on the complexity of their situation.

Henderson BA. *Essentials of Cataract Surgery, Second Edition (pp 341-350).*
© 2014 Taylor & Francis Group.

B. IOL Calculations

The most common method to determine IOL power is the *SRK formula*, which is:

$P = A - 2.5L - 0.9K$

where P is the IOL power for emmetropia, L is the length of eye, determined by A-scan ultrasonography, K is the average corneal curvature, determined by keratometry, and A is a constant specific for the type of lens.

After refractive surgery, standard keratometry measurements do not accurately measure central corneal power. Since keratometry is an important measurement in IOL power determination (see the SRK formula above), adjustment of keratometry or IOL formulas may be necessary.

IOL calculations following laser refractive surgery are often less predictable than in virgin corneas.[2] The reasons for this include instrument error, index of refraction error, and formula error.[3,4] First, the smaller effective central optical zone following refractive surgery causes both the keratometers and Placido disk-based corneal topography units to measure the corneal curvature farther away from the cornea's center. In other words, most keratometers measure the central corneal radius assuming that the cornea still has a sphero-cylinder shape. This leads to an overestimation of corneal refractive power ("hyperopic surprise") by 15% to 25% in eyes with a history of prior myopic refractive surgery. The relationship between the anterior and posterior curvature of the cornea may also be altered, since the cornea is flattened after myopic laser surgery, but the anterior chamber depth remains relatively unchanged. As a result, the actual keratometry is flatter than the IOLMaster (Carl Zeiss Meditec) keratometry measurement. Therefore, the IOLMaster underestimates the necessary IOL power.[5] Few IOL power formulas exist to determine IOL power after refractive surgery, and most require prerefractive surgery data. Overall, the results of various formulas should be compared with each other, and with standard keratometric readings, corneal topographic central power, and simulated K readings.

1. Example 1: The IOLMaster can underestimate IOL Power after myopic refractive surgery

A patient had an original prescription of $-5.00 - 1.00 \times 130$, which equates to a spherical equivalent (SEQ) of -5.50 diopters (D).

He underwent 5 D of flattening. His mean corneal curvature was 42.4 D preoperatively, which gives a corrected corneal curvature of K = 42.4 - 5.54 = 36.9 D postoperatively.

However, this patient's topography (precataract) reads 38.19 (Figure 30-1), which underestimates the flattening of the cornea and would underestimate the IOL power if this keratometry is used for lens calculation.

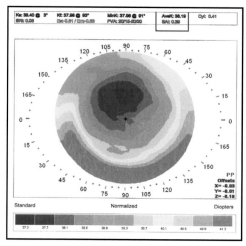

Figure 30-1. Average *K* reading via topography.

Thus, we must use an alternative strategy to calculate IOL power in these patients. The *post-keratorefractive calculator* (Figures 30-2 and 30-3) developed by Warren Hill, MD; Li Wang, MD, PhD; and Doug Koch, MD can be found at the American Society of Cataract and Refractive Surgery Web site (http://iol.ascrs.org/).

2. Example 2: Calculation using *K* and SEQ

The formula $K_{postop} = K_{preop} - (SEQ_{postop} - SEQ_{preop})$ requires knowing the *K* values and spherical equivalent prior to and after the refractive surgery, and is hence called the clinical history or historical method. The American Academy of Ophthalmology (AAO) has developed the K Card to assist in this calculation (http://one.aao.org/CE/GlobalONE/Default.aspx).

a. Preoperative

Average keratometry: 44.00 D
Spherical equivalent refraction (vertex distance 12 mm): –8.00 D
Refraction at the corneal plane: -8.00 D$/(1 - [0.012x - 8.00$ D$])$
$= -7.30$ D

b. Postoperative

Spherical equivalent refraction (vertex distance 12 mm) = –1.00 D
Refraction at the corneal plane= -1.00 D$/(1 - [0.012x - 1.00$ D$])$
$= -0.98$ D
Change in manifest refraction of the corneal plane: –7.30 D – (–0.98 D) = –6.32 D
Postoperative estimated keratometry: 44.00 D – 6.32 D = 37.68 D

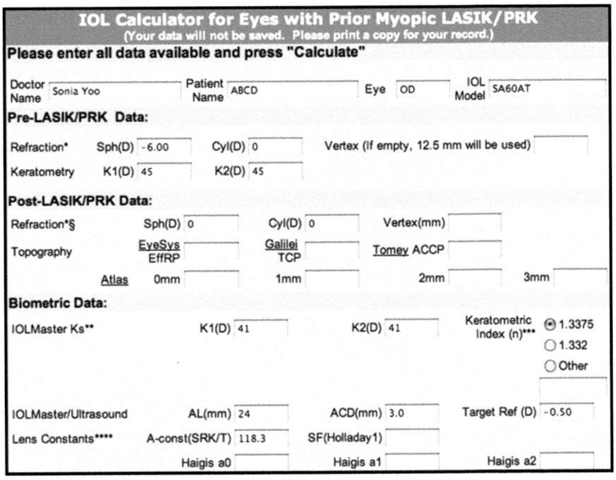

Figure 30-2. Screenshot for the ASCRS post-keratorefractive IOL calculator.

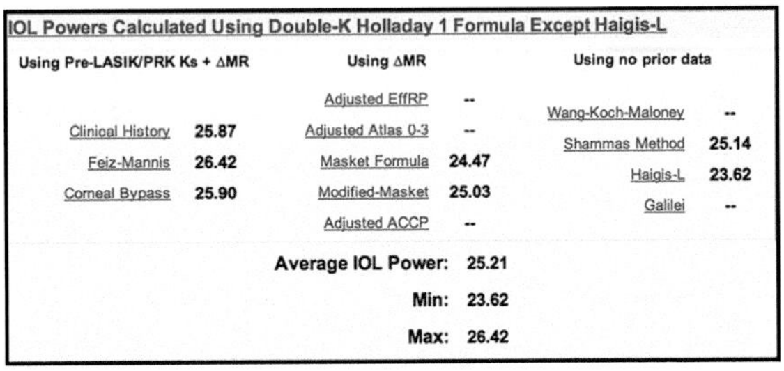

IOL Calculator for Eyes with Prior Myopic LASIK/PRK
(Your data will not be saved. Please print a copy for your record.)

Please enter all data available and press "Calculate"

Doctor Name: Sonia Yoo   Patient Name: ABCD   Eye: OD   IOL Model: SA60AT

Pre-LASIK/PRK Data:

Refraction* Sph(D) -6.00   Cyl(D) 0   Vertex (if empty, 12.5 mm will be used)
Keratometry K1(D) 45   K2(D) 45

Post-LASIK/PRK Data:

Refraction*§ Sph(D) 0   Cyl(D) 0   Vertex(mm)
Topography   EyeSys EffRP   Galilei TCP   Tomey ACCP
Atlas 0mm   1mm   2mm   3mm

Biometric Data:

IOLMaster Ks** K1(D) 41   K2(D) 41   Keratometric Index (n)*** ⊙ 1.3375 ○ 1.332 ○ Other

IOLMaster/Ultrasound AL(mm) 24   ACD(mm) 3.0   Target Ref (D) -0.50
Lens Constants**** A-const(SRK/T) 118.3   SF(Holladay1)
Haigis a0   Haigis a1   Haigis a2

Figure 30-3. IOL calculations using various formulae with the average, minimum and maximum IOL powers.

IOL Powers Calculated Using Double-K Holladay 1 Formula Except Haigis-L

Using Pre-LASIK/PRK Ks + ΔMR		Using ΔMR		Using no prior data	
		Adjusted EffRP	--	Wang-Koch-Maloney	--
Clinical History	25.87	Adjusted Atlas 0-3	--	Shammas Method	25.14
Feiz-Mannis	26.42	Masket Formula	24.47	Haigis-L	23.62
Corneal Bypass	25.90	Modified-Masket	25.03	Galilei	--
		Adjusted ACCP	--		

Average IOL Power: 25.21
Min: 23.62
Max: 26.42

For eyes with no preoperative information, the *contact lens overrefraction method* can be performed. This method requires a best-corrected acuity of at least 20/80, a plano hard contact lens with a known base curve, and a manifest refraction that is performed both before and after the contact lens is placed in the eye. If the refraction does not change after placing the contact lens, the cornea has the same power as the contact lens. If the contact lens makes the refraction more myopic, the contact lens is too powerful compared to the cornea (overrefraction), and the cornea's power is less.

3. Example 3: Contact lens over refraction method

If your current spherical equivalent manifest refraction is –2.00 D, and the contact lens has over refracted you to +2.00 D, then your change in refraction is +4.00 D. This number is added to the known power on the contact lens.

For example: if the power of the lens is 37.00 D, then your corneal power is 37.00 + 4.00 D = 41.00 D.

This method is more accurate in theory but not very useful in clinical practice due to its unreliability in patients with a cataract from poor vision and a possible myopic shift.[6]

The newer third- and fourth-generation formulas such as the *SRK/T* and *Holladay II* formulas allow surgeons to predict IOL powers with much greater accuracy.

III. RADIAL KERATOTOMY

Increased intraocular pressure during cataract surgery following radial keratotomy can result in compromise of globe integrity. RK incisions may contribute to changes in intraoperative fluid dynamics and subsequent corneal instability, and have been reported to rupture during cataract surgery.[7] Overall, these complications are likely due to the hyperopic fluctuations, the weakly healed RK incisions, and a weak globe, posing the risk of rupture with just half the force. Thus, any potential incisions that may be problematic require close monitoring, particularly incisions that are deep, near the limbus, gaped, or with epithelial plugs.[7]

Patients with previous RK surgery should be made aware of the increased possibility of requiring postoperative glasses or contact lens wear for best visual acuity, due to the unpredictability in refractive outcome following their RK. Postoperative hyperopic drift due to corneal instability warrants aiming for a more myopic target preoperatively. If patients do require refractive surgery, it may be better to perform a lens-based (IOL exchange or piggyback lens) surgery as opposed to further refractive surgery, and giving ample time (at least 3 months) until performing this operation to ensure stability of the corneal curvature. Some evidence suggests that corneal collagen crosslinking with riboflavin and UV light may be useful in stabilizing these post-RK corneas.[8] However, this has yet to be corroborated by others.

A. Surgical Considerations

There are several surgical points to consider for patients who have undergone prior RK. First, the incision size should be kept as small as possible to avoid corneal instability or astigmatism. Second, while performing the cataract surgery, avoiding areas with preexisting RK incisions can decrease the rate of complications such as irregular astigmatism, wound dehiscence, or leaks. In eyes with over 8 radial incisions, a scleral tunnel approach may be necessary. It has been recommended that a 1.7- to 2.2-mm clear cornea incision (CCI) be used to allow for microaxial phacoemulsification.[9]

Overall, with the advances in laser refractive surgery, RK is now seldom performed. The prospective evaluation of radial keratotomy (PERK) study showed that after 10 years, 43% of eyes had a progressive shift toward hyperopia of at least 1 D, which was worse for eyes with an optical zone of 3 mm or smaller.[10]

B. IOL Selection After Radial Keratotomy

RK results in a spherical aberration that makes simulated keratometry (sim K) an inaccurate method of calculating corneal power. Thus, formulas such as the Holladay method have greater accuracy in predicting the K-reading for post-RK patients.[11] Postoperative, unintentional hyperopia can be minimized by using the flatter K when calculating the IOL power.[11]

In addition, post-RK patients have lens restrictions. Traditional IOLs may further increase the spherical aberration and detract from both the visual acuity and contrast sensitivity in post-RK patients. Presbyopia-correcting lenses such as multifocal IOLs should be used with great caution in RK patients because they require an emmetropic refraction for optimal performance and may increase halo and glare in post-RK patients. A better IOL option might be one that has a negative spherical aberration or an aspheric lens.[9]

IOL centration is also an important factor, as lens decentration or tilt can further impair visual outcome. Evidence also suggests that for eyes with previous RK or myopic LASIK/PRK, the IOL power calculation can be performed using the central 2-mm total-mean corneal power, obtained by quantitative area topography on the Orbscan II (Bausch & Lomb).[12]

IV. PRK/LASIK

Prior to performing cataract surgery, it is important to obtain a thorough history in patients with prior PRK or LASIK to help the surgeon prepare for a potential intraoperative hazy view, variance in centration or corneal thickness, and IOL power adjustments. For patients with previous LASIK, hinge and flap location should be identified via the slit lamp to avoid flap disruption. Furthermore, the flap should be examined for evidence of epithelial ingrowth, which can lead to irregular astigmatism and refractive surprise after cataract surgery. In patients with a history of astigmatic incisions, the incision sites should also be identified to aid in cataract incision planning.

The literature suggests that wound healing after LASIK is a slow process that can impair the cornea's tensile strength.[13] The keratocyte response and preliminary incisional instability can last for up to 2 months until a scar forms to seal the incision site.[14-16] Thus, it is important to keep a few things in mind for these patients: the length and width of the corneal tunnel and its interaction with the LASIK flap, noting the type of incision (biplanar versus triplanar), LASIK treatment details (myopic versus hyperopic treatment, ablation depth, residual stroma), and iatrogenic changes, such as focal endothelial cell loss secondary to phacoemulsification, wound burns, and Descemet's tears.[14]

A. Haze

Although rare following PRK, the presence of haze is a sign to delay cataract surgery until the haze resolves and/or the cornea achieves stability. Sometimes mitomycin C may be used during PRK surgery to prevent this haze and regression.

B. Corneal Thickness

Cataracts may result in myopia and decreased BCVA. However, keratectasia following LASIK or PRK may also present as myopia. Thus, evaluation of keratometric stability, analysis of corneal curvature (anterior and posterior), and pachymetry may be useful in revealing the underlying cause of visual decline.[9]

V. CORNEAL SENSATION

Patients who have undergone LASIK and surface treatments for the correction of ametropia have transient, decreased corneal sensation and dry eye due to denervation. This is likely secondary to a neurotrophic effect, decreased goblet cell function, and altered corneal shape.[17] Hence, these patients are prone to suffer from dry eye symptoms, which may be reversed when the corneal sensitivity recovers. Of note, this recovery of corneal sensation is faster after PRK than LASIK. Studies suggest that corneal sensitivity and tear function can recover as early as 2 to 6 months after PRK and may take as long as 16 months following LASIK.[18-20] Furthermore, epi-LASIK-treated eyes have shown a faster rehabilitation of corneal sensitivity and tear function than LASIK-treated eyes.[21] A prolonged risk of decreased corneal sensation can also lead to neurotrophic keratitis, which should be monitored for during postoperative visits.

VI. INTRAOPERATIVE IMAGING

Even with the methods described previously, refractive surprises may occur after cataract surgery. Postrefractive patients, in particular, tend to have higher expectations and the desire to minimize their dependence on glasses after cataract surgery. Recent advances in intraoperative imaging allow for an objective measurement of the patient's refractive state and the optical aberrations of the patient's eye during surgery.

A. ORA Wavefront System

The ORA Wavefront System (WaveTec Vision) is an intraoperative aberrometer that is used before, during, and after surgery. Before surgery, preoperative measurements are entered into the ORA AnalyzOR system. The aberrometer is directly attached to the surgical microscope and during the procedure, wavefront images of the patient's eye are captured and used to calculate the refractive power of the patient's eye in the phakic, aphakic, or pseudophakic state. These real-time measurements allow the surgeon to adjust IOL power during surgery. Furthermore, it is potentially even more useful in patients who have previously undergone LASIK or other corneal refractive surgery that makes IOL power selection challenging. In measuring the wavefront aberrometry of the patient's eye, the ORA system also has the theoretical capability to allow for optimal axis placement during astigmatism-correcting surgery, such as the implantation of astigmatism-correcting IOLs or the creation of limbal relaxing incisions. It is also important to note that the accuracy of the intraoperative aberrometry depends on a number of factors including the intraocular pressure of the eye, parallax, status of the ocular surface, external pressure on the eye from the lid speculum, as well as corneal swelling from the surgery.[22]

B. Toric Lenses

Toric lenses are astigmatism-correcting lenses that are an increasingly popular technology for the refractive cataract surgeon. Currently, the process of toric IOL positioning is performed via a 3-step manual technique that consists of preoperative marking of the patient's eye (while the patient is seated upright to avoid cyclotorsion), intraoperative marking of the axis of astigmatism, and implantation and rotation of the IOL to the marked axis. This manual technique has been reported to result in a mean error in IOL alignment of 5 degrees, up to 10 degrees, which can reduce the effectiveness of astigmatic correction by 30%. Furthermore, ink marks can bleed or fade after the surgical preparation, limiting the accuracy of the IOL rotation.

C. Surgery Guidance 3000

The Surgery Guidance 3000 (SG3000; SensoMotoric Instruments) uses eye tracking and registration during surgery to facilitate and improve the precision in premium IOL positioning. The SG3000 consists of 2 units: a reference unit obtains preoperative measurements by acquiring a high-resolution digital image of the patient's eye and performing keratometry measurements.[23] The keratometry result is paired with the position and diameter of the limbus and pupil in a digital overlay, and this image is loaded into the surgery pilot unit. The surgeon can then perform preoperative planning of the incision location, capsulorrhexis size, and implantation axis. Intraoperative real-time imaging from the microscope is matched with the preoperative image, and eye tracking and registration allows for the correction of cyclotorsion during surgery. The incision, capsulorrhexis, and implantation axis are shown in an overlay, which is visible through the ocular end of the microscope, thus allowing the surgeon to precisely align the toric IOL. The SG3000 may also be used to center the capsulorrhexis over the undilated pupil and to achieve a precise capsulorrhexis diameter.[23] The accuracy and visual acuity outcomes of IOL implantation using intraoperative imaging has not yet been reported, but the technology appears to be promising.

KEY POINTS

1. Cataract surgery in patients with any history of refractive surgery is a generally more complex case, and the surgeon should be aware of details such as incision type, location of prior incisions, visualization, chamber stability, the need for sutures, and further ammetropia management.

2. After refractive surgery, standard keratometry measurements do not accurately measure central corneal power. Since keratometry is an important measurement in IOL power determination, adjustment of keratometry or IOL formulas may be necessary.

3. For patients that have undergone prior RK limit incision size to minimize corneal instability or astigmatism and avoid areas with preexisting cuts.

4. It is important to be aware of post-LASIK/PRK changes such as haze, change in corneal thickness, and decreased corneal sensation.

5. Newer technologies such as the ORA Wavefront provide real-time intraoperative measurements that allow the surgeon to adjust IOL power during surgery, while the SG3000 uses eye tracking and registration during surgery to facilitate and improve the precision in premium IOL positioning.

REFERENCES

1. Bellucci R, Scialdone A, Buratto L, et al. Visual acuity and contrast sensitivity comparison between Tecnis and AcrySof SA60AT intraocular lenses: a multicenter randomized study. *J Cataract Refract Surg.* 2005;31(4):712-717.

2. McCarthy M, Gavanski G, Paton K, et al. Intraocular lens power calculations after myopic laser refractive surgery: a comparison of methods in 173 eyes. *Ophthalmology.* 2011;118(5):940-944.

3. Hoffer KJ. Intraocular lens power calculations after previous laser refractive surgery. *J Cataract Refract Surg.* 2009;35:759-765.

4. Haigis W. Intraocular lens calculation after refractive surgery for myopia: Haigis-L formula. *J Cataract Refract Surg.* 2008;34:1658-1663.

5. Latkany RA, Chokshi AR, Speaker MG, et al. Intraocular lens calcifications after refractive surgery. *J Cataract Refract Surg.* 2005;31:562-770.

6. Hamilton DR, Hardten DR. Cataract surgery in patients with prior refractive surgery. *Curr Opin Ophthalmol.* 2003;14(1):44-53.

7. Behl S, Kothari K. Rupture of radial keratotomy incision after 11 years during clear corneal phacoemulsification. *J Cataract Refract Surg.* 2001;27:1132-1134.

8. Wollensak G, Wilsch M, Spoerl E, Seiler T. Collagen fiber diameter in the rabbit cornea after collagen crosslinking by riboflavin/UVA. *Cornea.* 2004;23:503-507.

9. Mifflin MD, Wolsey DH. Cataract surgery after refractive surgery. In: Henderson BA, ed. *Essentials of Cataract Surgery.* Thorofare, NJ: SLACK Incorporated; 2007.

10. Waring III GO, Lynn MJ, Gelender H, et al. Results of the prospective evaluation of radial keratomy (PERK) study one year after surgery. *Ophthalmology.* 1985;92:177-198, 307.

11. Chen L, Mannis MJ, Salz JJ, Garcia-Ferrer FJ, Ge J. Analysis of intraocular lens power calculation in post-radial keratotomy eyes. *J Cataract Refract Surg.* 2003;29(1):65-70.

12. Arce CG, Soriano ES, Weisenthal RW, et al. Calculation of intraocular lens power using Orbscan II quantitative area topography after corneal refractive surgery. *J Cataract Refract Surg.* 2009;25(12):1061-1074.

13. Philipp WE, Speicher L, Göttinger W. Histological and immunohistochemical findings after laser in situ keratomileusis in human corneas. *J Cataract Refract Surg.* 2003;29:808-820.

14. Cheng JC, Stark WJ. Wound instability and management after cataract surgery in a patient with prior laser in situ keratomileusis. *J Cataract Refract Surg.* 2009;33(7):1315-1317.

15. Rumelt S, Cohen I, Skandarani P, et al. Ultrastructure of the lamellar corneal wound after laser in situ keratomileusis in human eye. *J Cataract Refract Surg.* 2001;27:1323-1327.

16. McDonnell PJ, Taban M, Sarayba M, et al. Dynamic morphology of clear corneal cataract incisions. *Ophthalmology.* 2003;110:2342-2348.

17. Toda I. LASIK and the ocular surface. *Cornea.* 2008;27(suppl 1):S70-S76.

18. Perez-Santonja JJ, Sakla HF, Cardona C, et al. Corneal sensitivity after photorefractive keratectomy and laser in situ keratomileusis for low myopia. *Am J Ophthalmol.* 1999;127:497-504.

19. Lee HK, Lee KS, Kim HC, et al. Nerve growth factor concentration and implications in photorefractive keratectomy vs laser in situ keratomileusis. *Am J Ophthalmol.* 2005;139: 965-971.

20. Nejima R, Miyata K, Tanabe T, et al. Corneal barrier function, tear film stability, and corneal sensation after photorefractive keratectomy and laser in situ keratomileusis. *Am J Ophthalmol.* 2005;139:64-71.

21. Kalyvianaki MI, Katsanevaki VJ, Kavroulaki DS, et al. Comparison of corneal sensitivity and tear function following Epi-LASIK or laser in situ keratomileusis for myopia. *Am J Ophthalmol.* 2006;142(4):669-671.

22. Chen M. Correlation between ORange (Gen 1, pseudophakic) intraoperative refraction and 1-week postcataract surgery autorefraction. *Clin Ophthalmol.* 2011;5:197-199.

23. Visser N, Nuijts R. SG300 for toric lens implantation. *Cataract Refract Surg Today.* April 2011.

31

FEMTOSECOND LASER CATARACT SURGERY

Stephen G. Slade, MD, FACS

I. INTRODUCTION

We began our experience with femtosecond laser cataract surgery in February 2010 and continue to be impressed with the technology for use in cataract surgery. The primary advantages are precision and reproducibility, both of which provide direct benefits to the patient. By creating a reproducible benchmark, femtosecond lasers also give us the opportunity to learn more about the clinical significance of such surgical steps as precisely sized and positioned incisions and capsulotomies. The image guidance of these lasers is a key advantage; rather than simply create the incisions and capsulorrhexis, we can now plan, position, monitor, and measure these steps.

II. PATIENT SELECTION AND INDICATIONS/CONTRAINDICATIONS

In my practice, the vast majority of lens replacement surgeries are primarily performed for patients with cataracts rather than refractive lens exchanges. The presence of a cataract therefore is our major case-selection criterion. We select patients whose daily activities, based on our findings and their opinions, are reduced or impaired due to cataracts. Although we strive to provide the best possible refractive result and relative freedom from glasses postoperatively, safety and ocular health are our primary concerns and therefore drive our patient selection.

There are additional criteria for patient selection that are dictated by the laser, as not all patients are candidates for laser cataract surgery. The suction ring requires reasonable exposure and patient cooperation as well as a healthy cornea and conjunctiva. The surgeon should remember that docking the eye

Henderson BA. *Essentials of Cataract Surgery, Second Edition* (pp 351-369).
© 2014 Taylor & Francis Group.

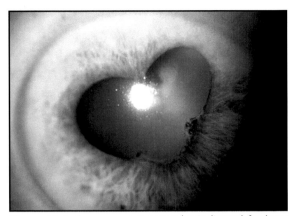

Figure 31-1. Some cases may not be indicated for laser refractive cataract surgery. Because the laser cannot pass through opaque media, in cases with small or misshapen pupils, such as the heart-shaped pupil pictured, the laser will not be able to make an effective capsulotomy or treat the lens. The laser can still be used to make the corneal incisions, including astigmatic cuts.

increases intraocular pressure (IOP), as is the case with LASIK. However, because the applanation lens is curved instead of flat, the increase in IOP will generally be lower than it is with LASIK. However pediatric patients or those adult patients with filtering blebs, compromised optic nerves, and extensive corneal scarring or previous surgery may not be good candidates for suction-ring placement.

This laser cannot pass through the iris, so patients whose eyes dilate poorly or who have misshapen or decentered pupils may not be the best candidates (Figure 31-1). The laser likewise cannot pass through a white cataract. In cases of white cataracts, we use the laser to make the corneal incisions, including any astigmatic cuts, and the capsulotomy, for which it does an excellent job. We will often still use capsular dye in the eye to ensure that the capsule is completely free before it is removed. Although the laser cannot penetrate a white cataract, it is able to impressively penetrate dark, hard nuclei, or "root beer" cataracts. In our experience, if the surgeon is able to see some retinal detail through the lens, even if highly colored, the laser can typically cut the nucleus.

The ocular coherence tomography (OCT) of the laser is a valuable tool in itself. We use the OCT images not only to guide the laser treatment but in surgery as well. We are able to precisely see if the lens is thick (Figure 31-2) or thin (Figure 31-3) as well as its density. An important safety concern during phaco sculpting is to know how deep to go. In the future, the lens density may be able to be quantified and fed directly into the phacoemulsification device

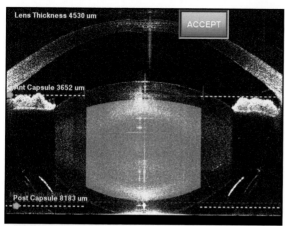

Figure 31-2. A thick lens as demonstrated by OCT imaging on a femtosecond laser.

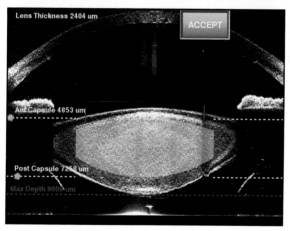

Figure 31-3. A thin lens with the OCT images of the femtosecond laser.

to efficiently optimize its settings for dense or less dense lenses. We are also able to see the occasional asymmetric lens. The importance of the OCT imaging was recognized in 2012 by Center for Medicare Services (CMS) in allowing surgeons to bill for this feature with premium IOLs.

III. Day of Surgery

We perform the procedure at our office-based ambulatory surgery center in Houston, TX. Each patient is examined and counseled in the clinic area one last time just before surgery, which gives us the chance to speak with him or her, perform a final slit-lamp examination to aid in surgical planning, review the numbers of the laser parameters, and answer any remaining questions that the patient or family members might have. The patient is then brought into the surgery center and placed on a rolling, electronic gurney (UFSK-International OSYS GmbH) in the preoperative area, which is next to the laser itself. He or she is prepared in the usual fashion, on the gurney, with particular attention paid to dilation.

When we are satisfied that maximal dilation is achieved, we move the patient, again on the gurney, to the laser. The data for the corneal incisions, any astigmatic cuts, and the capsulotomy and lens cuts are reviewed and entered. Next, the patient is placed under the laser, and the eye is docked. The incisions, capsulotomy, and nucleus fragmentation are then performed, and the patient is taken to the operating room (OR) for the remainder of the procedure. We try to minimize movement of the patient during the entire process, especially between the laser and the OR, by keeping the patient on the gurney. If there is an incomplete capsulotomy or a perforation of any corneal incision, the capsulorrhexis may be at risk during any movement. We have also designed our surgical center so that the preoperative area, the laser area, and the OR are as close together as possible.

IV. PREOPERATIVE MEDICATIONS

Preoperative medications used for laser cataract surgery are quite similar to those used for standard lens surgery. We sedate each patient, unless he or she declines, with oral sedatives, including Valium (diazepam; Roche Pharmaceuticals) or Versed (midazolam; Roche Pharmaceuticals). We also premedicate with antibiotics, steroids, and NSAIDS. We do pay more attention to the patient's dilation. The application of the suction ring and of the laser energy inside the eye tends to bring the dilated pupil down. To counteract this, we use Ocufen (flurbiprofen; Allergan, Inc) preoperatively, as well as 10% phenylephirine and 1% Mydriacyl (tropicamide; Alcon Laboratories, Inc) in every case. I also use intraocular Shugarcaine on every case as a routine.

V. DOCKING AND LASER TREATMENT

Once the patient is ready for surgery, fully dilated, and has provided informed consent, he or she is moved to the laser. The patient remains in the powered gurney from the preoperative area through the entire case—laser treatment, OR, and recovery—which allows him or her to remain stable and prone so that any forces on the eye are minimized.

The key to docking is to avoid tilt and have a flat, planar iris that is perpendicular to the laser beam (Figure 31-4). The patient interface needs to be well centered on the limbus. A tilted anterior segment, or decentered patient interface, will limit the surgical options, affect the placement of the primary incision at the limbus and the capsulotomy, and may require the lens cuts to be repositioned (Figure 31-5). If there is any question about placement or design of any of the cuts, they can simply be left off and performed manually.

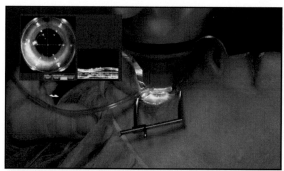

Figure 31-4. During the docking maneuver, as the patient interface approaches the eye, an overlay of a real-time OCT is shown.

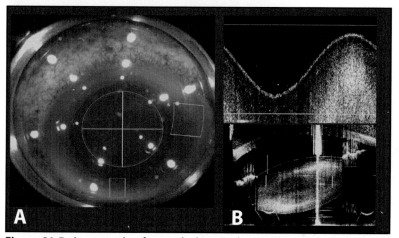

Figure 31-5. An example of poor docking is shown. The eye is decentered in the suction ring (A), which induces tilt of the lens and capsule (B), limiting and adversely affecting the rest of the surgery.

Often, the best option is to quit suction and reposition the suction ring. The design of the skirt of the LenSx ring makes repositioning easier than with a metal-ring interface of a manual microkeratome, for example. The LenSx Laser also has a very useful fixation light that helps with positioning. Each laser will have its own tips and techniques to maximize docking, and the surgeon should familiarize him- or herself with them and practice with the laser before his or her first cases.

The laser uses a real-time OCT imaging system to map the eye and place the incisions, capsulotomy, and nucleus cuts (Figure 31-6). During the laser treatment, it is important for the surgeon to carefully monitor the treatment as it progresses. Any poor placements or execution of laser cuts will affect the intraocular portion of the surgery. Decisions to modify or abort certain steps may need to be made during the treatment. We make it a point to have a staff

Figure 31-6. An image of the surgeon's view is overlaid with "drag and drop" incisions and the capsulotomy parameters (A); top right, an OCT section of the cornea in which a multiplane incision is planned and positioned, and bottom right, a section through the anterior segment showing the lens for planning and placement of the nucleus cuts (B).

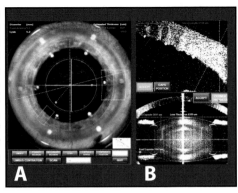

Figure 31-7. In this small pupil case, the diameter of the planned capsulotomy was reduced, but the pupil continued to come down and was contacted by the laser beam, which is also possible with patient movement. In our experience, this is self-limiting and does not affect the case.

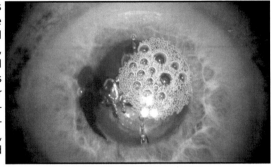

member hold the patient's hand and talk him or her through the surgery. Of course, the status of the suction ring also needs to be monitored so that any suction break will be recognized (Figure 31-7).

After the laser treatment, we typically move the patient immediately into the OR. We have not, however, found it necessary to rush the patient to the OR. As long as he or she remains relatively stationary, minutes or even hours can pass between the laser treatment and relocation to the operating room.

VI. THE INTRAOCULAR PORTION OF LASER REFRACTIVE CATARACT SURGERY

The key difference in the intraocular portion of laser cataract surgery is that the surgeon has to assess and recognize the steps that the laser has or has not completed before he or she begins the manual portion. In most instances, the laser has performed approximately half of the case (Figure 31-8). For example, rather than performing the primary incision, the surgeon evaluates the laser incision and determines whether or not its placement is correct, if it is complete and patent, and if any modifications are required (Figure 31-9).

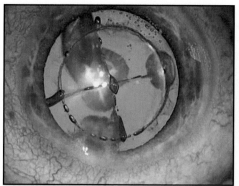

Figure 31-8. The eye as it presents in the operating room. Corneal incisions and the capsulotomy have been performed. In this case, a cross-shaped nuclear chop pattern is evident, as are gas bubbles behind the posterior aspect of the nucleus and in front of the posterior cortex and capsule.

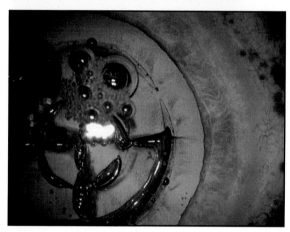

Figure 31-9. Although the lens chop has been completed, it is the surgeon's responsibility to notice the small bridge in the capsulotomy at 2:00.

VII. INCISIONS

Typically, there is no need to re-cut the main or side-port incisions. The entry sequence into the eye, however, is different in laser cataract surgery. It is important that the chamber is stabilized and there is no sudden loss of anterior chamber pressure. I simply verify that the incisions are open using a blunt instrument (Slade Laser Spatula, ASICO). First, I go in through the side port, put in the Shugarcaine, followed by the viscoelastic agent (Duovisc, Alcon Laboratories, Inc). When the anterior chamber has been stabilized, I open the primary incision with the same laser spatula. We currently use a 3-planed trapezoidal incision, designed with a 2.2-mm internal opening, a 2.4-mm external width, and a tunnel length of 2.0 mm. The control, reproducibility, and precision of a laser incision are evident. We are also able to directly compare the efficacy of a series of incisions with one set of parameters, then

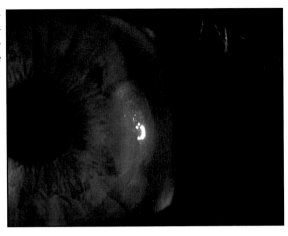

Figure 31-10. An incision that is too anterior will induce astigmatism and make the surgery more difficult.

change only one, and with the consistency of the laser, discover which parameters are best.

It is important that the main incision is placed at the limbus. We plan to place the incisions just within the vessels of the limbus. If the incision is too anterior, it will induce astigmatism and make the case more difficult to perform from an awkward angle (Figure 31-10). If the incision is too posterior, and on the sclera, it will not be patent, as the laser will not cut through opaque media and will need to be opened with a traditional blade.

VIII. THE CAPSULOTOMY

As in manual surgery, the capsulotomy is key to the success of the rest of the surgery (Figure 31-11). The surgeon should carefully inspect the capsulotomy for centration, completeness, and circularity, looking particularly for any tags. The surgeon should also be careful to ensure that the capsule is complete and without bridges or tags before removal to avoid any extension of an incomplete rhexis. I use a cystotome or forceps to confirm that the capsulotomy is free. I then use gentle hydrodissection under the edge of the capsule to detach the nucleus (Figure 31-12).

Although a laser capsulotomy may be as strong as or stronger than a standard manual capsulotomy, there are no guarantees against a radial tear or extension, so a gentle hydrodissection should be performed. There is also a possible increase in the chance of a capsular block syndrome, as there is more mass behind the lens in the form of gas, to push the lens forward. The anterior capsule is typically perfectly round and centered, therefore acting as a perfect seal when the nucleus rises up from irrigation fluid placed posteriorly. Again, smaller-bore cannulae and a carefully monitored technique are important.

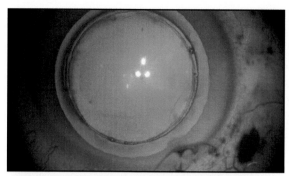

Figure 31-11. A complete, round, well-centered laser capsulotomy.

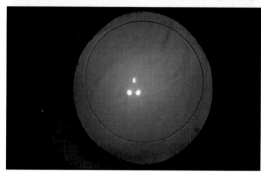

Figure 31-12. The size of the capsulotomy appears to effect the amount of lens tilt, such that a smaller diameter may result in less tilt in some lenses. The laser gives us the ability to customize the diameter and in the future, possibly the centration, of the capsulotomy to each individual lens and patient.

IX. THE LEARNING CURVE

All new technologies come with a learning curve, and the femtosecond laser is no exception. The procedure does, however, draw heavily on lessons learned from other ophthalmic surgeries, including LASIK and phacoemulsification. There are 2 parts to the procedure—the laser portion and the intraocular surgery. The laser portion involves planning the surgery, entering the patient data and treatment plan, and the laser treatment itself. Surgical planning is of utmost importance, and although no manual skill is needed, the lessons learned from examples of incorrect data entry in LASIK are powerful teachers. Of course, drawing on the experience of other users and a surgeon's own early cases can help with setting the laser parameters such as capsulotomy diameter, incision construction, and the lens chop and pattern. Docking is the main technical challenge with the laser portion of the surgery. The patient interface is different in design, and suction is applied longer at present; however, the technique can easily be learned. Certainly, all of the LASIK techniques used to achieve good exposure and suction and recognize suction breaks and movement become even more critical when intraocular surgery is performed.

The intraocular portion of the surgery requires the surgeon to learn to recognize what the laser has performed in each case and tailor the surgery accordingly, rather than actually performing the incisions, chops, etc. The laser certainly makes the procedure easier, as the incisions, capsulotomy, and lens chops are all completed. The surgical key then is to verify the incisions, ensure that the capsulotomy is complete, and take advantage of the lens chops. For example, the capsulotomy should be verified as complete before the primary incision is opened and the chamber is manipulated. Otherwise, capsular tags and incomplete cuts could extend in untoward directions. No additional manual skills are typically required, but the more cases a surgeon performs, the better he or she becomes at determining how to best manage each case. The laser shortens the intraocular portion of the case, as fewer steps are required, but the total time spent with the patient may increase with the addition of the laser portion.

Does the laser allow a less skilled surgeon to perform lens surgery or reduce the skills of an experienced surgeon? I do not believe either of these to be the case. Good surgery is the sum of one's manual skills, practice, experience, and judgment. The laser may reduce the number of manual capsulotomies the surgeon performs; however, the less frequently he or she performs capsulotomies, the less practice he or she will have for difficult cases such as small pupils or scarred corneas, so the skill level required is actually increased. In reality, a surgeon will have to maintain or increase his or her skill level to compensate for the lack of practice—certainly not allow his or her skills to decrease.

X. COMPLICATIONS

A. Vitreous Loss

The risk of a broken capsule leading to vitreous loss is a serious complication in cataract surgery. Although the incidence seems to be less than in manual cataract surgery, cases of vitreous loss have occurred in laser cataract surgery. We have carefully examined 3 cases that were presented to us, and in all 3, we found causes other than the laser. Our findings have agreed with the surgeons' impressions. For example, in 2 cases where there was a posterior capsule rupture during hydrodissection, careful viewing of the surgical video revealed the likely development of anterior capsular block syndrome. Anterior capsule block has been reported in the literature with manual cataract surgery. In anterior capsular block, a forceful hydrodissection pushes the nucleus up against the anterior capsular rim. If a seal at the rim is affected, then the pressure behind the nucleus can rise immediately and dramatically to the point of forcing a rupture in the posterior capsule. Interestingly, laser refractive cataract surgery may be more prone to this complication. In laser

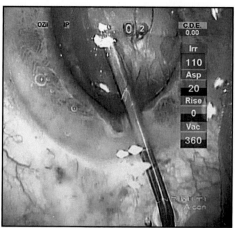

Figure 31-13. Hydrodissection with a large-gauge cannula and an iris block to the incision. This may allow a rapid, dramatic rise in pressure in the anterior chamber and posterior capsular rupture.

refractive cataract surgery, there is generally already pressure in the form of gas bubbles from the laser treatment behind the nucleus. As detailed previously, the perfectly round, centered laser capsulotomy may form a better, quicker, and stronger seal to allow the pressure to rise. It is therefore important to gently hydrodissect in these cases while making sure that fluid is escaping from behind the nucleus and out of the eye. As shown in Figure 31-13, if the iris is allowed to block the incision, then the pressure may rise to the point of capsular rupture. The largest published series showing this complication is that of Roberts et al (Table 31-1).

B. Phacoemulsification of the Nucleus

Surgeons often ask how the femtosecond laser will affect phacoemulsification. I think it is the perfect partner for phacoemulsification because it will allow us to optimize our phaco machines and techniques. We have used a variety of techniques to remove the fragmented nucleus—divide and conquer, vertical chop, horizontal chop—and the laser works well with them all (Figures 31-14 and 31-15). Currently, we are concentrating on optimizing our cataract surgeries using the INFINITI Vision System, OZil IP torsional ultrasound (Alcon Laboratories, Inc), with different tips and settings. I am impressed with this system's capacity for adjusting amplitude and flow rates in response to the varieties of nuclei. We are exploring how to adapt these technologies for combined use. For example, for soft nuclei, we can use a series of soft cylinders to liquefy the cataract, pick a specific phaco hand piece tip, and then perform irrigation/aspiration. We use the blend of femtosecond laser and phacoemulsification to improve our speed, safety, and outcomes.

TABLE 31-1. A REVIEW OF PUBLISHED COMPLICATIONS IN LARGE SERIES OF PHACOEMULSIFICATION CASES							
Authors	Study Design (N)	Surgery	AC tear	PC tear/No vit loss	+Vit loss	Lens Drop	TOTAL
Gimbel	R (18470)	M	–	0.24%	0.20%	0%	0.45%
Ta	R (2538)	M	–	–	3.6%	–	–
Androudi	R (543)	M	–	3.50%	4.05%	0%	7.55%
Muhtaseb	R (1441)	M	2.8%	–	1.7%	0.4%	2.2%
Hyams	R (1501)	M	–	0.99	1.93%	–	2.9%
Misra	P (1883)	M	–	0.16%	0.53%	0.11%	0.69%
Ang	R (2727)	M	–	1.7%	–	–	–
Chan	R (8230)	M	–	1.9%	–	–	–
Marques	R (2646)	M	0.79%	–	–	–	–
Unal	P (296)	M	5.1%	4.05%	6.4%	2.4%	10.4%
Olali	Case	M	0.56%	–	–	–	–
Zaidi	P/R (1000)	M	–	0.4%	1.1%	0.1%	1.5%
Mearza	R (1614)	M	–	–	2.66%	–	–
Agrawal	P (2984)	M	–	1.46%	–	–	–
Narendran	R (55567)	M	–	1.92%	0.18%	–	–
Greenberg	R (45082)	M	–	3.5%	–	–	–
Clark	POP (129982)	M	–	–	–	0.12%	–
Lundstorm	R (602553)	M	–	2.09%	–	–	–
Bali	P (200)	L	4%	0.5%	3%	2%	3.5%
Roberts	P (1300)	L	0.32%	0.08%	0.23%	0%	0.31%

Adapted from Friedman NJ, Palanker DV, Schuele G, et al. Femtosecond laser capsulotomy. *J Cataract Refract Surg.* 2011;37(7):1189-1198.; Roberts TV, Lawless M, Bali SJ, Hodge C, Sutton G. Surgical outcomes and safety of femtosecond laser cataract surgery: a prospective study of 1500 consecutive cases. *Ophthalmology.* 2013;120(2):227-233.

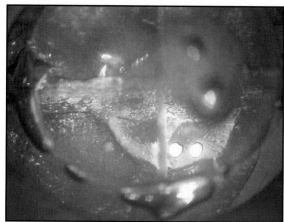

Figure 31-14. A high magnification view of a cross chop pattern in the lens. A layer of bubbles extends down through the depth of the nucleus, and gas bubbles are seen anterior to and beneath the posterior level of the nucleus.

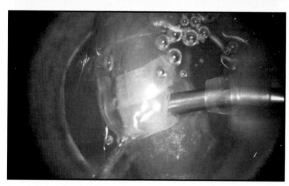

Figure 31-15. In this view, a cross section of the nucleus is shown. The chop pattern of opaque bubbles is seen to extend down to approximately the level of the posterior cortex.

XI. CURRENT NUCLEAR REMOVAL TECHNIQUE: CYLINDER CHOP

The current technique that we use, cylinder chop, is based on the latest software for the LenSx Laser. This software reduces the time for the laser portion of the surgery with intelligent ways to improve the efficacy of the capsulotomy, chop, and incisions and enables the cylinder chop technique. We have obtained our best results to date with this technique. In addition, it provides the most reproducible nucleus disassembly that we have seen with any technique, laser or nonlaser. The technique provides outstanding, consistent control over a wide range of nuclei.

The cylinder chop technique begins with a set of nested cylinders created in the center of the nucleus (Figure 31-16). The outer diameter of the largest cylinder is 3.5 mm but may be set to the surgeon's preference. A simple cross pattern is also programmed and can be seen (see Figure 31-13), with its outer diameter currently set at 5.5 mm. The nucleus pattern is brought up to just

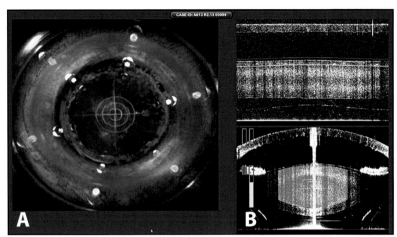

Figure 31-16. Laser settings in the cylinder chop technique. Note the set of nested cylinders and the radial chop being completed on the video camera view (A). The capsulotomy has been performed, evidenced by the ring of gas bubbles. The setting of the capsule cutting (upper right) and the depth and placement of the lens chop (lower right) can be seen on the OCT image (B).

below the anterior capsule and set a bit higher off the posterior capsule than in the past. This allows the gas bubbles to escape anteriorly and have less of an effect in pressurizing the nucleus as previously mentioned.

Once the laser treatment is complete and the patient is moved into the OR, the intraocular portion of the surgery proceeds differently as well. The first step is to check the completeness of the capsulotomy (Figure 31-17). Again, this should be done with as little change in the anterior chamber pressure as possible.

Once the capsule is verified and removed, the nucleus disassembly begins. We begin by using the OZil tip to core out the center portion that has been lasered with nested cylinders. In our experience, this central core comes out easily with a pre-phaco setting on the phacoemulsification unit with OZil energy only and low suction. Often, the quadrants defined by the cross-chop pattern will begin to come apart even this early in the procedure (Figure 31-18).

Once the central core is removed, the phaco tip and a second instrument are used in a "crossed swords" technique to complete the separation of the quadrants of the nucleus, if this has not been accomplished spontaneously in the previous step (Figure 31-19).

Once the quadrants are separated, the first section is brought out with the "chop" high-vacuum setting on the phacoemulsification unit. This higher-vacuum, lower-power setting, combined with a quadrant that has its apex removed for increased space, allows the first quadrant to be easily and

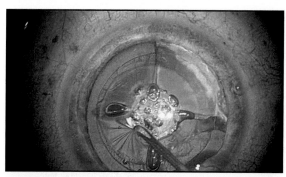

Figure 31-17. The capsule is checked to ensure that there are no tags or bridges.

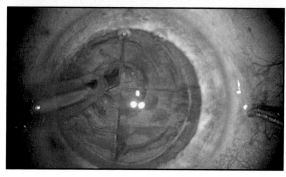

Figure 31-18. The angled OZil tip with a Kelman angle is used to core out the center portion of the nucleus to 80% depth. Gaps between the quadrants are evident, even at this early stage of the nucleus disassembly.

consistently brought up into the anterior chamber to be emulsified. The setting is then changed to "quadrant removal" for the emulsification of the quadrants and completion of the nucleus removal. "Quadrant removal" is a lower vacuum but higher-power setting designed to rapidly remove nuclear material. The remainder of the case, cortex removal and lens insertion, is carried out in a standard fashion.

The cylinder chop technique takes advantage of the laser's ability to work with phacoemulsification. We have adjusted and customized the settings of the 2 devices to complement each other in this technique for the first time. As the technologies develop, and we gain more experience, I believe we can look forward to increased synergy between the laser and phaco machine in ways that we can only imagine.

XII. CORTEX

The epinucleus is typically disengaged from the cortex from the LenSx Laser's gas hydrodissection and is easy to aspirate and emulsify. Likewise, the cortex has a well-defined edge and aspirates well, often in one piece. In some cases, however, the cortex may take longer to remove than the surgeon

Figure 31-19. The phaco tip and the second instrument may now be used to completely break apart the quadrants of the nucleus.

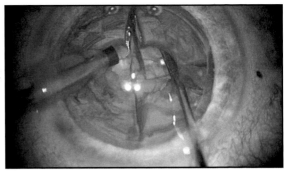

is accustomed to. There may be a smooth cut edge right at the capsulotomy rather than the more easily engaged tags in manual cataract surgery. In some cases, the gas pressure beneath the lens may push the cortex against the capsule, making the aspiration more challenging. In these cases, it often helps to try to hydrodissect the cortex more extensively from the capsule at the start, or after the nucleus is out, come back, and run fluid or viscoelastic agent under it.

XIII. TECHNIQUE AND SAFETY ADVANTAGES IN DIFFICULT CASES

Femtosecond lasers may also be advantageous in difficult cases, such as those of compromised zonules, traumatic cataracts, and pseudoexfoliation. In these cases, there may be added safety in a "no-touch" capsulorrhexis. By using the laser, we do not have to stress the zonules when making the capsulorrhexis or chopping the nucleus, which could yield fewer dislocated lenses and dropped nuclei. The laser also helps with white cataracts, dislocated lenses, and fibrous capsules. We are better able to optimize the dimensions and construction of the cataract incision and perform it repeatedly with the laser. This may lead to fewer wound leaks, improved lens stability, and lower infection rates. Better wounds could also lower induced astigmatism, resulting in fewer required secondary procedures and their associated risks.

XIV. SUMMARY

The femtosecond laser provides tremendous benefit to both patient and surgeon. The added precision of the arcuate cuts enables my postoperative patients to see well, and the laser can perform these cuts better than I can. The laser also adds precision to the capsulotomy, which, in most patients, it can also perform better than I can. It is a superb refractive machine, but make no mistake, the surgery must be completed by the surgeon. Does this diminish the role of the ophthalmic surgeon? Having used the laser since early 2010, I can report the answer is no. In fact, this surgery requires me to be a better surgeon than I was before. In the past, I had a lot of practice with capsulotomies and cracking different types of nuclei. Now, the capsules I manage are the difficult ones, or small pupils or incomplete rhexii, and the nuclei that I must crack completely are also small pupils, super hard, white, etc. I have had to learn to recognize what the laser has or has not done, and I have become a better observer and student of the surgery. Overall, the laser improves my refractive results and has truly enabled me to become a better cataract surgeon.

Key Points

1. Laser cataract surgery is a new use for femtosecond lasers that has promise in providing increased precision and accuracy to cataract surgery.

2. A primary advantage of laser cataract surgery is the accuracy of the capsulorrhexis. This in turn translates into an increased accuracy in the effective lens position and spherical component of the lens. The laser can also be used to treat astigmatism with arcuate incisions at the same time as the cataract procedure.

3. There are potential complications with laser cataract surgery, such as anterior capsular block. The surgeon must adapt his or her technique to avoid these complications. While the learning curve is short, it is important.

4. While laser cataract surgery may add safety to other cases as well, such as white cataracts, dense nuclei, and Fuchs', there are some cases that might be relatively contraindicated such as poor exposure or cooperation, small bound down pupils, or patients with corneal scarring that would block the laser.

Bibliography

Aykan U, Bilge AH, Karadayi K. The effect of capsulorhexis size on development of posterior capsule opacification: small (4.5 to 5.0 mm) versus large (6.0 to 7.0 mm). *Eur J Ophthalmol.* 2003;13:541-545.

Cekiç O, Batman C. The relationship between capsulorhexis size and anterior chamber depth relation. *Ophthalmic Surg Lasers.* 1999;30(3):185-190.

Holladay JT. IOL Power calculations for multifocal lenses. *Cataract Refract Surg Today.* 2007 August:71-73.

Holladay JT, Prager TC, Chandler TY. A three-part system for refining intraocular lens power calculations. *J Cataract Refract Surg.* 1988;13:17-24.

Holladay JT, Prager TC, Ruiz RS, Lewis JW. Improving the predictability of intraocular lens calculations. *Arch Ophthalmol.* 1986;104:539-541.

Hollick EJ, Spalton DJ, Meacock WR. The effect of capsulorhexis size on posterior capsular opacification: one-year results of a randomized prospective trial. *Am J Ophthalmol.* 1999;128:271-279.

Kezirian GM. Qualifying visual performance with the Crystalens. *Cataract Refract Surg. Today.* 2010;May(suppl):3-4.

Nagy Z. Intraocular femtosecond laser applications in cataract surgery: precise laser incisions may enable surgeons to deliver more reproducible outcomes. *Cataract Refract Surg Today.* 2009;9(9):29-30.

Nagy Z, Takacs A, Filkorn T, Sarayba M. Initial clinical evaluation of an intraocular femtosecond laser in cataract surgery. *J Refract Surg.* 2009;25(12):1053-1060.

Nagy, Z. Use of the femtosecond laser in cataract surgery. Paper presented at *the AAO Annual Meeting,* October 27, 2009, San Francisco, CA.

Nagy Z. Use of femtosecond laser system in cataract surgery. Paper presented at *the XXVII Congress of the ESCRS,* September 15, 2009, Barcelona, Spain.

Norrby S. Sources of error in intraocular lens power calculation. *J Cataract Refract Surg.* 2008;34(3):368-376.

Poll JT, Wang L, Koch DD, Weikert MP. Correction of astigmatism during cataract surgery: toric intraocular lens compared to peripheral corneal relaxing incisions. *J Refract Surg.* 2011;27(3):165-171.

Slade SG, Culbertson WW, Kreuger RR. Femtosecond lasers for refractive cataract surgery. *Cataract Refract Surg Today.* 2010;10(8):67-69.

Szigeti A, Kranitz K, Takacs A, et al. Comparison of long-term visual outcome and IOL position with a single-optic accommodating IOL after 5.5 or 6.0 mm femtosecond laser capsulotomy. *J Refract Surg.* 2012;28(9):609-614.

SUGGESTED READINGS

Precision

Friedman NJ, Palanker DV, Schuele G, et al. Femtosecond laser capsulotomy. *J Cataract Refract Surg.* 2011;37(7):1189-1198.

Masket S, Sarayba M, Ignacio T, Fram N. Femtosecond laser-assisted cataract incisions: architectural stability and reproducibility. *J Cataract Refract Surg.* 2010;36(6):1048-1049.

Nagy Z, Takacs A, Filkorn T, Sarayba M. Initial clinical evaluation of an intraocular femtosecond laser in cataract surgery. *J Refract Surg.* 2009;25(12):1053-1060.

Safety

Ecsedy M, Miháltz K, Kovács I, Takács A, Filkorn T, Nagy ZZ. Effect of femtosecond laser cataract surgery on the macula. *J Refract Surg.* 2011;27(10):717-722.

Friedman NJ, Palanker DV, Schuele G, et al. Femtosecond laser capsulotomy. *J Cataract Refract Surg.* 2011;37(7):1189-1198.

Nagy ZZ, Ecsedy M, Kovács I. Macular morphology assessed by optical coherence tomography image segmentation after femtosecond laser-assisted and standard cataract surgery. *J Cataract Refract Surg.* 2012;38(6):941-946.

Nagy ZZ, Kránitz K, Takacs A, Filkorn T, Gergely R, Knorz MC. Intraocular femtosecond laser use in traumatic cataracts following penetrating and blunt trauma. *J Refract Surg.* 2012;28(2):151-153.

Roberts TV, Lawless M, Bali SJ, Hodge C, Sutton G. Surgical outcomes and safety of femtosecond laser cataract surgery: a prospective study of 1500 consecutive cases. *Ophthalmology.* 2013;120(2):227-233.

Roberts TV, Sutton G, Lawless MA, Jindal-Bali S, Hodge C. Capsular block syndrome associated with femtosecond laser-assisted cataract surgery. *J Cataract Refract Surg.* 2011;37(11):2068-2070.

Takács AI, Kovács I, Miháltz K, Filkorn T, Knorz MC, Nagy ZZ. Central corneal volume and endothelial cell count following femtosecond laser-assisted refractive cataract surgery compared to conventional phacoemulsification. *J Refract Surg.* 2012;28(6):387-391.

Efficacy

Kránitz K, Miháltz K, Sándor GL, Takacs A, Knorz MC, Nagy ZZ. Intraocular lens tilt and decentration measured by Scheimpflug camera following manual or femtosecond laser-created continuous circular capsulotomy. *J Refract Surg.* 2012;28(4):259-263.

Kránitz K, Takacs A, Miháltz K, Kovács I, Knorz MC, Nagy ZZ. Femtosecond laser capsulotomy and manual continuous curvilinear capsulorrhexis parameters and their effects on intraocular lens centration. *J Refract Surg.* 2011;27(8):558-563.

Masket S, Sarayba M, Ignacio T, Fram N. Femtosecond laser-assisted cataract incisions: architectural stability and reproducibility. *J Cataract Refract Surg.* 2010;36(6):1048-1049.

Miháltz K, Knorz MC, Alió JL. Internal aberrations and optical quality after femtosecond laser anterior capsulotomy in cataract surgery. *J Refract Surg.* 2011;27(10):711-716.

Nagy ZZ, Kránitz K, Takacs AI, Miháltz K, Kovács I, Knorz MC. Comparison of intraocular lens decentration parameters after femtosecond and manual capsulotomies. *J Refract Surg.* 2011;27(8):564-569.

Review

Hodge C, Bali SJ, Lawless M. Femtosecond cataract surgery: A review of current literature and the experience from an initial installation. *Saudi J Ophth.* 2012;26(1):73-78.

Lawless Michael, Hodge C. Femtosecond Laser Cataract Surgery: An Experience From Australia. *APJO.* 2012;1(1):5-10.

Martin AI, Hodge C, Lawless M, Roberts T, Hughes P, Sutton G. Femtosecond laser cataract surgery: challenging cases. [published online November 15, 2013]. *Curr Opin Ophthalmol.* doi:10.1097/ICU.0000000000000018.

FINANCIAL DISCLOSURES

Dr. Maria Aaron has not disclosed any relevant financial relationships.

Dr. John D. Au has no financial or proprietary interest in the materials presented herein.

Dr. Joseph Bayes has not disclosed any relevant financial relationships.

Dr. Hilary Beaver is a member of the speakers bureau for Genzyme Corporation.

Dr. John P. Berdahl has not disclosed any relevant financial relationships.

Dr. Kathryn Bollinger has no financial or proprietary interest in the materials presented herein.

Dr. Geoffrey Broocker has no financial or proprietary interest in the materials presented herein.

Dr. David F. Chang has not disclosed any relevant financial relationships.

Dr. Dongmei Chen has no financial or proprietary interest in the materials presented herein.

Dr. Sherleen H. Chen has not disclosed any relevant financial relationships.

Dr. Jessica Chow has no financial or proprietary interest in the materials presented herein.

Dr. Jessica B. Ciralsky is a consultant for Alcon.

Dr. Kenneth L. Cohen has no financial or proprietary interest in the materials presented herein.

Dr. John J. DeStafeno has no financial or proprietary interest in the materials presented herein.

Dr. James P. Dunn has not disclosed any relevant financial relationships.

Dr. Bryan D. Edgington has no financial or proprietary interest in the materials presented herein.

Dr. Ryan Fante has not disclosed any relevant financial relationships.

Dr. Tamiesha A. Frempong has not disclosed any relevant financial relationships.

Dr. Michael H. Goldstein has no financial or proprietary interest in the materials presented herein.

Dr. B. David Gorman has not disclosed any relevant financial relationships.

Dr. Artem Grush has not disclosed any relevant financial relationships.

Dr. John C. Hart, Jr. has not disclosed any relevant financial relationships.

Dr. Bonnie An Henderson has not disclosed any relevant financial relationships.

Dr. A. Tim Johnson has no financial or proprietary interest in the materials presented herein.

Dr. Sandra M. Johnson has no financial or proprietary interest in the materials presented herein.

Dr. Carol L. Karp has no financial or proprietary interest in the materials presented herein.

Dr. Terry Kim is a consultant for Alcon, B&L, Ista, Ocular Therapeutix, OSI, Powervision, and SARcode Bioscience.

Dr. Lynda Z. Kleiman has not disclosed any relevant financial relationships.

Dr. Talia Kolin has no financial or proprietary interest in the materials presented herein.

Dr. Roger H. S. Langston has no financial or proprietary interest in the materials presented herein.

Dr. Francis S. Mah receives research support and consults for Alcon, Allergan, Bausch and Lomb, ForeSight, Nicox and Omeras.

Dr. Sankaranarayana Mahesh has not disclosed any relevant financial relationships.

Dr. *Jack Manns* has not disclosed any relevant financial relationships.

Dr. *Scott M. McClintic* has not disclosed any relevant financial relationships.

Dr. *Mario A. Meallet* has no financial or proprietary interest in the materials presented herein.

Dr. *Shahzad I. Mian* has no financial or proprietary interest in the materials presented herein.

Dr. *Kevin M. Miller* has not disclosed any relevant financial relationships.

Dr. *Eydie Miller-Ellis* is on the advisory board for Alcon, Allergan, Merck, ONO Pharma USA, and Sucampo.

Dr. *Wuqaas M. Munir* has no financial or proprietary interest in the materials presented herein.

Dr. *Ayman Naseri* is co-holder of a patent on cataract incision construction.

Dr. *Peter A. Netland* has received research support from Alcon for a prospective randomized trial of the EX-PRESS miniature glaucoma device compared with trabeculectomy.

Dr. *Thomas A. Oetting* has no financial or proprietary interest in the materials presented herein.

Dr. *Yuri S. Oleynikov* has no financial or proprietary interest in the materials presented herein.

Dr. *Lisa Park* has not disclosed any relevant financial relationships.

Dr. *Jeff Pettey* has not disclosed any relevant financial relationships.

Dr. *Roberto Pineda II* has not disclosed any relevant financial relationships.

Dr. *Saraswathy Ramanathan* has no financial or proprietary interest in the materials presented herein.

Dr. *Susannah Rowe* has not disclosed any relevant financial relationships.

Dr. Nisha V. Shah has not disclosed any relevant financial relationships.

Dr. Brett Shapiro has no financial or proprietary interest in the materials presented herein.

Dr. Stephen G. Slade has not disclosed any relevant financial relationships.

Dr. Scott D. Smith has no financial or proprietary interest in the materials presented herein.

Dr. Priyanka Sood has no financial or proprietary interest in the materials presented herein.

Dr. Clark Springs has no financial or proprietary interest in the materials presented herein.

Dr. Michael E. Sulewski has not disclosed any relevant financial relationships.

Dr. Geoffrey Tabin has not disclosed any relevant financial relationships.

Dr. Diamond Y. Tam has not disclosed any relevant financial relationships.

Dr. Robin R. Vann receives lecture honorariums and travel reimbursement as a member of Alcon Speakers Alliance.

Dr. Evan Waxman has no financial or proprietary interest in the materials presented herein.

Dr. Sonia H. Yoo has received consulting fees from Alcon, Bausch and Lomb, Carl Zeiss Meditec, Transcend Medical, and Optimedica and has received research grants from Allergan and Genentech.

Dr. Chi-Wah (Rudy) Yung has no financial or proprietary interest in the materials presented herein.

INDEX

nuclear removal technique, 363–
365
patient selection, 351–353
lashes, slit lamp exam, 16
LASIK (laser assisted in-situ
keratomileusis), 75, 341, 346–352,
359
lenses, 329–339
accommodating, 330
astigmatism, 334
compromise, 334
cost, 334
future, 336–338
future lenses, 336–338
need for enhancements, 334
patient selection, 333–334
slit lamp exam, 17
visual expectations, 334
visual potential, 334
LENSTAR, 159
lenticular astigmatism, 20
lidocaine, 207–208
lids, slit lamp exam, 16
LPI (laser peripheral iridotomy), 17

macula, optical coherence tomography, 21
macular edema, 293–303
diagnosis, 295–297
epidemiology, 294
pathophysiology, 294
prophylaxis, 300
risk factors, 294–295
treatment, 297–300
manual keratometry, 160
Marfan syndrome, 13, 271, 274, 277
material, IOL, 173–176
anterior capsular contraction, 176
biocompatibility, 175–176
chromatophores, 174
foldable optic materials, 174

haptic materials, 174
optic materials, 174
posterior capsular opacity, 176
YAG capsulotomy rates, 176
mature cataract, 249–269
maturity of cataract, 251–252
McCannel suture, 170, 195–197, 205
medical history, 12–13
steroids, 12
systemic diseases, 13
medications, 13–14, 25–30, 207–217
anticoagulants, 14
causing cataracts, 13
effect on cataract surgery, 13–14
perioperative medications, 207–
212
postoperative medications, 212–
215
miotics, 209
MMA (methylmethacrylate), 175
monocular patients, 5
monovision, 329
motility, 16
multifocal lenses, 330
multifocals, 331–333
mydriatics, 208

Nd:YAG (Neodymium:yttrium-alu-
minum-garnet), 76, 92, 96, 154,
156, 176, 331, 336
needle, 183–185
needle characteristics, 183–185
chord length, 185
curvature, 185
point cutting edge, 184
radius, chord, 185
round, 184–185
taper-point, 184–185
nepafenac, 300
neuropsychiatric exam, 18

Printed in the United States
by Baker & Taylor Publisher Services